Acceptance and Commitment Therapy and Mindfulness for Psychosis

Louise: To Mum and Dad, for your love and endless support, and to my boys – le gioie della mia vita

Joe: To my parents, José and Dennis, for all the love and support you've given me

Eric: To Liz, Matilda & Miles – every day I am grateful for your love and faith in me

Acceptance and Commitment Therapy and Mindfulness for Psychosis

Edited by

Eric M. J. Morris, Louise C. Johns
and Joseph E. Oliver

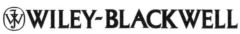

A John Wiley & Sons, Ltd., Publication

This edition first published 2013
© 2013 John Wiley & Sons, Ltd.

Wiley-Blackwell is an imprint of John Wiley & Sons, formed by the merger of Wiley's global Scientific, Technical and Medical business with Blackwell Publishing.

Registered Office
John Wiley & Sons, Ltd, The Atrium, Southern Gate, Chichester, West Sussex, PO19 8SQ, UK

Editorial Offices
350 Main Street, Malden, MA 02148-5020, USA
9600 Garsington Road, Oxford, OX4 2DQ, UK
The Atrium, Southern Gate, Chichester, West Sussex, PO19 8SQ, UK

For details of our global editorial offices, for customer services, and for information about how to apply for permission to reuse the copyright material in this book please see our website at www.wiley.com/wiley-blackwell.

The right of Eric M. J. Morris, Louise C. Johns and Joseph E. Oliver to be identified as the authors of the editorial material in this work has been asserted in accordance with the UK Copyright, Designs and Patents Act 1988.

Library of Congress Cataloging-in-Publication Data

Acceptance and commitment therapy and mindfulness for psychosis / edited by Louise C. Johns, Eric M.J. Morris, and Joseph E. Oliver.
    pages cm
  Includes bibliographical references and index.
  ISBN 978-1-119-95080-6 (cloth) – ISBN 978-1-119-95079-0 (pbk.)   1. Psychoses–Treatment.
2. Acceptance and commitment therapy.   I. Johns, Louise C., editor of compilation.
II. Morris, Eric M. J., editor of compilation.   III. Oliver, Joseph E., editor of compilation.
  RC512.A27 2013
  616.89–dc23
                                    2012039877
A catalogue record for this book is available from the British Library.

Cover design by Design Deluxe.

Set in 11/13pt Dante by SPi Publisher Services, Pondicherry, India

1   2013

Contents

About the Editors

Eric M. J. Morris is a chartered consultant clinical psychologist and the psychology lead for early intervention for psychosis, at the South London and Maudsley NHS Foundation Trust, UK.

Eric Morris completed training as a clinical psychologist in 1995 at Murdoch University, Western Australia, specialising in psychological interventions for psychosis. On qualifying he worked in a pioneering service for early intervention for psychosis in Perth, Western Australia, before moving to the UK in 1999 to work for the National Health Service in Hampshire and South London. Eric has been a practising Acceptance and Commitment Therapy (ACT) for more than ten years, and is a highly experienced trainer and supervisor of therapists using contextual cognitive behavioural therapies. Eric is completing a PhD at the Institute of Psychiatry, King's College London, researching psychological flexibility and auditory hallucinations, as well as the investigation of ACT as a workplace intervention. He is a founding member and former chair for the Acceptance and Commitment Therapy Special Interest Group of the British Association for Behavioural and Cognitive Psychotherapies.

Eric is a co-director of Contextual Consulting, an independent consultancy specialising in providing training in contextual cognitive behavioural therapies.

Louise C. Johns is a chartered consultant clinical psychologist with the Psychological Interventions Clinic for Oupatients with Psychosis (PICuP), South London and Maudsley NHS Foundation Trust, UK. PICuP provides bespoke training and supervision in cognitive behaviour therapy (CBT) and family intervention for psychosis, as well as a specialist clinical service. Louise is also an honorary lecturer at the Institute of Psychiatry, King's College London, UK, and a tutor and supervisor on the Postgraduate Diploma in CBT for Psychosis, King's College London.

Louise received a BA (Hons) in natural sciences, specialising in psychology, at Cambridge University in 1991, and went on to complete a Doctor of Philosophy

(DPhil) at the University of Oxford. Her Doctorate in Clinical Psychology (DClinPsy) was completed in 1998 at the Institute of Psychiatry, London. She has a Postgraduate Certificate in Academic Practice from King's College London, and is an accredited cognitive behavioural therapist with the British Association of Behavioural and Cognitive Psychotherapies (BABCP).

Since qualifying as a clinical psychologist, Louise has worked continuously in a clinical and research capacity in the field of psychosis. She has extensive experience of delivering therapy and of training and supervising staff across all stages of presentation of psychosis. She has published over 50 articles on psychosis, covering development and psychopathology of symptoms as well as cognitive behavioural treatments. She has led on the first UK funded studies to evaluate ACT for psychosis in group settings.

Joseph E. Oliver is a clinical psychologist working in the Lambeth Early Onset (LEO) Psychosis Service, South London & Maudsley NHS Foundation Trust. He is also co-director of Contextual Consulting, an ACT-based consultancy that offers contextual-CBT training, supervision and psychological therapy.

Joseph graduated from Victoria University, Wellington, New Zealand, receiving a BA (Hons) before going on to complete his postgraduate diploma in clinical psychology and PhD in 2003. His PhD research investigated the psychological processes of stress and wellbeing within the workplace. Alongside his clinical work, specialising in the area of psychosis, Joseph carries out research at the Institute of Psychiatry, King's College London, being involved in a number of trials investigating the use of ACT with people with psychosis and within the workplace. He has published numerous scientific articles and book chapters in the clinical application of ACT and is currently leading on an RCT comparing ACT and mindfulness-based stress reduction interventions for workplace wellbeing.

Joseph is also current chair of the British Association of Behavioural and Cognitive Psychotherapies (BABCP) ACT Special Interest Group, which promotes and develops ACT within the UK, by offering professional development opportunities, grants and training workshops. In addition, he regularly provides ACT and contextual-CBT training, both nationally and internationally.

Joseph is particularly interested in service user involvement as a method to both promote recovery and improve services. He chairs a group of service user consultants and psychologists who aim to promote and increase effective, recovery based service user involvement. Finally, Joseph has an interest in disseminating ACT ideas and concepts to other professionals and to the general public. In addition to organising ACT events for the wider public, Joseph has also been developing ACT-based animations as teaching tools for training and within therapy. He has produced a number of animations that illustrate key ACT metaphors and has developed a free YouTube channel to promote these.

List of Contributors

Patty Bach, PhD
Psychology Clinic Director, Clinical Assistant Professor, Department of Psychology, University of Central Florida, Orlando, FL, USA

Andrew M. Busch, PhD
Assistant Professor, Department of Psychiatry & Human Behavior, Warren Alpert Medical School of Brown University and Centers for Behavioral and Preventive Medicine, The Miriam Hospital, Providence, RI, USA

Majella Byrne, BA (Hons), MA, MSc, PhD, DClinPsy
Clinical Psychologist, Department of Psychosis Studies, King's College London and Outreach and Support in South London (OASIS), South London and Maudsley NHS Foundation Trust, Lonon, UK

Isabel Clarke, MA Cantab, BA (OU), CClinPsychol
Consultant Clinical Psychologist, Intensive Support Programme Lead, Southern Health NHS Foundation Trust, Hampshire, UK

Lyn Ellett, PhD, DClinPsy
Lecturer in Clinical Psychology, Royal Holloway, University of London, London, UK

John Farhall, BA(Hons), MA(Clin Psychol), PhD
Senior Lecturer, School of Psychological Science, La Trobe University, and Consultant Clinical Psychologist, North Western Mental Health, Melbourne Health, Melbourne, Australia

Daniel Freeman, PhD, DClinPsy, FBPsS
Professor of Clinical Psychology and UK Medical Research Council (MRC) Senior Clinical Fellow, Department of Psychiatry, Oxford University, and Oxford Health NHS Foundation Trust; Fellow of University College, Oxford, UK

José Manuel García Montes, PhD
Professor of Theories and Processes of Personality, Departamento de Psicología, University of Almería, Almería, Spain

Brandon A. Gaudiano, PhD
Assistant Professor, Department of Psychiatry & Human Behavior, Warren Alpert Medical School of Brown University, and Psychosocial Research Program, Butler Hospital, Providence, RI, USA

Mark Hayward, BA (Hons), DClinPsy, PhD
Director of Research, Sussex Partnership NHS Foundation Trust, and Visiting Senior Lecturer, Department of Psychology, University of Sussex, Brighton, UK

Claire Hepworth, PhD, DClinPsy
Clinical Psychologist, South London and Maudsley NHS Foundation Trust, London, UK

Louise C. Johns, MA, DPhil, DClinPsy
Consultant Clinical Psychologist, Psychological Interventions Clinic for Outpatients with Psychosis (PICuP), South London and Maudsley NHS Foundation Trust, London, UK; Honorary Lecturer, Department of Psychology, Institute of Psychiatry, King's College London, London, UK

Candice Joseph, BSc, MSc
Trainee Clinical Psychologist, School of Psychology, University of East London, UK

Amy McArthur, BA (Hons), DClinPsychol
Clinical Psychologist, NHS Fife, Department of Psychology, Lynebank Hospital, Fife, UK

Helena B. McGuinness, BA, MA
Design Lecturer and Service User, UK

Gordon Mitchell, BSc, MSc
Consultant Clinical Psychologist, Psychological Interventions for Psychosis Service (PIPs) NHS Fife, Department of Clinical Psychology, Stratheden Hospital, Cupar, Fife, UK

Eric M. J. Morris, BAppSc, GradDipAppSc, MAppPsych (Clinical), CPsychol, AFBPsS
Psychology Lead for Early Intervention, Psychosis Clinical Academic Group, South London and Maudsley NHS Foundation Trust, London, UK

Joseph E. Oliver, BA (Hons), PGDipClinPsyc, PhD
Clinical Psychologist, Early Intervention Service, South London and Maudsley NHS Foundation Trust, London, and Clinical Tutor, Department of Psychology, Institute of Psychiatry, King's College London, London, UK

Marino Pérez Álvarez, PhD
Professor of Clinical Psychology, Facultad de Psicología, University of Oviedo, Oviedo, Spain

Salvador Perona Garcelán, Psychologist Specialist in Clinical Psychology
Clinical Psychologist, Virgen del Rocío University Hospital in Seville, and Associate Professor, Department of Personality, Evaluation and Psychological Treatment, University of Seville School of Psychology, Seville, Spain

Fran Shawyer, BSc (Hons), PhD
Research Fellow, School of Psychology and Psychiatry, Faculty of Medicine, Nursing and Health Sciences, Monash University, Melbourne, Australia

Helen Startup, DPhil, DClinPsy
Principal Clinical Psychologist, South London and Maudsley NHS Foundation Trust, London, and Department of Psychiatry, Oxford University, Oxford, UK

Clara Strauss BA (Hons), DPhil, DClinPsych, PGDip (Cognitive Therapy)
Clinical Psychologist & Research Lead, Sussex Mindfulness Centre, Sussex Partnership NHS Foundation Trust and Acting Research Director, Clinical Psychology Training Programme, University of Surrey, Surrey, UK

Neil Thomas, BSc (Hons), DClinPsy, CPsychol, MAPS, AFBPsS
Senior Clinician, Monash Alfred Psychiatry Research Centre, The Alfred, and Brain and Psychological Sciences Research Centre, Swinburne University, Melbourne, Australia

Ross White, BSc, DClinPsy, PhD
University Teacher, Institute of Health and Well-being, University of Glasgow, and Honorary Principal Clinical Psychologist, NHS Greater Glasgow and Clyde, UK

Acknowledgements

We would like to acknowledge the people in the field who have inspired us to learn about and practise ACT and mindfulness, in particular Steve Hayes, Paul Chadwick, Kelly Wilson, Patty Bach, Brandon Gaudiano, Gordon Mitchell and Amy McArthur. We have admired their work and approach to working with people with psychosis and other mental health problems.

We would also like to acknowledge our colleagues, mentors and friends in the area of Cognitive Behaviour Therapy (CBT) for psychosis. We are extremely fortunate to have worked closely with so many experts and pioneers in this field, both in the UK and overseas. In addition to authors in this volume, we have been particularly influenced over the years by Elizabeth Kuipers, Philippa Garety, Til Wykes, Emmanuelle Peters, Suzanne Jolley, Juliana Onwumere, Lucia Valmaggia, Richard Bentall, Gillian Haddock and Tony Morrison. We have learned a great deal from working with these psychologists, which has shaped our understanding of psychosis, our research interests and clinical practice.

It is important for us to acknowledge other colleagues and mentors in the South London and Maudsley NHS Foundation Trust and at the Institute of Psychiatry, King's College London, who have supported us and our work over the years. There are too many to list them all here, but we would particularly like to mention Adrian Webster, Emmanuelle Peters and Suzanne Jolley, who have supervised and managed our work with sound judgement and with compassion when we have erred.

We acknowledge our co-authors for their excellent contributions to this volume and for meeting all the deadlines in a timely fashion, which made our role as editors much easier. We also acknowledge the publisher Wiley-Blackwell for their original interest and for assistance and patience along the way.

Lastly, we would like to acknowledge our respective friends and families for their on-going love and support, which has enabled us to pursue our common value of making a positive difference to the lives of people with psychosis.

Foreword: Acceptance, Mindfulness and Psychotic Disorders
Creating a New Place to Begin

An editorial in the *British Journal of Psychiatry* (Morrison *et al.*, 2012) asks in its title, 'Anti-psychotics: Is it Time to Introduce Patient Choice?' The article is powerful, well-argued and disturbing all at the same time, but it was the title that stopped me cold in my tracks. In any other area of health or service delivery, such a title would completely dumbfound the reader. In any other area of health or service delivery, anyone reading such a thing would force out a mumbled 'Don't we have that now?!' Could we imagine a title in a major journal that read, 'Back Surgeries: Is it Time to Introduce Patient Choice?' or 'Prolonged Exposure: Is it Time to Introduce Patient Choice?'

Those experiencing psychotic disorders are amongst the most stigmatised people on the planet. They are frequently objectified and dehumanised by society. Their unusual experiences and actions are often objects of ridicule or fear. Steps are regularly taken to remove them from society, and their liberties are constantly at risk in ways large and small.

That is a terrible state of affairs, but it is not the worst of it. The cruellest blow is that the treatment delivery system itself often objectifies them as well. This happens in multiple ways. People experiencing psychotic disorders are told cartoon stories about genetics, the brain or neurotransmitters as the certain sources of their difficulties, when the true state of knowledge is far more ambiguous. Horizons and expectations are lowered excessively, and patients are no longer treated as whole human beings. The benefits of medication are overstated and the likelihood of long-term side effects and neurobiological opponent processes from these medications are understated. But the biggest betrayal of all is that patients are offered such a limited range of treatment options.

Fortunately, development of psychosocial interventions has continued. Researchers and clinicians have continued to seek out and find new ways to be helpful. Where there were few options, they have created more choice.

You hold in your hands one of the results. This is the first volume to summarise the literature on modern acceptance and mindfulness based-approaches to psychosis, particularly acceptance and commitment therapy (ACT) and related methods such as person-centred cognitive therapy (PBCT) and emotional processing and metacognitive awareness (EPMA). These new methods are breaking ground, challenging long-held assumptions and offering real choices.

A practitioner or clinical researcher drawn to this area of work needs to know that it is young. While there are now several successful randomised trials, these are not turnkey approaches. The purpose of a volume like this is not to provide final answers – it is to open new avenues to explore. A dedicated student or professional reading these pages can be part of creating a path forward. The field is new enough that innovations occur on a regular basis. Treatment development is rapid and ongoing.

Everything a practitioner or a clinical researcher needs to begin to explore this area clinically and empirically is here: rationale, data, assessment tools, protocols and expert guidance. The adjustments needed for specific subpopulations and problem areas (dealing with delusions, auditory hallucinations, the emotional upheaval following psychotic breaks, managing first episodes, acute episodes and so on) are described in detail. Different formats and specific approaches are laid out. The book properly gives voice to end users themselves. The editors have carefully chosen a group of well-prepared chapter authors – this truly is a state-of-the-art volume. There is nothing else like it in the world's scientific and practical literature.

I am writing this foreword with a sense of humbled excitement. It is humbling how much we have to learn and how far we have to go. There are many implications of work in acceptance, mindfulness and values which are yet to be tested, and we don't know how they will work out. The social need for progress is enormous and growing, and we don't know if we can meet this challenge. Even as we develop real treatment alternatives, we are aware that the systems of care are often difficult to change, and at times it may be hard to insert real choice into the current system.

The excitement comes because we have begun in earnest. It now seems undeniable that there is conceptual and clinical progress being made by those interested in ACT, and acceptance and mindfulness methods generally, in understanding and treating these debilitating conditions. We have a long way to go but there is something important in this work. Researchers and clinicians need to tease it out, by studying the processes that give rise to these problems and the processes of change that acceptance and mindfulness methods engage. They need to continue to develop new procedures that foster positive change in these processes, and learn how to integrate them with other methods of known value. We need a new model of psychotic symptoms and a new approach to intervention. No one is speaking of a panacea, but these pages show the field that there is now another place to begin.

Steven C. Hayes
University of Nevada
Co-developer of ACT and author of
Get Out of Your Mind and Into Your Life

Reference

Morrison, A., Hutton, P., Shiers, D. & Turkington, D. (2012). Antipsychotics: is it time to introduce patient choice? *British Journal of Psychiatry*, 201, 83–84.

1

Introduction to Mindfulness and Acceptance-based Therapies for Psychosis

Joseph E. Oliver, Candice Joseph, Majella Byrne, Louise C. Johns and Eric M. J. Morris

1.1   Introduction to Psychosis

'Psychosis' is an umbrella term covering a range of associated symptoms, including perceptual, cognitive, emotional and behavioural disturbances. The term tends to refer to 'positive' symptoms of unusual beliefs (delusions), anomalous perceptual experiences (illusions and hallucinations) and disturbances of thought and language (formal thought disorder) (described in Peters *et al.*, 2007). These are invariably accompanied by emotional difficulties such as anxiety and depression (Birchwood, 2003; Freeman & Garety, 2003; Johnstone *et al.*, 1991). In addition, a significant proportion of people diagnosed with a psychotic disorder, particularly schizophrenia, are likely to experience 'negative' symptoms such as avolition and anhedonia (described in Kuipers *et al.*, 2006). The median incidence of psychotic disorders is estimated at 15.2 per 100 000, with estimates ranging between 7.7 and 43.0 per 100 000 (McGrath *et al.*, 2004), indicating a high degree of variability in incidence across geographic regions. The reported lifetime risk remains at approximately 1% (Saha *et al.*, 2005).

One of the diagnostic peculiarities of psychosis is that two individuals can receive the same diagnosis but have completely different sets of symptoms that have no overlap or commonality. This perhaps points to some of the complexities of the disorder, which the current accumulated evidence suggests is likely a manifold interaction between a range of genetic, biological, psychological and social factors, with probable multiple aetiological pathways (Oliver & Fearon, 2008).

Acceptance and Commitment Therapy and Mindfulness for Psychosis, First Edition.
Edited by Eric M. J. Morris, Louise C. Johns and Joseph E. Oliver.
© 2013 John Wiley & Sons, Ltd. Published 2013 by John Wiley & Sons, Ltd.

Furthermore, psychotic symptoms are not exclusively reported by those with a diagnosis of psychotic disorder (such as schizophrenia, schizoaffective disorder or delusional disorder), but also occur in varying degrees in other mental-health problems, including bipolar affective disorder, mood disorders and personality disorders (particularly borderline personality disorder (BPD)). Additionally, some authors have vigorously criticised the schizophrenia diagnosis, arguing that the associated breadth and diversity of clinical phenomenology actually represents a lack of construct validity and reliability (Bentall, 2003; Boyle, 2002).

The mere presence of psychotic symptoms, no matter how apparently bizarre they may be, is not sufficient to warrant a diagnosis. Key to a psychotic disorder is recognition that the symptoms must co-occur with significant interruption to the individual's life. Schizophrenia is associated with significant long-term disability (Thornicroft *et al.*, 2004; World Health Organization, 2001) and, in addition to positive and negative psychotic symptoms, depressive symptoms are also strong predictors of poor quality of life in this client group (Saarni *et al.*, 2010). For those who continue to live with distressing psychotic symptoms and emotional disturbance, advances in treatments for psychosis are of paramount importance.

Alongside the devastation that psychosis can cause to the lives of individuals and their families, there are also significant economic costs. Estimates suggest that in 2002 the direct (e.g. service charges) and indirect (e.g. unemployment) costs associated with psychotic disorders were approximately \$62.7 billion in the United States (Wu *et al.*, 2005). Similar estimates within the United Kingdom have indicated costs of approximately £4 billion (McCrone *et al.* 2008).

1.2   Interventions

The first line of treatment for psychosis is almost always antipsychotic medication. However, there are limitations to pharmacological treatments, including issues of compliance, intolerable side effects and poor symptomatic response to antipsychotic medication (Curson *et al.*, 1988; Kane, 1996; Lieberman *et al.*, 2005). These findings, in conjunction with the recognition of the importance of social and psychological factors in psychosis (Bebbington & Kuipers, 1994; Garety *et al.*, 2001; van Os, 2004), have contributed to the development of psychological interventions for people with psychosis. Such interventions include family therapy, cognitive behavioural therapy (CBT) and social and cognitive rehabilitation. They are not proposed as alternatives to medication, but are used as adjunctive therapies.

1.2.1   Cognitive Behavioural Therapy

The main assumption underlying CBT is that psychological difficulties are maintained by vicious cycles involving thoughts, feelings and behaviours (Beck *et al.*, 1979). Therapy aims to break these cycles by helping people to learn more adaptive ways of thinking and coping, which leads to a reduction in distress. In the 1980s and 1990s, research on psychotic symptoms led to treatments that adapted the successful use of CBT for anxiety and depression to the more complex problems of psychosis (Fowler *et al.*, 1995; Kingdon & Turkington, 1991). Cognitive models of psychotic symptoms (e.g. Garety *et al.*, 2001; Morrison, 2001) have informed the development of therapeutic approaches, highlighting that it is not the unusual experiences themselves that are problematic, but the appraisal of them as external and personally significant. CBT for psychosis (CBTp) aims to increase understanding of psychosis and its symptoms, reduce distress and disability arising from psychotic symptoms, promote coping and self-regulation and reduce hopelessness and counter-negative appraisals (of self and illness) (see Johns *et al.*, 2007 for an overview).

Evidence from randomised controlled trials (RCTs) has shown that CBT delivered on a one-to-one basis is efficacious for individuals with psychosis, particularly those with persistent positive symptoms (Smith *et al.*, 2010; Wykes *et al.*, 2008; Zimmerman *et al.*, 2005). A meta-analysis of 33 studies by Wykes *et al.* (2008) revealed a modest overall effect size of 0.40 for target symptoms and effect sizes ranging between 0.35 and 0.44 for positive symptoms, negative symptoms, functioning, mood and social anxiety. A recent study identified CBTp as being most effective when the full range of therapy procedures, including specific cognitive and behavioural techniques, are implemented (Dunn *et al.*, 2011). While CBTp offers symptom improvement in some areas for a number of people, it is not a panacea.

1.2.2   Developments in CBT: Contextual Approaches

Additional developments in the field of behavioural and cognitive therapy approaches have led to the evolution of a cluster of therapies termed 'contextual CBTs' (Hayes *et al.*, 2011). This evolution has been in response to several anomalies present within the CBT model, including debate about whether cognitive change/restructuring is actually the necessary component of therapy (Hayes, 2004; Longmore & Worrell, 2007). While not ignoring the importance of cognition, contextual approaches emphasise the historical and situational context an organism is situated within as a means for focusing upon central processes to be targeted to effect behavioural change. Critically, contextual approaches deemphasise the importance of changing the content and frequency of cognition, moving instead towards the use of acceptance and mindfulness procedures to alter the context in which these experiences occur, thereby increasing behavioural flexibility.

A number of approaches fall under the umbrella of contextual CBT, including dialectical behaviour therapy (DBT) (Linehan, 1987), functional analytic psychotherapy (FAP) (Kohlenberg & Tsai, 1991), mindfulness-based cognitive therapy (MBCT) (Teasdale *et al.*, 1995), integrative behavioural couples therapy (IBCT) (Jacobson & Christensen, 1996), Acceptance and Commitment Therapy (ACT) (Hayes *et al.*, 1999), metacognitive therapy (MCT) (Wells, 2000) and person-based cognitive therapy

(PBCT) for psychosis (Chadwick, 2006). These therapies include components such as mindfulness, experience with the present moment, acceptance, values and greater emphasis on the therapeutic relationship. While they may incorporate more traditional behavioural and cognitive techniques, they tend to be more experiential in nature and involve second-order strategies of change as well as first-order ones. Within these therapies, ACT, PBCT and mindfulness groups have mostly been implemented in the psychological treatment of psychosis.

1.2.3   Acceptance and Commitment Therapy

ACT is a modern behavioural approach that incorporates acceptance and mindfulness to help people disentangle from difficult thoughts and feelings in order to facilitate engagement in behavioural patterns that are guided by personal values. It has firm roots in behavioural traditions and is underpinned by a behavioural analytic account of language: relational frame theory (RFT) (Blackledge *et al.*, 2009). Broadly, the ACT stance focuses on changing one's relationship to internal experiences (thoughts, feelings) rather than altering the form or frequency of these experiences (Hayes *et al.*, 1999). The approach is transdiagnostic and uses the same theoretical model to formulate and target common processes underlying a wide range of symptomatically diverse problems (such as depression, BPD and diabetes).

ACT's six core theoretical processes are set out visually in a hexagonal shape (known colloquially as the 'hexaflex'; see Figure 1.1) and move in synchrony towards increasing psychological flexibility or 'the ability to contact the present moment more fully as a conscious human being, and to change or persist in behaviour when doing so serves valued ends' (Hayes *et al.*, 2006, p. 7). These processes are highly interrelated and, although represented as distinct entities in the model, share considerable overlap. More recently, the processes have been clustered into

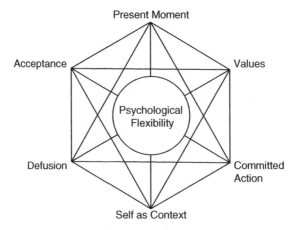

Figure 1.1   The ACT model of psychological flexibility

Table 1.1   Central ACT processes (adapted from Luoma *et al.*, 2007)

Process	Definition
Open	
Acceptance	The active and aware embrace of private events that are occasioned by our history, without unnecessary attempts to change their frequency or form, especially when doing so would cause psychological harm.
Defusion	The process of creating nonliteral contexts in which language can be seen as an active, ongoing relational process that is historical in nature and present in the current context.
Aware	
Self as Context	A continuous and secure 'I' from which events are experienced, but which is also distinct from those events.
Present Moment	Ongoing, nonjudgmental contact with psychological and environmental events as they occur.
Active	
Values	Verbally constructed, global, desired and chosen life directions.
Committed Action	Step-by-step process of acting to create a whole life, a life of integrity, true to one's deepest wishes and longings.

three broader sets of response styles: open, aware and active (Hayes *et al.*, 2011) (see Table 1.1).

1.2.3.1   Open

The processes of acceptance and defusion work synergistically to build the broader skill of developing openness towards internal content that occurs 'under the skin' (thoughts, emotions, memories, perceptions). Psychotic symptoms, by their nature, have a number of qualities that tend to increase the likelihood that people will respond to them with suppression or avoidance. Symptoms, such as voices, are often highly distressing, critical and personally salient (Close & Garety, 1998; Nayani & David, 1994). Experiences associated with delusional ideation have been shown to be highly linked with appraisals of shame, humiliation and entrapment (Birchwood *et al.*, 2000) and therefore much more likely to lead to experiential avoidance. Research bears this out, demonstrating that people with distressing psychosis tend to utilise more suppression and avoidance and less acceptance strategies (Morrison *et al.*, 1995; Perry *et al.*, 2011). Conversely, psychotic experiences can be extremely engaging, in that they can be magical, interesting and have high personal meaning, especially in the context of a life devoid of meaningful activity and social connection. As such, these experiences may be used as a method to escape a dreary, mundane existence, but this may come at high personal cost in the long term.

Acceptance is the process by which clients are encouraged to embrace their thoughts and feelings without trying to resist, avoid or suppress them via 'experiential avoidance'. This is not merely a process of tolerance or resignation, but a full willingness to step towards and make space for psychological phenomena, including psychotic symptoms, without engaging in unworkable struggle against them.

Alongside the process of acceptance, building of defusion further supports an open stance towards internal experience. Defusion aims to help clients step back from internal experiences such as thoughts, memories or appraisals of external experiences (voices or other anomalous experiences) and see them for what they are, rather than what they say they are, thereby reducing unhelpful literal, rule-based responding to internal events. From an ACT perspective, fusion increases the likelihood of a narrowing of an individual's behavioural repertoire in the face of such experiences, thereby limiting opportunities for values-based actions. Defusion works to expand and add to that repertoire by undermining adherence to thoughts and verbal rules that promote restriction, narrowing or avoidance. For example, an ACT therapist might usefully work on defusion related to a thought such as 'I can't tolerate this paranoia' that occurs in the context of high anxiety and avoidance of valued activities such as connecting with friends. An intervention might focus on assisting the client to first notice this as a thought and then develop a more defused stance towards it, so that subsequent actions are guided more by values (actively connecting with friends) rather than fusion ('I must avoid situations that lead to paranoia'). This is contrasted with more traditional cognitive approaches, in which interventions target the veracity of thoughts or appraisals and, where distorted, adjust or correct them.

1.2.3.2   Aware

The self as context is the perspective from which all internal experiences are observed and in which they are held. By promoting an awareness of this particular perspective, detachment to distressing thoughts, images, beliefs or hallucinations that may arise is cultivated through a mindful contact with the present moment. The idea that language gives humans a sense of 'self' and perspective explains the inclusion of spirituality in human existence, because the 'mind' has no boundaries (Hayes, 1984). Mindfulness can help individuals learn to notice, but not judge, passing thoughts, feelings or images, in order to develop a more centred stance towards internal experiences, so as to support engagement with core values.

1.2.3.3   Active

The heart of ACT work is in assisting clients to become more engaged with and active in their lives, through a process of identifying and constructing sets of values and using them to inform the development of goals and specific action plans. Goals are set in ways that increase the likelihood they will be met, for example by setting initial small, measureable, meaningful tasks, which are increasingly built into larger and larger patterns of committed action. To use a sailing metaphor, the verbal construction and articulation of values is comparable to the setting of sails, which are then used to 'catch the wind', or the natural reinforcement that occurs as values-directed behaviour is engaged in. In sailing, catching the wind can be both exhilarating and scary; so can taking steps towards values. The therapist's job is to help the client cue into these sensations and to assist in ongoing adjustments to help the client stay on course.

At the time of publication, there are four RCTs evaluating the use of acceptance and mindfulness approaches for people with psychosis (Bach & Hayes, 2002; Gaudiano & Herbert, 2006; Shawyer *et al.*, 2012; White, 2011). Although they have modest sample sizes, the findings are promising, and indicate that such interventions are efficacious for people with distressing psychosis.

1.2.4   Mindfulness and Person-based Cognitive Therapy for Psychosis

Over the last 10–15 years, mindfulness approaches have become increasingly prominent in the psychological literature (Hayes *et al.*, 2005), and have been applied in an increasingly broad range of difficulties. An evidence base has developed to indicate that mindfulness is effective for a wide variety of problems, including eating disorders, affective disorders, anxiety, stress and substance-misuse problems, and as a complementary treatment for physical disorders (Baer, 2003; Hayes *et al.*, 2006).

Mindfulness can be described as 'paying attention in a particular way: on purpose, in the present moment and non-judgementally' (Kabat-Zinn, 1994, p. 3). It can involve a focusing of attention and an acceptance of present-moment experiences (Linehan, 1993), as contrasted with cognitive processes such as rumination, worry, planning and automatic engagement with activity without awareness (Baer *et al.*, 2004).

Evidence is emerging to indicate that mindfulness can be useful for people with distressing symptoms of psychosis. Chadwick (2006) has developed a mindfulness-based therapy programme which has the aim of influencing how people relate to their psychotic experiences. The programme focuses on facilitating awareness of the body, mindfulness (with prompting), introducing homework audiotapes and emphasing the therapeutic process. Two small trials have provided some initial evidence that mindfulness can be helpful with this group (Chadwick *et al.*, 2005, 2009). A qualitative study carried out by Abba *et al.* (2007) helped to illuminate the processes by which mindfulness can help with the experience of psychosis. A three-stage process was identified. The first stage involved learning to maintain a centred awareness alongside the experience of psychosis as an alternative to becoming lost in the experience; this process developed a new position – the person and the presence of the voice, paranoia or thought/image. The second stage involved a focus on allowing voices, thoughts and images to come and go without reaction or struggle. The final stage emphasised a reclaiming of power through acceptance: observing that all unpleasant experiences happen in the same way as other human experiences – they are just one part of human experience.

Alongside this work, Chadwick (2006) integrated mindfulness into a broader CBT to develop the PBCT protocol for distressing psychosis. This aims to alleviate the distress associated with clients' reactions to their psychotic experiences and move towards their acceptance of these experiences and improved well-being. The therapy is deeply embedded in Rogerian therapy, in particular Rogerian acceptance (Rogers, 1961). It also involves an integration of cognitive therapy and mindfulness with Vygotsky's 'zones of proximal development' (ZoPD) (Vygotsky, 1978) as the structure of the therapeutic process. This model, and its application within group settings, is more comprehensively described in Chapter 10.

1.3   Conclusion

This volume aims to draw together current thinking and developments in the use of contextual CBTs with people who experience distressing psychosis. The various contributions represent theories and practice as they have developed, often independently, across a variety of locations, including the United Kingdom, Spain, Australia and the United States. The reader will gain an understanding of how the problems related to psychosis are conceptualised and treated using acceptance- and mindfulness-based therapy approaches, with a particular emphasis on ACT and PBCT, in both individual and group formats. In addition, there are chapters on the development of experiential interventions for paranoia and understanding and on working with spirituality from a metacognitive perspective, as well as on the experiences of service users (clients/patients) in engaging in these forms of therapy. Many of the chapters describe protocols demonstrated through case studies and vignettes of contemporary contextual CBTp. Finally, many of the common experiential exercises used in these therapies, and referred to in the chapters, are described in the appendices at the end of the volume.

References

Abba, N., Chadwick, P. & Stevenson, C. (2008). Responding mindfully to distressing psychosis: a grounded theory analysis. *Psychotherapy Research*, 18, 77–87.

Bach, P. & Hayes, S. C. (2002). The use acceptance and commitment therapy to prevent the rehospitalisation of psychotic patients: a randomised controlled trial. *Journal of Consulting and Counselling Psychology*, 70, 1129–1139.

Baer, R. A. (2003). Mindfulness training as a clinical intervention: a conceptual and empirical review. *Clinical Psychology: Science and Practice*, 10, 125–143.

Baer, R. A., Smith, G. T. & Allen, K. B. (2004). Assessment of mindfulness by report. The Kentucky Inventory of Mindfulness Skills. *Assessment*, 11, 191–206.

Bebbington, P. & Kuipers, L. (1994) The predictive utility of expressed emotion in schizophrenia: an aggregate analysis. *Psychological Medicine*, 24, 707–718.

Beck, A. T., Rush, A. J., Shaw, B. F. & Emery, G. (1979) *Cognitive Therapy of Depression*. New York: Guildford Press.

Bentall, R. P. (2003) *Madness Explained: Psychosis and Human Nature*. London: Penguin Books.

Birchwood, M. (2003). Pathways to emotional dysfunction in first-episode psychosis. *The British Journal of Psychiatry*, 182, 373–375.

Birchwood, M., Iqbal, Z., Chadwick, P. & Trower, P. (2000). Cognitive approach to depression and suicidal thinking in psychosis. I. Ontogeny of post-psychotic depression. *British Journal of Psychiatry*, 177, 516–521.

Blackledge, J. T., Ciarrochi, J. and Deane, F. P. (2009). *Acceptance and Commitment Therapy Contemporary Theory, Research and Practice*. Australian Academic Press.

Boyle. M. (2002). *Schizophrenia: A Scientific Delusion?* (2nd edn). London: Routledge.

Chadwick, P. (2006). *Person Based Cognitive Therapy for Distressing Psychosis*. Chichester: John Wiley & Sons.

Chadwick, P., Newman Taylor, K. & Abba, N. (2005). Mindfulness groups for people with psychosis. *Behavioural and Cognitive Psychotherapy*, 33, 351–359

Chadwick, P., Hughes, S., Russell, D., Russell, I. & Dagnan, D. (2009). Mindfulness groups for distressing voices and paranoia: a replication and randomised feasibility trial. *Behavioural and Cognitive Psychotherapy*, 37, 403–412

Close, H. & Garety, P. (1998). Cognitive assessment of voices: Further developments in understanding the emotional impact of voices. *British Journal of Clinical Psychology*, 37, 173–188.

Curson, D. A., Patel, M., Liddle, P. F. *et al.* (1988) Psychiatric morbidity of a long-stay hospital population with chronic schizophrenia and implications for future community care. *British Medical Journal*, 297, 819–822.

Dunn, G., Fowler, D., Rollinson, R., Freeman, D., Kuipers, E., Smith, B., Steel, C., Onwumere, J., Jolley, S., Garety, P. & Bebbington, P. (2011) Effective elements of cognitive behaviour therapy for psychosis: results of a novel type of subgroup analysis based on principal stratification. *Psychological Medicine*, 42, 1057–1068

Fowler, D. G., Garety, P. & Kuipers, E. (1995) *Cognitive Behaviour Therapy for Psychosis: Theory and Practice*. Chichester: John Wiley & Sons.

Freeman, D. & Garety, P. A. (2003) Connecting neurosis and psychosis: the direct influence of emotion on delusions and hallucinations. *Behaviour Research & Therapy*, 41, 923–947.

Garety, P. A., Kuipers, E., Fowler, D., Freeman, D. & Bebbington, P. E. (2001). A cognitive model of the positive symptoms of psychosis. *Psychological Medicine*, 31, 189–195.

Gaudino, B. A. & Herbert, J. D. (2006). Acute treatment of inpatients with psychotic symptoms using acceptance and commitment therapy: pilot results. *Behaviour Research and Therapy*, 44, 415–437.

Hayes, S. C. (1984). Making sense of spirituality. *Behaviourism*, 12, 99–110.

Hayes, S. C. (2004). Acceptance and commitment therapy, relational frame theory, and the third wave of behavioural and cognitive therapies. *Behaviour Therapy*, 35, 639–665.

Hayes, S. C., Strosahl, K. & Wilson, K. G. (1999). *Acceptance and Commitment Therapy: An Experiential Approach to Behavior Change*. New York: Guilford Press.

Hayes, S. C., Follette, V. M. & Linehan, M. M. (2004). *Mindfulness and Acceptance: Expanding the Cognitive-behavioral Tradition*. New York: Guilford Press.

Hayes, S. C., Luoma, J. B., Bond, F. W., Masuda, A. & Lillis, J. (2006). Acceptance and commitment therapy: model, processes and outcomes. *Behaviour Research and Therapy*, 44, 1–25.

Hayes, S. C., Villatte, M., Levin, M. & Hildebrandt, M. (2011). Open, aware and active: contextual approaches as an emerging trend in the behavioral and cognitive therapies. *Annual Review of Clinical Psychology*, 7, 141–168.

Jacobson, N. S. & Christenson, A. (1996). *Integrative Couple Therapy: Promoting Acceptance and Change*. New York: Norton.

Johns L. C., Peters, E. R. & Kuipers, E. (2007). Psychosis: treatment. In S. J. Lindsay & G. E. Powell (eds). *The Handbook of Clinical Adult Psychology 3rd Edition*. London: Brunner-Routledge.

Johnstone, E. C., Owens, D. G. C., Frith, C. D. & Leavy, J. (1991). Clinical findings: abnormalities of mental state and their correlated. The Northwick Park follow-up study. *British Journal of Psychiatry*, 159, 21–25.

Kabat-Zinn, J. (1994). *Wherever You Go, There You Are: Mindfulness Meditation in Everyday Life*. New York: Hyperion.

Kane, J. M. (1996). Drug therapy: schizophrenia. *New England Journal of Medicine*, 334, 34–41.

Kingdon, D. G. & Turkington, D. (1991) *Cognitive-behavioral Therapy of Schizophrenia*. Hove: LEA.

Kohlenberg, R. J. & Tsai, M. (1991). *Functional Analytic Psychotherapy: Creating Intense and Curative Therapeutic Relationships*. New York: Plenum.

Kuipers, E., Peters, E. & Bebbington, P. (2006). Schizophrenia. In A. Carr & M. McNulty (eds). *The Handbook of Adult Clinical Psychology: An Evidence-based Practice Approach*. New York: Routledge / Taylor & Francis Group.

Lieberman, J. A., Stroup, T. S., McEvoy, J. P. *et al.* for CATIE Investigators (2005). Effectiveness of antipsychotic drugs in patients with schizophrenia. *New England Journal of Medicine*, 353, 1209–1223.

Linehan, M. M. (1987). Dialectical behavioural therapy: a cognitive behavioural approach to parasuicide. *Journal of Personality Disorders*, 1, 328–333.

Linehan, M. (1993). *Cognitive-behavioral Treatment of Borderline Personality Disorder*. New York: Guilford Press.

Longmore, R. J. & Worrell, M. (2007) Do we need to challenge thoughts in cognitive behavior therapy? *Clinical Psychology Review*, 27, 173–187.

McCrone, P., Dhanasiri, S., Patel, A., Knapp, M. & Lawton-Smith, S. (2008). *Paying the Price. The Cost of Mental Health Care in England to 2006*. London: King's Fund.

McGrath, J. J., Saha, S., Welham, J., El-Saadi, O., MacCauley, C. & Chant, D. C. (2004). A systematic review of the incidence of schizophrenia: the distribution of rate items and the influence of methodology, urbanicity, sex and migrant status. *Schizophrenia Research*, 67, 65–66.

Morrison, A. P. (2001). The interpretation of intrusions in psychosis: an integrative cognitive approach to hallucinations and delusions. *Behavioural & Cognitive Psychotherapy*, 29, 257–276.

Morrison, A. P., Haddock, G. & Tarrier, N. (1995). Intrusive thoughts & auditory hallucinations: a cognitive approach. *Behavioural and Cognitive Psychotherapy*, 23, 265–265.

Nayani, T. & David, A. S. (1996). The auditory hallucination: a phenomenological survey. *Psychological Medicine*, 26, 177–189.

Oliver, E. A. & Fearon, P. (2008). Schizophrenia: epidemiology and risk factors. *Psychiatry*, 7, 410–414.

Perry, Y., Henry, J. D. & Grisham, J. R. (2011). The habitual use of emotion regulation strategies in schizophrenia. *British Journal of Clinical Psychology*, 50, 217–222.

Peters, E. R., Linney, Y., Johns, L. C. & Kuipers, E. (2007). Psychosis: investigation. In S. J. Lindsay & G. E. Powell (eds). *The Handbook of Clinical Adult Psychology* 3rd Edition. London: Brunner-Routledge.

Rogers, C. (1961). *On Becoming a Person: A Therapist's View of Psychotherapy*. London: Constable.

Saha, S., Chant, D., Welham, J. & McGrath, J. (2005). A systematic review of the prevalence of schizophrenia. *PLoS Medicine*, 2(5), e141.

Saarni, S., Viertiö, S., Perälä, J., Koskinen, S., Lönnqvist, J. & Suvisaari, J. (2010). Quality of life of people with schizophrenia, bipolar disorder and other psychotic disorders. *British Journal of Psychiatry*, 197, 386–394.

Shawyer, F., Farhall, J., Mackinnon, A., Trauer, T., Sims, E., Ratcliff, K., Larner, C., Thomas, N., Castle, D., Mullen, P. & Copolov, D. (2012). A randomised controlled trial of acceptance-based cognitive behavioural therapy for command hallucinations in psychotic disorders. *Behaviour Research and Therapy*, 50, 110–121.

Smith, B., O'Sullivan, B., Watson, P., Onwumere, J., Bebbington, P., Garety, P., Freeman, D., Fowler, D. & Kuipers, E. (2010). Individual cognitive behavioural therapy of auditory-verbal hallucinations. In F. Laroi & A. Aleman (eds). *Hallucinations: A Guide to Treatment and Management*. New York: Oxford University Press.

Teasdale, J. D., Segal, Z. V. & Williams, J. M. G. (1995). How does cognitive therapy prevent depressive relapse and why should attentional control (mindfulness) training help? *Behaviour Research and Therapy*, 33, 25–39.

Van Os, J. (2004). Does the urban environment cause psychosis? *British Journal of Psychiatry*, 184, 287–288.

Vygotsky, L. S. (1978). *Mind and Society: The Development of Higher Mental Processes*. Cambridge, MA: Harvard University Press.

Wells, A. (2000). *Emotional Disorders and Metacognition: Innovative Cognitive Therapy*. Chichester: John Wiley & Sons.

White, R. G., Gumley, A. I.., McTaggart, J., Rattrie, L., McConville, D., Cleare, S. & Mitchell, G. (2011) A feasibility study of Acceptance and Commitment Therapy for emotional dysfunction following psychosis. *Behaviour Research and Therapy*, 49, 901–907.

World Health Organization (2001). The World Health Report 2001. Mental health: new understanding, new hope. Geneva: World Health Organization.

Wu, E. Q., Birnbaum, H. G., Shi, L., Ball, D. E., Kessler, R. C., Moulis, M. & Aggarwal, J. (2005). The economic burden of schizophrenia in the United States in 2002. *Journal of Clinical Psychiatry*, 66, 1122–1129.

Wykes, T., Steel, C., Everitt, B. & Tarrier, N. (2009). Cognitive behavioural therapy for schizophrenia: effect sizes, clinical models, and methodological rigor. *Schizophrenia Bulletin*, 34, 523–537.

Zimmermann, G., Favrod, J., Trieu, V. H. & Pomini, V. (2005). The effect of cognitive behavioral treatment on the positive symptoms of schizophrenia spectrum disorders: a meta-analysis. *Schizophrenia Research*, 77, 1–9.

2

Theory on Voices

Fran Shawyer, Neil Thomas, Eric M. J. Morris
and John Farhall

2.1   Phenomenology

Auditory hallucinations are experienced by more than two-thirds of those who receive a diagnosis of schizophrenia. They are by far the most common modality of hallucination in schizophrenia and perhaps the symptom that is most recognised (Larøi *et al.*, 2012). Auditory hallucinations are prevalent in residual as well as acute phases, persisting in approximately a third of people, despite therapeutic doses of medication (Carr, 1988; Curson *et al.*, 1988).

Overwhelmingly, auditory hallucinations are reported as verbal hallucinations, usually described as a voice or voices. Although most commonly associated with schizophrenia, they can also occur in other conditions and in psychologically and medically healthy individuals in the general population (Barrett & Caylor, 1998; Daalman *et al.*, 2011; Johns, 2005; Wiles *et al.*, 2006).

In psychotic disorders, voices may be experienced as coming from inside or outside the head, but are distinguished from thoughts by having an auditory quality that is often not under the voice hearer's control (Copolov *et al.*, 2004b; Hoffman *et al.*, 2008; Oulis *et al.*, 1995). The voices may or may not sound like people known to the hearer. They may be male or female, although most often they are reported to be male. The majority of voice hearers hear multiple voices: Nayani & David (1996) reported that two-thirds of their sample heard more than one voice, with a mean of 3.2 voices reported. Reports of loudness and clarity vary greatly but voices are often described as similar to normal conversation (Nayani & David, 1996; Oulis *et al.*, 1995). The frequency of voices is often high, usually several times a day (Hustig & Hafner, 1990; Junginger & Frame, 1985; Oulis *et al.*, 1995), while the duration of discrete

Acceptance and Commitment Therapy and Mindfulness for Psychosis, First Edition.
Edited by Eric M. J. Morris, Louise C. Johns and Joseph E. Oliver.
© 2013 John Wiley & Sons, Ltd. Published 2013 by John Wiley & Sons, Ltd.

experiences of hearing a voice ranges from a few seconds to several hours, with some individuals experiencing voices as continuously present (Nayani & David, 1996).

As well as their verbal form, a striking characteristic of auditory hallucinations is that their content is almost always self-referent, talking to or about the person, their activities or their concerns (Leudar *et al.*, 1997). Typically, voices address the percipient in the second person (e.g. 'You're weak!'), but the experience of hearing voices in the third person commenting on one's behaviour or conversing with each other is relatively common. The content of voices is varied – commands, questions, criticism, supportive comments, frightening content, arguments – but themes are predominantly negative (Carter *et al.*, 1996; Close & Garety, 1998; Copolov *et al.*, 2004a; Farhall & Gehrke, 1997; Johns *et al.*, 2002; Soppitt & Birchwood, 1997), such as verbal abuse (Linn, 1977; Nayani & David, 1996) and false accusations (Linn, 1977). Voices that give orders or issue directives, commonly referred to as command hallucinations, are typically more stressful than noncommands (Mackinnon *et al.*, 2004). If present, command hallucinations can range from trivial to life-threatening directives (Beck-Sander *et al.*, 1997; Shawyer *et al.*, 2003, 2008). Given the bias of voice content towards negative, emotive and self-referent material, it is not surprising that many patients are distressed by their experience of voices.

2.2 Mechanisms and Origins of Hearing Voices

Although the precise mechanisms of auditory hallucinations have not been agreed upon, most researchers consider that they occur when self-generated mental events are wrongly attributed to an external source (Waters *et al.*, 2012). A common proposal has been that hallucinations reflect a misinterpretation of inner speech or processes related to speech production, resulting in internally generated verbal material appearing alien (Allen *et al.*, 2007; Frith, 1992; Jones & Fernyhough, 2007; Leudar *et al.*, 1997; Waters *et al.*, 2011). However, considering hallucinations as a manifestation of inner speech does not fully explain the distinct content of hallucinatory experience, in particular why it is usually in the form of the second or third person and so frequently includes critical, threatening or commanding themes. Alternative models have suggested that particular types of verbal material intruding into consciousness may account for the content of voices (Beck & Rector, 2003; Hoffman, 1986; Morrison *et al.*, 1995; Steel *et al.*, 2005; Waters *et al.*, 2006). For example, Morrison (2001; Morrison & Baker, 2000) noted that hallucinations are similar to intrusive thoughts in a number of ways, such as being repetitive, unintended and having content viewed as unacceptable. He argued that the cognitive dissonance associated with intrusive thoughts motivates the person to disown such intrusive thoughts, attributing them to an external source. Meanwhile, Waters *et al.* (2006) have proposed that auditory hallucinations arise from a combined deficit in intentional inhibition (the deliberate suppression of information from consciousness after deciding it is irrelevant) and context memory (the cues that enable differentiation between memories). They present evidence to suggest that deficits in these two domains result in the production of uncontrollable and unwanted thoughts which are not recognised due to the loss of contextual cues. Thus, the content of voices may be reproductions of speech and other sounds heard in the past, accounting for features such as the voice often being known, the speech being in the second or third person, the voice having age, affect and gender characteristics and the voice seeming so personal.

In line with the possible role of memory, there have been increasing reports of associations between hallucinatory content and broader cognitive structures and personal history. For example, there is increasing recognition of the frequency of past trauma exposure in psychotic disorders, particularly childhood sexual abuse (Bendall *et al.*, 2010; Cutajar *et al.*, 2010). Auditory hallucinations are also found at elevated levels in trauma-exposed groups, often being reported, for example, in borderline personality disorder (BPD) (Kingdon *et al.*, 2010; Sar, 2007). Additionally, the content of voices may reflect past emotional events and relationships, although seemingly at a thematic level rather than as a 'replaying' of specific memories (Hardy *et al.*, 2005; Steel *et al.*, 2005).

Other theorists have considered the meaning of auditory hallucinations from an evolutionary perspective. Gilbert *et al.* (2001) hypothesised that traumatic events in development can lead to the limbic-based threat system dominating the interpretation of emotional signals. Evolved processes of hostile dominant–subordinate interactions that are played out socially can also be played internally in this sensitised system, and they proposed that voices represent such an interaction. Evolutionary theorists have been particularly struck by a central question of schizophrenia: if this highly heritable condition confers such negative effects on fitness, why has it not been selected out (Kellenher *et al.*, 2010)? This has led some to formulate psychosis as one end of the spectrum of a fundamental genetic variation common to *Homo sapiens* (Burns, 2004; Crow, 1997; Kellenher *et al.*, 2010). For example, Crow (1997) has argued that it developed as part of the brain changes associated with the evolution of language, especially its lateralisation. As such, it is an extreme of variation in the general population as old as our species: 'the price that *Homo sapiens* pays for language' (p. 127). Symptoms such as voices are proposed to relate to a failure to establish clear lateral hemispheric dominance, most specifically in the breakdown of the fundamental 'I' and 'you' structure of language on which communication relies and which forms part of the hemispheric specialisation (Crow, 2004).

2.3   Meaning Given to Voice Experience

In actively attempting to make sense of the experience of hearing voices, the person will typically form a set of explanatory beliefs for their symptoms (Nayani & David, 1996). In keeping with the perceptual experience of voices as externally caused, it is typical for the person to develop beliefs that their voices originate from sentient others located in external reality, as opposed to being a mentally generated phenomenon. Chadwick & Birchwood (1994) highlighted that people readily form beliefs about the identity and motives of these perceived beings. If voices sound like people the hearer knows, they are likely to be attributed to those people; other voices may be perceived as coming from God, the devil, machines and so on (Nayani & David, 1996). Most people additionally report their voice to be very powerful, a belief that is significantly correlated with depression and anxiety (Chadwick & Birchwood, 1994; Chadwick *et al.*, 2000a; Close & Garety, 1998; Mawson *et al.*, 2010; van der Gaag *et al.*, 2003). The beliefs formed about voices may also be influenced by core personal and autobiographical beliefs, for example cognitions about differences between self and others in terms of social rank (Birchwood *et al.*, 2000). In this way, there may arise a series of beliefs related to the experience of hallucinations, which further reinforce their sense of being external and real.

Of course, the meaning imposed upon voices may be influenced by other psychotic symptoms, in particular the person's awareness of their difficulties and delusional beliefs. A number of reasoning biases have been demonstrated to be present to a greater degree in psychosis compared to healthy controls, including a tendency to attach blame for negative events to external factors (Laroi & Van der Linden, 2005) a tendency to 'jump to conclusions' on the basis of relatively little evidence (Barkus *et al.*, 2007; Garety *et al.*, 1991) and a poorer ability to generate alternative explanations for experiences (Freeman *et al.*, 2004).

A further relationship with psychosis more broadly is the role of assignment of personal meaning and salience to both external events and internal experiences. Kapur (2003) describes the attribution of salience as 'a process whereby events and thoughts come to grab attention, drive action, and influence goal-directed behavior because of their association with reward or punishment' (p. 14). This process is ordinarily regulated by dopamine, which has a central role in motivating behaviour by attributing salience to events that are likely to be rewarding or punishing based on prior experience. Kapur argues that, in psychosis, dopamine transmission becomes dysregulated – that is, dopamine release is no longer governed by relevant contextual factors but is stimulus-independent. Rather than being a mediator of contextually appropriate saliences, dopamine becomes 'a creator of saliences, albeit aberrant ones' (p. 15). This may lead to the content of hallucinations and related thoughts about voices taking on particular importance. The message from the brain is essentially, 'this is important for your survival – think about nothing else', leading to increased attention and preoccupation.

2.4 Responses to Voices

Given that the characteristics of voices are similar to heard speech, it is unsurprising that most voice hearers describe talking back to their voices, either aloud or silently, as they would another person (Leudar *et al.*, 1997). This may give rise to a dialogue-like interchange, which may immerse the person further in their private experience and reinforce hallucinatory activity. Indeed, people can describe responding to their voices in terms similar to those of normal interpersonal relationships (Benjamin, 1989).

In considering different types of response to voices, Chadwick & Birchwood (1995) describe contrasting responses of either resisting voices or engaging with them. These seem to be predicted by the interpersonal meaning which the voice hearer imposes upon the experience (Chadwick & Birchwood, 1995) and can be understood as reciprocal responses to perceived hostile or affiliative voice behaviour (Thomas *et al.*, 2009). Engagement may also incorporate submissive responses to voices, which may involve compliance or appeasement behaviours in response to command hallucinations (Braham *et al.*, 2004; Shawyer *et al.*, 2005, 2008).

Research on different responses to voices has also examined voice hearers' responses from the perspective of attempts to cope with them as a potentially stressful experience. The majority of patients are able to identify coping methods they have spontaneously developed in an attempt to cope with the symptom (Falloon & Talbot, 1981; Farhall & Gehrke, 1997; Farhall & Voudouris, 1996; Farhall *et al.*, 2007; Nayani & David, 1996; O'Sullivan, 1994). These may include responses specific to coping with hearing voices, such as listening to music or wearing earplugs, but more often involve general methods of coping not specific to hallucinations, such as increasing activity. In line with the interpersonal literature, analyses of coping responses have also elicited themes of engagement with voices and rejection of or resistance to voices; however, additional factors identified have included both passive and active forms of acceptance of the phenomenon (Farhall & Gehrke, 1997; Farhall *et al.*, 2007; O'Sullivan, 1994).

Following the common theme of resistance and engagement as responses to voices, we consider their impact in more detail, and look at the potential role of acceptance as an alternative.

2.4.1   Resistance

Resistance may be defined as an effortful attempt at regulation or control of voices with the aim of directly eliminating or reducing the voices themselves or their impact. Borrowing from evolutionary psychology, resistance to hostile voices can be divided into the fundamental 'fight' (attempts to confront) and 'flight' (attempts to escape, avoid or suppress) responses (Gilbert *et al.*, 2001). In an exploration of these mechanisms in voice hearers, Gilbert *et al.* (2001) found that both these responses were associated with powerful voices and also with feeling trapped and depressed. They speculated that 'voice hearers probably do not think they can easily defeat their voices, but also do not willingly or affiliatively subordinate themselves to their voices and may feel more like angry subordinates' (p. 1122). This may be why, although resistance to command hallucinations is common, it is of limited effectiveness in reducing compliance, especially if the voice is considered powerful (Shawyer *et al.*, 2005, 2008). If efforts to resist ongoing auditory hallucinations are experienced as futile, it is understandable that depression is the outcome. Some have suggested that this process may contribute to the high rate of suicide in schizophrenia (Drake & Cotton, 1986; Harris & Barraclough, 1998).

Findings from the auditory hallucination coping literature also point to the often ineffectual and potentially harmful nature of resistance. 'Fight' strategies such as shouting back at the voices or arguing with them have been identified as an inadequate method of coping (Falloon & Talbot, 1981; Farhall & Voudouris, 1996; McInnis & Marks, 1990; Romme & Escher, 1989) and are associated with poorer emotion control (Farhall & Gehrke, 1997). 'Flight' responses have also been associated with poor coping levels (Romme *et al.*, 1992), depression (Escher *et al.*, 2003), distress (Vaughan & Fowler, 2004) and reduced self-esteem (Haddock *et al.*, 1998). Flight strategies may also have the effect of maintaining auditory hallucinations, and the power of auditory hallucinations, in the longer term (Morrison & Haddock, 1997). The use of 'safety behaviours', for example, which are designed to prevent a feared outcome associated with delusional interpretations of voices, may prevent the assessment of true risk and subsequent disconfirmation of the interpretation (Hacker *et al.*, 2008; Morrison, 1998; Morrison & Renton, 2001; Yusupoff & Tarrier, 1996).

Actively hostile, negative and nonaccepting attitudes towards one's voices may contribute to increases in voice frequency and reduced coping through the increased physiological arousal created by these emotions (Al-Issa, 1995; Gilbert *et al.*, 2001; Romme & Escher, 1989). The role of stress and arousal in exacerbating auditory hallucinations has been postulated for many years (Slade, 1972, 1973, 1976). In support of this interaction, there is evidence that anxiety predicts hallucination intensity (Delespaul *et al.*, 2002) and that emotions increase the bias towards the external attribution of thoughts, the process thought to be at the heart of the formation of auditory hallucinations (Morrison & Haddock, 1997).

2.4.2   Engagement

Engagement describes the most direct, contrasting response to resistance and is defined as 'elective listening, willing compliance, and doing things to bring on the voices' (Chadwick & Birchwood, 1994). At its most basic, engagement involves listening to the voices and accepting what they say (Falloon & Talbot, 1981; Farhall & Gehrke, 1997; Farhall & Voudouris, 1996; Frederick & Cotanch, 1995). At a more complex level, it may involve a capacity for discrimination: accepting the 'good' voices and rejecting the 'bad' ones (Frederick & Cotanch, 1995; Romme & Escher, 1989), or in the case of directives, considering their worth rather than blocking or ignoring them (Leudar *et al.*, 1997). In the auditory hallucinations literature, the term 'acceptance' has not infrequently been used to mean the same thing as 'engagement' (Birchwood & Chadwick, 1997; Farhall & Voudouris, 1996; Lucas & Wade, 2001; Pembroke, 1998), though acceptance in this sense is narrowly confined to accepting, to some degree, the content of the voices. In the coping literature, this form of engaged acceptance has been rated as a moderately useful natural coping strategy (Falloon & Talbot, 1981; Farhall & Voudouris, 1996) which may potentially lead to greater control of hallucinations (Falloon & Talbot, 1981; Farhall & Gehrke, 1997; Frederick & Cotanch, 1995)

However, engagement with voices has the potential to become overly 'intimate' and has hidden costs in terms of flexibility, privacy, confidence, adherence to treatment and social adaptation (Benjamin, 1989; Birchwood & Chadwick, 1997; Falloon & Talbot, 1981). Favrod *et al.* (2004) found, for example, that those who had a positive relationship with their voices and engaged with them experienced poorer social functioning and cooperation with treatment. Vaughan & Fowler (2004) also found a strong positive correlation between helplessness and dependency on voices and benevolence, suggesting that 'people submit to a voice when they trust it' (p. 151). Engagement is also likely to result in problems for the majority of people with psychosis who experience exclusively negative voices, such as derogatory comments, and is of greatest concern for those who experience harmful command hallucinations. Viewing voices as positive has been linked to compliance with harmful commands (Beck-Sander *et al.*, 1997; Fox *et al.*, 2004; Shawyer *et al.*, 2008), particularly when the commands are supported by congruent delusions, since the 'logical' basis for action is stronger (Junginger, 1990; Shawyer *et al.*, 2008).

2.5   Implications for the Role of Acceptance and Mindfulness in Voices

Our survey of the literature suggests the following important points in understanding the experience of auditory hallucinations. First, there are a number of ways in which hallucinations are an unusually compelling verbal experience for people with psychosis:

(1)   They are often intrusive, uncontrollable and inescapable.
(2)   Their content typically involves self-referent and often negative and emotive material.
(3)   While models of auditory hallucinations are varied, they converge on the idea that voices originate in cognitive activity that would ordinarily be experienced as normal verbal thought, but which ends up being experienced as if originating in external reality.
(4)   Through its interpersonal-like characteristics and potentially through the aberrant assignment of salience to it, additional meaning may be imposed upon voice experience, making it appear especially important to attend to.

Second, the responses often elicited by this phenomenon may end up both reinforcing the experience and compounding related distress and/or disability. In the face of this adverse interpersonal experience, voice hearers develop attempts to cope as best they can based on their beliefs about the voices and their more general beliefs about social relationships. However, the main forms of response – engagement and resistance – tend to compound the problem. While engagement has the potential to promote unhealthy involvement in voices, resistance can have harmful repercussions and appears to be of limited effectiveness in controlling voices. Both forms of response are associated with poorer adaptation, probably because they perpetuate the relationship with voices through continued involvement with them. This continued preoccupation may come at the cost of pursuing important life goals and directions.

Over the past 2–3 decades, acceptance as a potentially more adaptive response to voices has been an emerging theme in the auditory hallucinations literature. Over a quarter of a century ago, for example, Cohen (1985) identified acceptance as a 'do nothing' coping response used by some patients with schizophrenia, which suggested they had learned to live with symptoms such as voices. He distinguished this response from a less healthy alternative 'do nothing' strategy which involved helplessness and giving up. This new form of acceptance, involving a general orientation to voices, rather than the simple acceptance of content highlighted in the previous section, has been incorporated into therapeutic interventions for its potential to improve adaptation to voices.

One of the most established ways of seeking to promote acceptance of voices through therapeutic interventions has been to attempt to cultivate 'insight'. This form of acceptance has been central to some forms of cognitive behaviour therapy (CBT) for psychosis (Kingdon & Turkington, 1991, 1994; Morrison & Renton, 2001; Sensky *et al.*, 2000), and interventions here typically include nonconfrontational and personalised discussions of alternative illness-based models, along with other efforts to challenge beliefs about voices and ultimately reattribute voices to the self using belief-modification techniques (Bentall *et al.*, 1994; Garety *et al.*, 2000; Kingdon & Turkington, 1991). By coming to accept voices as being part of an illness rather than as coming from real people, it is hoped that such interventions will result in improved adaptation and disengagement from voices (Chadwick & Birchwood, 1994; van der Gaag, 2006).

However, the available data suggest that, despite CBT interventions, improvements in insight often either fail to occur (Chadwick *et al.*, 2000b; Newton *et al.*, 2005), fluctuate (Bentall *et al.*, 1994) or are not maintained (Valmaggia *et al.*, 2005). There may be a number of reasons for this, such as cognitive inflexibility (Garety *et al.*, 1997; McGowan *et al.*, 2005) or defence of self-esteem (Bentall, 1990). Perhaps more fundamentally, illness models and self-attribution may be resisted because they do not tally with the compelling nature of the ongoing, subjective experience of auditory hallucinations (Gray *et al.*, 1991; Kapur, 2003). Thus, even where an illness model is 'accepted' to some degree, allegiance to the delusional explanation may persist (McGowan *et al.*, 2005).

Another approach has been pioneered in the work of Romme and colleagues (Romme & Escher, 1989, 1993a, 1993b; Romme *et al.*, 1992), who suggest that acceptance of voices can be achieved by exploring their personal meaning, acknowledging their positive aspects and learning to incorporate them into one's life, rather than by attempting to eliminate them. This work has been influential with consumer groups, such as the UK Hearing Voices Network, who promote a theme of accepting voices, including via self-help publications and peer-support groups (Baker, 1995; Coleman & Smith, 2002). However, to date there have been no controlled studies published which directly evaluate the impact of this method (Ruddle *et al.*, 2011).

Though quite different in approach, these therapeutic forms of acceptance have in common a dependence upon the voice hearer adopting a particular point of view – in particular, 'accepting' some particular explanation for their voices. Thus, therapeutic interventions incorporating this approach are narrowly reliant on the person adhering to a verbally based narrative about the experience. It is assumed that these explanations will then result in less distress and life disruption. While these explanations may inform the use of certain coping strategies, neither specifically encompasses skills for accepting voices as they occur. This is important because, as noted earlier, the 'on-line' experience of voices often remains real and engulfing despite an ability to rationally reflect upon them after the event. In the face of the salience of the voice experience as it occurs, alternative explanations may be of limited effectiveness and may sit in opposition to other important sources of meaning for the person.

The recent developments in what has been called the 'third wave' of behaviour therapy (Hayes, 2004), such as mindfulness-based cognitive therapy (MBCT) (Segal *et al.*, 2002) and acceptance and commitment therapy (ACT) (Hayes *et al.*, 2012), have highlighted a form of acceptance that may provide a more adaptive alternative response to both engagement and resistance, which fosters skills that can be applied 'on-line' as the voices occur. This form of acceptance – what might be termed 'mindful acceptance' – is neither a coping strategy nor a process of providing meaning, but rather a particular style of relating to aversive and uncontrollable psychological events such as voices. It involves two main sets of skills: (1) non-judgemental awareness – deliberately observing voices as they occur without judging them as good or bad and without reacting to them; and (2) disengagement (detachment) from the literal meaning of the content of voices and associated appraisals – that is, distinguishing the actual experience (sounds/words) from what it represents (literal reality): 'seeing things the way they really are' (Marlett *et al.*, 2004, p. 267).

This represents a distinct approach to acceptance of voices from that of CBT for psychosis (CBTp) or the one advocated by Romme *et al.* There is no attempt either to explore or modify the content of the voices or to foster a better understanding of their origins or meaning. Likewise, there is no attempt to change their occurrence or form. Instead, these approaches focus on changing the person's *relationship* to these experiences (Pérez-Álvarez *et al.*, 2008).

Mindful acceptance is increasingly being trialled in psychosis in various forms. Mindfulness training, specifically adapted for psychosis, has been assessed both on its own (Abba *et al.*, 2008; Ashcroft *et al.*, 2011; Chadwick *et al.*, 2005, 2009; Davis *et al.*, 2007; Ellett *et al.*, 2008; Jacobsen *et al.*, 2010; Langer *et al.*, 2012; Newman Taylor *et al.*, 2009) and incorporated into broader CBT models, in particular person-based cognitive therapy (PBCT) (Dannahy *et al.*, 2011). These approaches are reviewed in Chapters 10 and 16, where it is noted that their formal evaluation is only at a very preliminary stage, with no large, well-controlled trials yet published. However, anecdotal case studies and other qualitative data from voice hearers offer potential insights into how mindfulness may be of benefit in reducing the impact of voices through nonjudgemental acceptance of their presence (Abba *et al.*, 2008; Ashcroft *et al.*, 2011; Chadwick *et al.*, 2005) and reduced belief in what they say (Newman Taylor *et al.*, 2009).

The application of mindful acceptance to psychosis in the form of ACT is a little more advanced in terms of evaluation. In applying ACT to voices, the process of mindful acceptance is supported by a number of practical skills, including *cognitive defusion* – a method of letting go of the literal reality of the content of voices and associated appraisals without having to undertake the difficult task of directly challenging their veracity or replacing them with a new narrative; *present moment, self-as-context* – a method of developing the dispassionate stance of a mindful observer of voice experience and the capacity to redirect attention to real-world activity; and *values, committed action* – a means of fostering an attitude of willingness to experience voices while pursuing valued action. Two randomised controlled trials (RCTs) assessing the effect of a brief version of ACT on symptoms and rehospitalisation in samples of inpatients have been conducted. These show promising findings, especially in relation to auditory hallucinations (Bach & Hayes, 2002; Gaudiano & Herbert, 2006a). Shawyer *et al.* (2012) have also compared an ACT-CBT hybrid treatment with befriending as an intervention for command hallucinations. Although power was low, the results showed that both interventions had strong benefits compared to waitlist on specific and general symptom measures, especially confidence in coping with command hallucinations (effect size = 1.07).

While a specific model for the application of mindfulness to psychotic symptoms has been proposed (see Chapter 10), comprehensive models of ACT or Relational Frame Theory (RFT) for psychosis in general and the phenomena of voices in particular have yet to be developed (Bach *et al.*, 2012; McLeod, 2009). ACT, however, is a transdiagnostic treatment approach based on the core assumption that human suffering is ubiquitous, as it arises predominantly from language (Hayes *et al.*, 2012). The general treatment principles of ACT as described in the hexaflex are therefore considered to be as applicable to hallucinations – particularly to responses to hallucinations – as to other problematic verbally mediated events (Hayes *et al.*, 2012; McLeod, 2009), albeit with pragmatic adaptations (detailed in Chapter 7), with acknowledgement of the extraordinary fusion and entanglement frequently engendered by the experience.

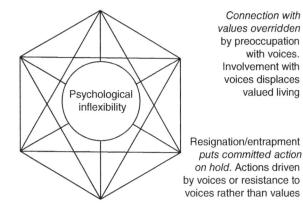

Loss of attentional flexibility as the
salience of voices as sentient beings
captures attention.
Perceived interpersonal dynamics activate
automatic engagement or resistance
reactions, impeding connection with the current
context within the external world

Experiential avoidance
Investment in struggle, escape and avoidance (resistance) prevents positive action

Cognitive fusion
Beliefs about voices and voice content are responded to as if literally true, triggering engagement or resistance and negatively impacting on functional activity

Connection with values overridden by preoccupation with voices. Involvement with voices displaces valued living

Resignation/entrapment *puts committed action on hold.* Actions driven by voices or resistance to voices rather than values

Psychological inflexibility

Domination of self as content, defined by self-referential voices and other beliefs (e.g. powerless, inferior, flawed, mad), interferes with the ability to make useful life changes. Lack of decentred awareness (diminution of 'I/here/now' perspective) leads to being lost in habitual reactions and engulfment with voices

Figure 2.1   An ACT model of problematic voice hearing

Figure 2.1 provides a hexaflex representation of the ACT model of treatment as applied to voices. Within this model, the association of resistance and engagement with poorer outcomes can be readily understood as a key expression of experiential avoidance and cognitive fusion. Making hallucinations the target of experiential avoidance through resistance efforts to control or eliminate them results in maintenance of the voices and negative consequences (Hayes *et al.*, 1996). Responding literally to hallucinations (i.e. fusion with the content) leads to narrowing of the response repertoire, resulting in reduced contact with direct contingencies (Hayes, 1989), such as when voices are used as a guide for actions or a source of meaning/knowledge, obeyed (in the case of command hallucinations) or indeed resisted.

However, despite the potentially detrimental effects of resisting or engaging with voices, it is important that these responses are understood within the *functional contextual framework* embodied by the hexaflex as a whole – that is, what is 'workable' within the context of the explicit articulation of, and commitment to, personal values and goals that cultivate real-world involvement. Within this framework, beliefs about voices and responses to voices, *including* engagement and resistance, are neither right nor wrong; the question is how these behaviours function in context. There is no attempt to impose a particular narrative on the voices; rather, the focus is on whether the beliefs and responses of the person help them to live their chosen way of life. The pragmatic lens of the functional contextual framework provides an alternate method of evaluating actions in relation to voice hearing, including narratives about the experience (sense-making). The voice hearer's personal values contextualise the impact of auditory hallucinations, by considering the various responses to voices as *functional classes of behaviour* (i.e. approach, escape, avoidance, sense-making) rather than by topographical categories (such as resistance and engagement). Thus, as described earlier, responses of resistance may be similar to engagement in terms of the functional consequences of reduced contact with meaning (reinforcement) in important life areas. For example, when examining with the patient how different ways of handling the voices work for them in family relationships, they may report that it is difficult to fully engage with their partner or children, whether they listen to the voices, argue back to them or try to work out what they mean. In the context of desiring strong family relationships, each of these responses to the voices has the same functional consequence of deflecting the person from their valued life path.

The constructional approach that underpins ACT (Goldiamond, 1974) means that focus is upon helping the voice hearer develop additional ways of coping, in order to increase behavioural flexibility and contact with life meaning (values). Thus, rather than the voice hearer being discouraged from using certain coping strategies, there is an emphasis on trying an increased range of different methods – especially alternative acceptance and other underused coping methods – and promoting choice in actions while hearing voices. ACT promotes pragmatic efforts to engage in valued actions in a broad range of environments and to notice when the experience of voice hearing appears to act as a barrier to engaging in these actions. This emphasis of personal values also means that the voice hearer's own experience of the workability of coping methods becomes central to the process of therapy. Personal values may also form a critical alternative to delusional reference systems associated with hearing voices, which may be of special relevance in preventing compliance to harmful command hallucinations (Shawyer *et al.*, 2008). For example, tuning into spiritual, moral or family values may counteract paranoia associated with commands to harm others and support a stance of noncompliance.

While there is some outcome evidence to support the applicability of ACT to auditory hallucinations, the implementation of any model of ACT in this area should ultimately rest on evidence that connects the theoretically important elements of the model to health or pathology (Hayes *et al.*, 2012). To date, very little has been published to demonstrate such links. A central role of cognitive fusion in understanding the negative effects of hallucinations is suggested by the finding that the distress they cause is mediated by reductions in their believability (Gaudiano & Herbert, 2006b; Gaudiano *et al.*, 2010). In addition, psychological flexibility and nonjudgemental awareness have been found to correlate negatively with depression and anxiety in a sample of distressed voice hearers, and to significantly account for the variance in disruption related to voice hearing (Morris *et al.*, submitted). Finally, a specific measure of acceptance and avoidance-based processes in auditory and command hallucinations, the Voices Acceptance and Action Scale (VAAS), has shown strong associations with measures of well-being and coping with command hallucinations, as well as a capacity to discriminate compliance with harmful command hallucinations from noncompliance (Shawyer *et al.*, 2007).

To conclude, the 'on-line' application of mindful acceptance and its overarching functional–contextual theoretical framework has arguably been a missing link in the psychological treatment of auditory hallucinations – a field in which the potential value of acceptance has been recognised for many years. Together, ACT and mindfulness provide:

(1)   A means of distancing from intrusive, inescapable and salient experiences.
(2)   A way of defusing from the literal content of voices and associated appraisals.
(3)   An alternative to being preoccupied with voices and drawn into unworkable responses.

By reducing struggle with voices on the one hand, and engagement with voices on the other, key responses that tend to compound the hallucinatory experience, such as arousal, attention and activation of brain areas, are hypothesised to be reduced. By developing alternative coping responses, attentional and behavioural flexibility is potentially increased so as to better reflect personal values and goals.

However, ACT for psychosis and other mindfulness-based interventions are at an early stage of development and evaluation in terms of both outcome and process, and as such it cannot be regarded as an evidence-based treatment for either auditory hallucinations or psychosis. Nevertheless, a number of potential synergies exist between ACT and other theoretical frameworks, including the development of language and brain asymmetry postulated by evolutionary genetic theory, the domination of threat–response systems highlighted by evolutionary psychology and the central role of suppression and avoidance mechanisms highlighted by several cognitive theories. These synergies, together with efforts to build on the existing experimental findings related to ACT-specific processes, may be fruitful lines of investigation to pursue in further understanding the application of ACT to voices.

References

Abba, N., Chadwick, P. & Stevenson, C. (2008). Responding mindfully to distressing psychosis: a grounded theory analysis. *Psychotherapy Research*, 18(1), 77–87.
Al-Issa, I. (1995). The illusion of reality or the reality of illusion: hallucinations and culture. *British Journal of Psychiatry*, 166, 336–373.

Allen, P., Aleman, A. & Mcguire, P. K. (2007). Inner speech models of auditory verbal hallucinations: Evidence from behavioural and neuroimaging studies. *International Review of Psychiatry*, 19(4), 407–415.

Ashcroft, K., Barrow, F., Lee, R. & MacKinnon, K. (2011). Mindfulness groups for early psychosis: a qualitative study. *Psychology and Psychotherapy: Theory, Research and Practice*, doi: 10.1111/j.2044-8341.2011.02031.x.

Bach, P. & Hayes, S. C. (2002). The use of Acceptance and Commitment Therapy to prevent rehospitalization of psychotic patients: a randomized controlled trial. *Journal of Consulting and Clinical Psychology*, 70(5), 1129–1139.

Bach, P., Hayes, S. C. & Gallop, R. (2012). Long-term effects of brief acceptance and commitment therapy for psychosis. *Behavior Modification*, 36(2), 165–181.

Baker, P. (1995). *The Voice Inside. A Practical Guide to Coping with Hearing Voices*. Manchester: Handsell Publications.

Barkus, E., Stirling, J., Hopkins, R., McKie, S. & Lewis, S. (2007). Cognitive and neural processes in non-clinical auditory hallucinations. *British Journal of Psychiatry*, 191, s76–s81.

Barrett, T. R. & Caylor, M. R. (1998). Verbal hallucinations in normals, V: perceived reality characteristics. *Personality and Individual Differences*, 25(2), 209–221.

Beck, A. T. & Rector, N. A. (2003). A cognitive model of hallucinations. *Cognitive Therapy and Research*, 27(1), 19–52.

Beck-Sander, A., Birchwood, M. & Chadwick, P. (1997). Acting on command hallucinations: a cognitive approach. *British Journal of Clinical Psychology*, 36(1), 139–148.

Bendall, S., Jackson, H. J. & Hulbert, C. A. (2010). Childhood trauma and psychosis: review of the evidence and directions for psychological interventions. *Australian Psychologist*, 45, 299–306.

Benjamin, L. S. (1989). Is chronicity a function of the relationship between the person and the auditory hallucination? *Schizophrenia Bulletin*, 15(2), 291–310.

Bentall, R. P. (1990). The illusion of reality: a review and integration of psychological research on hallucinations. *Psychological Bulletin*, 107(1), 82–95.

Bentall, R. P., Haddock, G. & Slade, P. D. (1994). Cognitive behaviour therapy for persistent auditory hallucinations: from theory to therapy. *Behaviour Therapy*, 25, 51–66.

Birchwood, M. & Chadwick, P. (1997). The omnipotence of voices: testing the validity of a cognitive model. *Psychological Medicine*, 27(6), 1345–1353.

Birchwood, M., Meaden, A., Trower, P., Gilbert, P. & Plaistow, J. (2000). The power and omnipotence of voices: subordination and entrapment by voices and significant others. *Psychological Medicine*, 30, 337–344.

Braham, L. G., Trower, P. & Birchwood, M. (2004). Acting on command hallucinations and dangerous behavior: a critique of the major findings in the last decade. *Clinical Psychology Review*, 24, 513–528.

Burns, J. K. (2004). An evolutionary theory of schizophrenia: cortical connectivity, metarepresentation, and the social brain. *Behavioral and Brain Sciences*, 27, 831–885.

Carr, V. (1988). Patients' techniques for coping with schizophrenia: an exploratory study. *British Journal of Medical Psychology*, 61(4), 339–352.

Carter, D. M., Mackinnon, A. & Copolov, D. L. (1996). Patients' strategies for coping with auditory hallucinations. *The Journal of Nervous and Mental Disease*, 184(2), 159–164.

Chadwick, P. & Birchwood, M. (1994). The omnipotence of voices: a cognitive approach to auditory hallucinations. *British Journal of Psychiatry*, 164, 190–201.

Chadwick, P. & Birchwood, M. (1995). The omnipotence of voices II: the Beliefs About Voices Questionnaire (BAVQ). *British Journal of Psychiatry*, 166, 773–776.

Chadwick, P., Lees, S. & Birchwood, M. (2000a). The revised Beliefs about Voices Questionnaire (BAVQ-R). *The British Journal of Psychiatry*, 177, 229–232.

Chadwick, P., Sambrooke, S., Rasch, S. & Davies, E. (2000b). Challenging the omnipotence of voices: group cognitive behaviour therapy for voices. *Behaviour Research and Therapy*, 38(10), 993–1003.

Chadwick, P., Newman Taylor, K. & Abba, N. (2005). Mindfulness groups for people with psychosis. *Behavioural and Cognitive Psychotherapy*, 33(3), 351–359.

Chadwick, P., Hughes, S., Russell, D., Russell, I. & Dagnan, D. (2009). Mindfulness groups for distressing voices and paranoia: a replication and feasibility trial. *Behavioural and Cognitive Psychotherapy*, 37, 403–412.

Close, H. & Garety, P. (1998). Cognitive assessment of voices: further developments in understanding the emotional impact of voices. *British Journal of Clinical Psychology*, 37(2), 173–188.

Cohen, C. I. & Berk, L. A. (1985). Personal coping styles of schizophrenic outpatients. *Hospital and Community Psychiatry*, 36(4), 407–410.

Coleman, R. & Smith, M. J. (2002). *Working with Voices. Victim to Victor 1.* Wellington: Keepwell.

Copolov, D., Mackinnon, A. & Trauer, T. (2004a). Correlates of the affective impact of auditory hallucinations in psychotic disorders. *Schizophrenia Bulletin*, 30(1), 163–171.

Copolov, D., Trauer, T. & Mackinnon, A. (2004b). On the non-significance of internal versus external auditory hallucinations. *Schizophrenia Research*, 69(1), 1–6.

Crow, T. J. (1997). Is schizophrenia the price that *Homo sapiens* pays for language? *Schizophrenia Research*, 28, 127–141.

Crow, T. (2004). Auditory hallucinations as primary disorders of syntax: an evolutionary theory of the origins of language. *Cognitive Neuropsychiatry*, 9(1–2), 125–145.

Curson, D. A., Patel, M., Liddle, P. F. & Barnes, T. R. (1988). Psychiatric morbidity of a long stay hospital population with chronic schizophrenia and implications for future community care. *British Medical Journal*, 297(6652), 819–822.

Cutajar, M. C., Mullen, P. E., Ogloff, J. R. P., Thomas, S. D., Wells, D. L. & Spataro, J. (2010). Schizophrenia and other psychotic disorders in a cohort of sexually abused children. *Archives of General Psychiatry*, 67, 1114–1119.

Daalman, K., Boks, M. P., Diederen, K. M., de Weijer, A. D., Blom, J. D., Kahn, R. S. & Sommer, I. E. (2011). The same or different? A phenomenological comparison of auditory verbal hallucinations in healthy and psychotic individuals. *Journal of Clinical Psychiatry*, 72(3), 320–325.

Dannahy, L., Hayward, M., Strauss, C., Turton, W., Harding, E. & Chadwick, P. (2011). Group person-based cognitive therapy for distressing voices: pilot data from nine groups. *Journal of Behavior Therapy and Experimental Psychiatry*, 42(1), 111–116.

Davis, L. W. P., Strasburger, A. M. M. A. & Brown, L. F. B. A. (2007). Mindfulness: an intervention for anxiety in schizophrenia. *Journal of Psychosocial Nursing & Mental Health Services*, 45(11), 23–29.

Delespaul, P., deVries, M. & van Os, J. (2002). Determinants of occurrence and recovery from hallucinations in daily life. *Social Psychiatry and Psychiatric Epidemiology*, 37(3), 97–104.

Drake, R. E. & Cotton, P. G. (1986). Depression, hopelessness and suicide in chronic schizophrenia. *British Journal of Psychiatry*, 148, 554–559.

Ellett, L., Freeman, D. & Garety, P. A. (2008). The psychological effect of an urban environment on individuals with persecutory delusions: the Camberwell walk study. *Schizophrenia Research*, 99(1–3), 77–84.

Escher, S., Delespaul, P., Romme, M., Buiks, A. & van Os, J. (2003). Coping defence and depression in adolescents hearing voices. *Journal of Mental Health*, 12(1), 91–99.

Falloon, I. R. H. & Talbot, R. E. (1981). Persistent auditory hallucinations: coping mechanisms and implications for management. *Psychological Medicine*, 11(2), 329–339.

Farhall, J. & Gehrke, M. (1997). Coping with hallucinations: exploring stress and coping framework. *British Journal of Clinical Psychology*, 36(2), 259–261.

Farhall, J. & Voudouris, N. (1996). Persisting auditory hallucinations: prospects for non-medication interventions in a hospital population. *Behaviour Change*, 13(1), 112–123.

Farhall, J., Greenwood, K. M. & Jackson, H. J. (2007). Coping with hallucinated voices in schizophrenia: a review of self-initiated strategies and therapeutic interventions. *Clinical Psychology Review*, 27(4), 476–493.

Favrod, J., Grasset, F., Spreng, S., Grossenbacher, B. & Hodé, Y. (2004). Benevolent voices are not so kind: the functional significance of auditory hallucinations. *Psychopathology*, 37(6), 304–308.

Fox, J. R. E., Gray, N. S. & Lewis, H. (2004). Factors determining compliance with command hallucinations with violent content: the role of social rank, perceived power of the voice and voice malevolence. *The Journal of Forensic Psychiatry & Psychology*, 15(3), 511–531.

Frederick, J. & Cotanch, P. (1995). Self-help strategies for auditory hallucinations in schizophrenia. *Issues in Mental Health Nursing*, 16(3), 213–224.

Freeman, D., Garety, P., Fowler, D., Kuipers, E., Bebbington, P. E. & Dunn, G. (2004). Why do people with delusions fail to choose more realistic explanations for their experiences? *Journal of Consulting and Clinical Psychology*, 72, 671–680.

Frith, C. D. (1992). *The Cognitive Neuropsychology of Schizophrenia*. London: LEA.

Garety, P. A., Hemsley, D. & Wessely, S. (1991). Reasoning in deluded schizophrenic and paranoid patients: biases in performance on a probabilistic inference task. *The Journal of Nervous and Mental Disease*, 179, 194–201.

Garety, P., Fowler, D., Kuipers, E., Freeman, D., Dunn, G., Bebbington, P., Hadley, C. & Jones, S. (1997). London-East Anglia randomized controlled trial of cognitive-behavioural therapy for psychosis. II: predictors of outcome. *British Journal of Psychiatry*, 171, 420–426.

Garety, P., Fowler, D. & Kuipers, E. (2000). Cognitive-Behavioral Therapy for medication-resistant symptoms. *Schizophrenia Bulletin*, 26(1), 73–86.

Gaudiano, B. A. & Herbert, J. D. (2006a). Acute treatment of inpatients with psychotic symptoms using Acceptance and Commitment Therapy: pilot results. *Behaviour Research and Therapy*, 44(3), 415–437.

Gaudiano, B. A. & Herbert, J. D. (2006b). Believability of hallucinations as a potential mediator of their frequency and associated distress in psychotic inpatients. *Behavioural and Cognitive Psychotherapy*, 34(4), 497–502.

Gaudiano, B. A., Herbert, J. D. & Hayes, S. C. (2010). Is it the symptom or the relation to it? Investigating potential mediators of change in acceptance and commitment therapy for psychosis. *Behavior Therapy*, 41(4), 543–554.

Gilbert, P., Birchwood, M., Gilbert, J., Trower, P., Hay, J., Murray, B., Meaden, A., Olsen, K. & Miles, J. N. V. (2001). An exploration of evolved mental mechanisms for dominant and subordinate behaviour in relation to auditory hallucinations in schizophrenia and critical thoughts in depression. *Psychological Medicine*, 31(6), 1117–1127.

Goldiamond, I. (1974). Toward a constructional approach to social problems: ethical and constitutional issues raised by applied behavior analysis. *Behaviorism*, 2(1), 1–84.

Gray, J. A., Feldon, J., Rawlins, J. N. P., Hemsley, D. R. & Smith, A. D. (1991). The neuropsychology of schizophrenia. *Behavioral and Brain Sciences*, 14(1), 56–84.

Hacker, D., Birchwood, M., Tudway, J., Meaden, A. & Amphlett, C. (2008). Acting on voices: omnipotence, sources of threat, and safety-seeking behaviours. *British Journal of Clinical Psychology*, 47(2), 201-213.

Haddock, G., Slade, P. D., Bentall, R. P., Reid, D. & Faragher, E. B. (1998). A comparison of the long-term effectiveness of distraction and focusing in the treatment of auditory hallucinations. *British Journal of Medical Psychology*, 71, 339–349.

Hardy, A., Fowler, D., Freeman, D., Smith, B., Steel, C., Evans, J., Garety, P., Kuipers, E., Bebbington, P. & Dunn, G. (2005). Trauma and hallucinatory experience in psychosis. *The Journal of Nervous and Mental Disease*, 193(8), 501–507.

Harris, C. & Barraclough, B. (1998). Excess mortality of mental disorder. *British Journal of Psychiatry*, 173, 11–53.

Hayes, S. C. (1989). *Rule-governed Behavior: Cognition, Contingencies, and Instructional Control*. New York: Plenum Press

Hayes, S. C. (2004). Acceptance and Commitment Therapy, Relational Frame Theory, and the third wave of behavior therapy. *Behavior Therapy*, 35(4), 639–665.

Hayes, S. C., Wilson, K. G., Gifford, E. V., Follette, V. M. & Strosahl, K. (1996). Experiential avoidance and behavioral disorders: a functional dimensional approach to diagnosis and treatment. *Journal of Consulting and Clinical Psychology*, 64(6), 1152–1168.

Hayes, S. C., Strosahl, K. & Wilson, K. G. (2012). *Acceptance and Commitment Therapy. The Process and Practice of Mindful Change*. New York: Guilford Press.

Hoffman, R. E. (1986). Verbal hallucination and language production processes in schizophrenia. *The Behavioural and Brain Sciences*, 9, 503–548.

Hoffman, R. E., Varanko, M., Gilmore, J. & Mishara, A. L. (2008). Experiential features used by patients with schizophrenia to differentiate 'voices' from ordinary verbal thought. *Psychological Medicine*, 38(8), 1167–1176.

Hustig, H. H. & Hafner, J. (1990). Persistent auditory hallucinations and their relationship to delusions and mood. *The Journal of Nervous and Mental Disease*, 178(4), 264–267.

Jacobsen, P., Morris, E. & Johns, L. C. (2010). Mindfulness groups for psychosis: key issues for implementation on an inpatient unit. *Behavioural and Cognitive Psychotherapy*, 39, 349–353.

Johns, L. C., Hemsley, D. & Kuipers, E. (2002). A comparison of auditory hallucinations in a psychiatric and non-psychiatric group. *British Journal of Clinical Psychology*, 41(1), 81–86.

Johns, L. (2005). Hallucinations in the general population. *Current Psychiatry Reports*, 7(3), 162–167.

Jones, S. R. & Fernyhough, C. (2007). Thought as action: inner speech, self-monitoring, and auditory verbal hallucinations. *Consciousness and Cognition*, 16(2), 391–399.

Junginger, J. (1990). Predicting compliance with command hallucinations. *The American Journal of Psychiatry*, 147(2), 245–247.

Junginger, J. & Frame, C. L. (1985). Self-report of the frequency and phenomenology of verbal hallucinations. *The Journal of Nervous and Mental Disease*, 173(3), 149–155.

Kapur, S. (2003). Psychosis as a state of aberrant salience: a framework linking biology, phenomenology, and pharmacology in schizophrenia. *American Journal of Psychiatry*, 160(1), 13–23.

Kellenher, I., Jenner, J. A. & Cannon, M. (2010). Psychotic symptoms in the general population – an evolutionary perspective. *The British Journal of Psychiatry*, 197, 167–169.

Kingdon, D. G. & Turkington, D. (1991). The use of cognitive behaviour therapy with a normalising rationale in schizophrenia. *The Journal of Nervous and Mental Disease*, 179(4), 207–211.

Kingdon, D. G. & Turkington, D. (1994). *Cognitive-Behavioral Therapy of Schizophrenia*. New York: Guilford Press.

Kingdon, D. G., Ashcroft, K., Bhandari, B., Gleeson, S., Warikoo, N. M. S. et al. (2010). Schizophrenia and borderline personality disorder:similarities and differences in the experience of auditory hallucinations, paranoia, and childhood trauma. *Journal of Nervous and Mental Disease*, 198(6), 399–403.

Langer, Á. I., Cangas, A. J., Salcedo, E. & Fuentes, B. (2012). Applying mindfulness therapy in a group of psychotic individuals: a controlled study. *Behavioural and Cognitive Psychotherapy*, 40(1), 105–109.

Laroi, F. & Van der Linden, M. (2005). Megacognitions in proneness towards hallucinations and delusions. *Behaviour Research amd Therapy*, 43, 1425–1441.

Larøi, F., Sommer, I. E., Blom, J. D., Fernyhough, C., Ffytche, D. H., Hugdahl, K. et al. (2012). The characteristic features of auditory verbal hallucinations in clinical and nonclinical groups: state-of-the-art overview and future directions. *Schizophrenia Bulletin*, doi:10.1093/schbul/sbs061.

Leudar, I., Thomas, P., McNally, D. & Glinski, A. (1997). What voices can do with words: pragmatics of verbal hallucinations. *Psychological Medicine*, 27(4), 885–898.

Linn, E. L. (1977). Verbal auditory hallucinations: mind, self, and society. *The Journal of Nervous and Mental Disease*, 164(1), 8–17.

Lucas, S. & Wade, T. (2001). An examination of the power of the voices in predicting the mental state of people experiencing psychosis. *Behaviour Change*, 18(1), 51–57.

Mackinnon, A., Copolov, D. L. & Trauer, T. (2004). Factors associated with compliance and resistance to command hallucinations. *The Journal of Nervous and Mental Disease*, 192(5), 357–362.

Marlett, G. A., Witkiewitz, K., Dillworth, T. M., Bowen, S. W., Parks, G. A., Macpherson, L. M. et al. (2004). Vipassana meditation as a treatment for alcohol and drug use disorders. In S. C. Hayes, V. M. Follette & M. M. Linehan (eds). *Mindfulness and Acceptance: Expanding the Cognitive-Behavioral Tradition*. New York: Guildford Press, pp. 261–286.

Mawson, A., Cohen, K. & Berry, K. (2010). Reviewing evidence for the cognitive model of auditory hallucinations: the relationship between cognitive voice appraisals and distress during psychosis. *Clinical Psychology Review*, 30(2), 248–258.

McGowan, J. F., Lavender, T. & Garety, P. (2005). Factors in outcome of cognitive-behavioural therapy for psychosis: users' and clinicians' views. *Psychology and Psychotherapy: Theory, Research and Practice*, 78, 513–529.

McInnis, M. & Marks, I. (1990). Audiotape therapy for persistent auditory hallucinations. *British Journal of Psychiatry*, 157, 913–914.

McLeod, H. J. (2009). ACT and CBT for psychosis: comparisons and contrasts.
In J. T. Blackledge, J. Ciarrochi & F. Deane (eds). *Acceptance and Commitment Therapy: Contemporary Theory Research and Practice*. Bowen Hills: Australian Academic Press, pp. 263–279.

Morris, E. M. J., Garety, P. A. & Peters, E. R. (submitted). Psychological flexibility and auditory hallucinations: relationship with distress and coping responses.

Morrison, A. P. (1998). A cognitive analysis of the maintenance of auditory hallucinations: are voices to schizophrenia what bodily sensations are to panic? *Behavioural and Cognitive Psychotherapy*, 26(4), 289–302.

Morrison, A. P. (2001). The interpretation of intrusions in psychosis: an integrative cognitive approach to hallucinations and delusions. *Behavioural and Cognitive Psychotherapy*, 29, 257–276.

Morrison, A. P. & Baker, C. A. (2000). Intrusive thoughts and auditory hallucinations: a comparative study of intrusions in psychosis. *Behaviour Research amd Therapy*, 38, 1097–1106.

Morrison, A. P. & Haddock, G. (1997). Cognitive factors in source monitoring and auditory hallucinations. *Psychological Medicine*, 27(3), 669–679.

Morrison, A. P. & Renton, J. C. (2001). Cognitive therapy for auditory hallucinations: a theory-based approach. *Cognitive and Behavioral Practice*, 8(2), 147–160.

Morrison, A. P., Haddock, G. & Tarrier, N. (1995). Intrusive thoughts and auditory hallucinations: a cognitive approach. *Behavioural and Cognitive Psychotherapy*, 23, 265–280.

Nayani, T. H. & David, A. S. (1996). The auditory hallucination: a phenomenological survey. *Psychological Medicine*, 26(1), 177–189.

Newman Taylor, K., Harper, S. & Chadwick, P. (2009). Impact of mindfulness on cognition and affect in voice hearing: evidence from two case studies. *Behavioural and Cognitive Psychotherapy*, 37(4), 397–402.

Newton, E., Landau, S., Smith, P., Monks, P., Shergill, S. & Wykes, T. (2005). Early psychological intervention for auditory hallucinations: an exploratory study of young people's voices groups. *The Journal of Nervous and Mental Disease*, 193(1), 58–61.

O'Sullivan, K. (1994). Dimensions of coping with auditory hallucinations. *Journal of Mental Health*, 3(3), 351–361.

Oulis, P. G., Mavreas, V. G., Mamounas, J. M. & Stefanis, C. N. (1995). Clinical characteristics of auditory hallucinations. *Acta Psychiatrica Scandinavica*, 92(2), 97–102.

Pembroke, L. (1998). Echoes of me. *Nursing Times*, 94(4), 30–31.

Pérez-Álvarez, M., García-Montes, J. M., Perona-Garcelán, S. & Vallina-Fernández, O. (2008). Changing relationship with voices: new therapeutic perspectives for treating hallucinations. *Clinical Psychology and Psychotherapy*, 15(2), 75.

Romme, M. & Escher, A. (1989). Hearing voices. *Schizophrenia Bulletin*, 15(2), 209–216.

Romme, M. & Escher, S. (1993a). *Accepting Voices*. London: Mind.

Romme, M. & Escher, S. (1993b). The new approach: a Dutch experiment. In M. Romme & S. Escher (eds). *Accepting Voices*. London: Mind, pp. 11–27.

Romme, M., Honig, A., Noorthoorn, E. O. & Escher, A. D. (1992). Coping with hearing voices: an emancipatory approach. *British Journal of Psychiatry*, 161, 99–103.

Ruddle, A., Mason, O. & Wykes, T. (2011). A review of hearing voices groups: evidence and mechanisms of change. *Clinical Psychology Review*, 31(5), 757–766.

Sar, V., Koyuncu, A., Ozturk, E., Yargic, L. I., Kundakci, T., Yazici, A., Kuskonmaz, E. & Aksüt, D. (2007). Dissociative disorders in the psychiatric emergency ward. *General Hospital Psychiatry*, 29(1), 45–50.

Segal, Z. V., Williams, J. M. G. & Teasdale, J. D. (2002). *Mindfulness-Based Cognitive Therapy for Depression*. New York: Guildford Press.

Sensky, T., Turkington, D., Kingdon, D., Scott, J. L., Scott, J., Siddle, R., O'Carroll, M. & Barnes, T. R. E. (2000). A randomized controlled trial of cognitive-behavioural therapy for persistent symptoms in schizophrenia resistant to medication. *Archives of General Psychiatry*, 57(2), 165–172.

Shawyer, F., Mackinnon, A., Farhall, J., Mullen, P., Sims, E., Blaney, S. *et al.* (2003). Risk factors for compliance with harmful command hallucinations in psychotic disorders. *Schizophrenia Research*, 60(Suppl.), 25–26.

Shawyer, F., Farhall, J., Sims, E. F. & Copolov, D. (2005). Command hallucinations in psychosis: Acceptance and disengagement as a focus of treatment. In M. Jackson & G. Murphy (eds). *Theory and Practice in Contemporary Australian Cognitive and Behaviour Therapy: Proceedings of the 28th National AACBT Conference*. Melbourne: Australian Association for Cognitive Behaviour Therapy, pp. 5–14.

Shawyer, F., Ratcliff, R., Mackinnon, A., Farhall, J., Hayes, S. C. & Copolov, D. (2007). The Voices Acceptance and Action Scale (VAAS): pilot data. *Journal of Clinical Psychology*, 63(6), 593–606.

Shawyer, F., Mackinnon, A., Farhall, J., Sims, E., Blaney, S., Yardley, P. *et al.* (2008). Acting on harmful command hallucinations in psychotic disorders: an integrative approach. *The Journal of Nervous and Mental Disease*, 196(5), 390–398.

Shawyer, F., Farhall, J., Mackinnon, A., Trauer, T., Sims, E., Ratcliff, R. *et al.* (2012). A randomised controlled trial of acceptance-based cognitive behavioural therapy for command hallucinations in psychotic disorders. *Behaviour Research and Therapy*, 50, 110–121.

Slade, P. D. (1972). The effects of systematic desensitization on auditory hallucinations. *Behaviour Research and Therapy*, 10(1), 85–91.

Slade, P. D. (1973). The psychological investigation and treatment of auditory hallucinations: a case report. *British Journal of Medical Psychology*, 46(3), 293–296.

Slade, P. D. (1976). Towards a theory of auditory hallucinations: outline of an hypothetical four-factor model. *British Journal of Social and Clinical Psychology*, 15(4), 415–423.

Soppitt, R. W. & Birchwood, M. (1997). Depression, beliefs, voice content and topography: a cross-sectional study of schizophrenic patients with auditory verbal hallucinations. *Journal of Mental Health*, 6(5), 525–532.

Steel, C., Fowler, D. & Holmes, E. A. (2005). Trauma-related intrusions and psychosis: an information processing account. *Behaviour and Cognitive Psychotherapy*, 33, 139–152.

Thomas, N., McLeod, H. J. & Brewin, C. R. (2009). Interpersonal complementarity in responses to auditory hallucinations in psychosis. *British Journal of Clinical Psychology*, 48(4), 411–424.

Valmaggia, L. R., van der Gaag, M., Tarrier, N., Pijnenborg, M. & Slooff, C. J. (2005). Cognitive-behavioural therapy for refractory psychotic symptoms of schizophrenia resistant to atypical antipsychotic medication. *British Journal of Psychiatry*, 186, 324–330.

van der Gaag, M. (2006). A neuropsychiatric model of biological and psychological processes in the remission of delusions and auditory hallucinations. *Schizophrenia Bulletin*, 32(S1), S113–S122.

van der Gaag, M., Hageman, M. C. & Birchwood, M. (2003). Evidence for a cognitive model of auditory hallucinations. *The Journal of Nervous and Mental Disease*, 191, 542–545.

Vaughan, S. & Fowler, D. (2004). The distress experienced by voice hearers is associated with the perceived relationship between the voice hearer and the voice. *The British Journal of Clinical Psychology*, 43(Pt 2), 143–153.

Waters, F., Badcock, J., Michie, P. & Mayberry, M. (2006). Auditory hallucinations in schizophrenia: intrusive thoughts and forgotten memories. *Cognitive Neuropsychiatry*, 11(1), 65–83.

Waters, F., Woodward, T., Allen, P., Aleman, A. & Sommer, I. (2011). Self-recognition deficits in schizophrenia patients with auditory hallucinations: a meta-analysis of the literature *Schizophrenia Bulletin*, doi:10.1093/schbul/sbq144.

Waters, F., Allen, P., Aleman, A., Fernyhough, C., Woodward, T. S. *et al.* (2012). Auditory hallucinations in schizophrenia and nonschizophrenia populations: a review and integrated model of cognitive mechanisms. *Schizophrenia Bulletin*, doi: 10.1093/schbul/sbs045.

Wiles, N. J., Zammit, S., Bebbington, P., Singleton, N., Meltzer, H. & Lewis, G. (2006). Self-reported psychotic symptoms in the general population. *The British Journal of Psychiatry*, 188(6), 519–526.

Yusupoff, L. & Tarrier, N. (1996). Coping strategy enhancement for persistent hallucinations and delusions. In G. Haddock & P. D. Slade (eds). *Cognitive-Behavioural Interventions with Psychotic Disorders*. London: Routledge, pp. 86–102.

3

Emotional Processing and Metacognitive Awareness for Persecutory Delusions

Claire Hepworth, Helen Startup and Daniel Freeman

3.1 Introduction

In recent years there has been increasing recognition of the direct contribution of negative affect and related processes to the development and maintenance of persecutory delusions. Thus, one potential target for intervention is direct enhancement of emotional processing. This chapter describes our recent work examining this. A brief intervention, emotional processing and metacognitive awareness (EPMA), was developed and piloted with patients who had persistent persecutory delusions (Hepworth *et al.*, 2011). The results indicate that encouraging patients to talk about their delusional experiences in a structured intervention such as EPMA may have therapeutic benefits.

3.2 Persecutory Delusions

A delusion is of the persecutory type when 'the individual believes both that harm is occurring, or is going to occur, to him or her, and that the persecutor has the intention to cause harm' (Freeman & Garety, 2000). Typical examples of the types of belief seen in clinical practice are: that the neighbours and council are in collusion to evict you, that your ex-partner has hired a hit man to kill you and that the

Acceptance and Commitment Therapy and Mindfulness for Psychosis, First Edition.
Edited by Eric M. J. Morris, Louise C. Johns and Joseph E. Oliver.
© 2013 John Wiley & Sons, Ltd. Published 2013 by John Wiley & Sons, Ltd.

police wish to poison you by contaminating the water supply to your home. Sartorius *et al.* (1986) report that persecutory delusions are the second most common symptom of psychosis after delusions of reference, occurring in almost 50% of first-episode cases. However, it is well established that there is a spectrum of paranoid thoughts in the general population (Freeman, 2007; van Os *et al.*, 2000).

3.3   Improving Treatments for Persecutory Delusions

Given the modest effect sizes for the first-generation cognitive behavioural therapy (CBT) for psychosis approaches (e.g. $d = 0.47$ in Pfammater *et al.*, 2006; $d = 0.35$ in Zimmerman *et al.*, 2005; $d = 0.40$ in Wykes *et al.*, 2008; National Institute for Health and Clinical Excellence, 2009), a number of developments of the intervention are underway (e.g. Foster *et al.*, 2010; Myers *et al.*, 2011; Ross *et al.*, 2011; Trower *et al.*, 2004; Waller *et al.*, 2011). These new approaches explicitly focus on one type of psychotic symptom and target one putative causal factor at a time (see Freeman, 2011). The results have been very encouraging.

In the research literature, one broad class of factor recently identified as playing a role in the development and maintenance of delusions has been negative affective processing. One notable emotional process implicated has been worry. In a series of studies, we have shown worry to predict the occurrence and persistence of paranoid thoughts (e.g. Freeman *et al.*, 2008, 2011; Startup *et al.*, 2007) and chronic worry to be evident in many patients with persecutory delusions, associated with the level of distress of delusional experience (e.g. Freeman & Garety, 1999; Bassett *et al.*, 2009). Importantly, we found that an intervention that directly targeted worry reduced levels of persecutory delusions and associated distress (Foster *et al.*, 2010).

One influential view in the emotional literature is that worry and rumination maintain distress by impeding emotional processing (Borkovec & Costello, 1993). Worry and rumination both involve repetitive negative thinking (Ehring & Watkins, 2008) and a predominance of verbal linguistic processing of emotional material (e.g. Borkovec *et al.*, 1998; McLaughlin *et al.*, 2007). Imaginal thoughts elicit a greater cardiovascular response than those retained at the verbal/linguistic level; thus, retaining information at the verbal level may inhibit activation of the complete fear structure (Vrana *et al.*, 1986), which impedes the habituation typically understood to be needed in order for anxiety modification to occur (Foa & Kozak, 1986).

Facilitating emotional processing, for example in treatments such as written emotional expression, can alleviate symptoms (Gortner *et al.*, 2006; Watkins, 2004). It is just such an approach that might be expected to have utility in the reduction of delusion-related distress. In this chapter, we therefore describe a novel approach to intervention for individuals with persecutory delusions, which focuses on enhancing emotional processing.

3.4   Development of the Intervention

The clinical intervention literature describes a range of techniques that have been used to enhance emotional processing. Examination of the focus of these interventions, and study of the theoretical literature, identified three key mechanisms that might impede emotional processing: (1) emotional inhibition; (2) a lack of metacognitive awareness; and (3) nonacceptance (avoidance) of internal experiences. When developing EPMA, we drew from several of the approaches that target these mechanisms (see Table 3.1).

The greatest influence on the development of the intervention was the literature on expressive writing. Emotional expression (or emotional disclosure) (Pennebaker, 1989) is a technique that has been reported to have success in enhancing emotional adaptation, with a range of beneficial health and well-being outcomes. A meta-analytic review by Smyth (1998) reported a mean improvement in outcome of 23% ($d = 0.47$). Markowicz (2007) found that written emotional expression of potential problems reduced worry at a 1-month post-intervention follow-up, but only in those individuals who consistently wrote about the same worry. Watkins (2004) examined the role of expressive writing in recovery from an upsetting event (an induced experience of failure). Following completion of a failure-inducing problem-solving task, study participants were asked to complete three essays on their experience of it: one immediately after, one prior to going to bed and one the following day. However, the participants were randomised to two conditions, in which the nature of the writing was different. Those in the first condition were encouraged to write in a self-evaluative, brooding way ('Why did you feel this way?') and those in the second were asked to write in an experiential, descriptive way ('How did you feel moment to moment?'). Those with high levels of trait rumination who were allocated to the brooding condition reported greater negative affect and a higher frequency of cognitive intrusions about the event 12 hours later. The experiential, expressive writing, however, appeared to serve as a buffer against the distressing impact of failure even in those who were high trait ruminators. This study indicates the positive effects of expressing emotion in an experiential rather than an evaluative way. Furthermore, Gortner *et al.* (2006) reported that the use of expressive writing lowered depressive symptoms, and that this change was mediated by a change in 'brooding' but not 'reflective rumination'. In addition to simple expression of emotion, the process or mode by which it is expressed may be important. Encouraging an individual to engage in adaptive emotional expression using an experiential rather than an evaluative focus would be predicted to reduce the distressing impact of paranoid thoughts.

However, we considered it likely, based on clinical experience, that many patients with psychosis would not take to writing exercises, and therefore we adapted the intervention to involve verbal expression of experiences, rather than written tasks. It is important to tailor interventions specifically to the needs of this client group.

Table 3.1 Sources of the components of EPMA

Mechanism to be targeted	Therapeutic techniques of EPMA	Literature base
Emotional inhibition	*Increasing access to emotional experience: exposure* Patients are encouraged to verbally express, in minute detail, the thoughts, images and sensations associated with a distressing persecutory delusion. Focusing on their most worrying persecutory delusion, patients are encouraged to elaborate upon this using an experiential rather than evaluative focus. That is, they are encouraged to describe their current experience as it is nonjudgementally and with present focus, rather than make an attempt to understand or problem-solve the experience. *Reducing verbal-linguistic processing* Participants are encouraged to use gestalt techniques to create distance from thoughts. They are invited to describe thoughts, images and sensations in terms of their physical characteristics – for example, their shape, weight and colour – in order to help them adopt an observer perspective.	Smyth (1998) produced a meta-analysis showing emotional expression has a wide range of positive health and well-being outcomes. Gortner et al. (2006) reported that expressive writing lowered depressive symptoms, and this change was mediated by a change in 'brooding' but not 'reflective rumination'. Watkins (2004) argued that experiential (but not evaluative) emotional expression served as a buffer against the distressing impact of induced failure in college students, even in those who were high trait ruminators. Markowitz (2007) reported a reduction in worry after written emotional expression about a single potential problem. Hayes (2005) suggests that objectifying a thought or feeling – for example, describing the colour, shape and weight of a thought – may alter its literality and thus enhance adaptation. Masuda et al. (2004) suggest that cognitive defusion techniques might be used 'to reduce the functions of thoughts by altering the context in which they occur, rather than attempting to alter the form, frequency, or situational sensitivity of the thoughts themselves'. They report findings which suggest that 'repetition of negative self-referential words, at least when combined with a clinical rationale, can reduce their believability and their negative emotional impact'. That is, defusion techniques reduce believability and distress. Blackledge (2007) report cognitive defusion techniques can be used to disrupt verbal processes in acceptance and commitment therapy (ACT). Levin et al. (2012) produced a meta-analysis of the impact of treatment components suggested by the psychological flexibility model, reporting a moderate effect size (using Hedge's g) for defusion techniques ($g = 0.77$) on targeted outcomes.

Metacognitive awareness	*Enhancing metacognitive insight* Participants are encouraged to recognise thoughts as thoughts rather than facts. They are encouraged to label thoughts, emotions, sensations, memories and images, and reflect on their natures, similarities and differences, with a particular focus on their transience and the interrelationships between internal experiences. *Taking a decentred perspective* Participants are encouraged to label and write down thoughts, feelings, sensations, images and memories in order to assist them in decentring from them.	Interventions that increase metacognitive awareness have been found to reduce rumination (MBCT; Segal *et al.*, 2002) and worry (metacognitive therapy for worry; Wells & King, 2006). According to Evans *et al.* (2008), individuals with generalised anxiety disorder (GAD) reported significant reductions in anxiety and depression following completion of mindfulness-based cognitive therapy.
Acceptance	*Noticing without judgement* Techniques are included to help participants focus on the present moment, with full awareness, nonjudgementally. They are encouraged to: • observe, accept and let go of worrying thoughts; • stay with anxious thoughts, and notice that they are fleeting and temporary, and dissipate naturally; • increase their awareness of the current environment, using all senses to notice sounds, sensations, thoughts, images (eyes closed and open); • describe these experiences as they are in the moment. Participants are encouraged to consciously (with deliberate intent) make an active choice to accept situations, thoughts or affective experiences as they are, with full participation and engagement, in order to act effectively. This is the opposite of experiential avoidance.	Becker & Zayfert (2001) describe the effectiveness of incorporating techniques from dialectical behaviour therapy (DBT), including radical acceptance, into exposure therapy for post-traumatic stress disorder (PTSD). This technique is used in DBT and ACT. Lynch *et al.* (2007) report that DBT has been found to be efficacious for the treatment of borderline personality disorder (BPD) (where individuals present with difficulties in emotion regulation, affective instability, reactivity etc.) in seven randomised controlled trials (RCTs), across four independent research teams, thus meeting the criteria for a 'well-established treatment intervention' outlined by Chambless & Ollendick (2001). Levin *et al.* (2012) conducted a meta-analysis reporting a large effect size (*g* = 0.8) for acceptance techniques on targeted outcomes.

Patients may be experiencing distracting and intrusive internal experiences, so it can be helpful to use clear and concrete (rather than abstract) language, to keep exercises brief and to provide prompts to bring mindful attention to task. Patients with psychosis may benefit from a greater level of coaching and guidance in accessing the emotional experience and tolerating emotional exposure, especially when experiencing distressing thoughts. Therefore, explicit as well as implicit attempts to increase metacognitive awareness were incorporated, in order to aid understanding of the difference between thoughts and facts. This therapy used practical and tangible experiential exercises to explain metaphors; for example, the leaves-on-the-stream metaphor (see Appendix B) was made into a concrete exercise involving writing down thoughts and feelings on paper 'leaves'. EPMA may hold its greatest potential as a therapeutic technique in complementing and enhancing other worry intervention approaches being developed for delusions (Foster *et al.*, 2010).

3.5   The EPMA Intervention

The basic elements of the therapy and their evidence base are summarised in Table 3.1. There were three sessions, each following the same format and each lasting 60 minutes. A summary of the session format is provided in Table 3.2.

During each session, participants were asked first to focus on a recent positive experience, in order to practise the techniques, and then to repeat the procedure with a recent experience of the persecutory delusion. In each session, participants recalled the positive experience twice, first in a narrative form to promote initial exposure, then in an experiential way. (These will be described in detail shortly.) The reported experience was then broken down into components to promote metacognitive insight and a decentred perspective. This procedure was repeated using

Table 3.2   Summary of session format

Target		Techniques: practised first with a positive experience, then with a distressing paranoid experience
1	Emotional inhibition: exposure	Narrative recall of experience
2	Emotional inhibition: experiential recall	Third-person experiential recall of experience
3	Metacognitive awareness: metacognitive insight	Labelling components of experience
4	Metacognitive awareness: decentred perspective	Decentred labelling of experience using 'paper leaves'
5	Acceptance	Nonjudgemental description of experience
6	Emotional inhibition: reducing verbal-linguistic processing	Objectification and defusion techniques used with salient distressing words

a recent experience of paranoid thinking, and then defusion and objectification techniques were used to reduce verbal-linguistic processing of particularly salient and distressing internal experiences.

To promote initial access to the experience, participants were encouraged to retell a recent positive experience in a narrative form, with as much detail and context as possible. Examples of positive experiences recalled by participants included 'playing football with my son', 'going for a walk by the river' and 'having a visit from a friend'. Notably, even those who felt most restricted and disabled by their delusional experiences were able to identify and recall positive experiences when prompted, such as having a cup of tea in the kitchen and noticing the warmth of the sunshine through the window or hearing a favourite song on the radio. When this exercise was repeated using a paranoid experience, one participant was asked to recall by the therapist the narrative of an occasion on which he believed that he was going to be violently attacked by his neighbour: 'I am aware that one of your specific worries is that your neighbour is trying to hurt you. I am going to ask you to tell me about a specific time when you thought that your neighbour was going to attack you. I am going to ask you to tell me a bit about what happened first, where you were at the time that you had the thought, what the was weather was like, who you were with and other such details – to, describe the scene in as much detail as possible. I am then going to guide you to focus on the feelings that you had in the same way that you just did for your positive memory.'

Participants were then encouraged to retell the narrative a second time, in an experiential rather than an evaluative manner, in order to promote exposure to the full fear structure and habituation of the arousal. This was done in the first-person present tense (e.g. 'I am thinking that he is looking at me' rather than 'Why is he looking at me?'). For example, 'When you feel that you have a clear picture in your mind, I am going to ask you to tell me about the memory, as though it is happening right now. Tell me how you are feeling, what you are thinking, what you notice as it happens.'

Participants were asked to describe any images and sensations. They were then asked to describe what they noticed about the experience, whether emotions were stronger at some points than at others, whether they noticed that thoughts and images were temporary. They were also asked to rate their distress.

The experience was then broken down and the patients were encouraged to identify and label the thoughts, feelings, sensations, memories and images that they experienced (to promote metacognitive insight). It was notable that many participants did not find it easy to label the different elements of cognitive experience. Guidance was given to aid differentiation, for example between a thought ('He is watching me') and an emotion ('I am afraid').

Participants were encouraged to write down their thoughts and feelings and observe and describe them from a decentred perspective. The metaphor of leaves on the stream was used in a concrete, tangible way to promote the idea of acceptance: noticing and labelling thoughts and feelings, and not engaging with them.

Participants were encouraged to take a step back and use an observer perspective to reflect on the 'leaves' that they had written for their positive and negative experiences: for example, noticing any similar body sensations or rating the strength of the emotion that they experienced. They were encouraged to describe the components of the experience, without judgement, in order to enhance acceptance. For example, one participant, when recalling a game of football with his son, observed that his experience of the sensation of his heart racing was as strong when playing football as it was when feeling anxious when he believed that he was being followed by a stranger. He also described his surprise that he had rated the strength of the emotion 'pride' during the positive memory equal to that of his 'fear' during the delusional experience. Furthermore, he was able to observe that it was as easy for him to evoke the imagery associated with the positive scenario as that of the delusion; both were equally salient. Participants were encouraged to observe the transient nature of thoughts (to promote acceptance and defusion). Several participants observed that on recall they were able to evoke the same positive emotions that they had experienced at the time, and that when accessing these memories, the delusional experience had faded.

Finally, objectification and defusion techniques were used to reduce verbal-linguistic processing, where particular thoughts and emotions were particularly powerful and distressing (e.g. 'I am vulnerable', 'shame', 'humiliation'). These tried to break the individual's 'literalisation', which refers to the tendency to take as literal the content of thoughts expressed in language, a concept drawn from acceptance and commitment therapy (ACT) (Hayes *et al.*, 1999). For example, one client was encouraged to describe the shape, weight and colour of the word 'weak' until he observed that the word no longer felt as 'powerful' and meaningful to him.

For homework, participants were asked to practise using the techniques. The feedback often given to the therapist was that it felt safe to recall the delusion narrative knowing that a positive experience could also be recalled, which enhanced feelings of control.

3.6   The EPMA Pilot Study

The EPMA intervention was piloted with 12 patients (Hepworth *et al.*, 2011). The entry criteria were: a current persecutory delusion, as defined by Freeman & Garety (2000); persecutory delusions that had persisted for 6 months or longer despite treatment with neuroleptic medication; a primary case note diagnosis of schizophrenia, schizoaffective disorder or delusional disorder; and age between 18 and 65. The intervention took place across three 1-hour sessions, arranged as closely together as possible (this was typically over 3 weeks). In addition to the intervention, all participants continued to receive their standard treatment as usual.

Delusional distress and persecutory delusions were assessed using the Psychotic Symptoms Rating Scale – Delusions (PSYRATS) (Haddock *et al.*, 1999) at four time points (baseline, pre-therapy, post-therapy and follow-up). Secondary outcome measures of worry (Penn State Worry Questionnaire, PSWQ; Meyer *et al.*, 1990), rumination (Ruminative Response Scale of the Response Styles Questionnaire (Nolen-Hoeksema & Morrow, 1993), anxiety and depression (Depression Anxiety Stress Scales, DASS; Lovibond & Lovibond, 1995) were assessed once before the intervention and then again after the intervention. In this initial evaluation there was no control group and assessments were not blind.

It was found that EPMA particularly reduced levels of delusional distress, and that this was maintained at follow-up. The effect size was large (= 1.03) and changes were maintained at follow-up. Nine of the twelve patients reported a >25% reduction in their level of delusional distress. There were also significant reductions in levels of worry and depression.

This is therefore an approach that shows potential as part of a programme to improve treatment for delusions. More rigorous evaluation using a randomised controlled trial (RCT) with blind assessments is now required.

3.7   Case Study

The details of this case study have been anonymised. Ms Cooper was a 36-year-old white British female who had experiences diagnosed as schizophrenia. She had developed persecutory beliefs following a violent relationship with her former partner. She believed that her ex-partner was following her as he wished to rape and humiliate her. She believed that this person was on every street corner, and had commanded others to hurt her too. She believed that the ex-partner was obtaining information about her and had cars following her. Ms Cooper avoided leaving the house and socialising, as she believed that others had conspired with her ex-partner to hurt her. Ms Cooper also heard voices, which gave a commentary of her life, and made critical comments about her physical appearance. Ms Cooper was prescribed two antipsychotics and one antidepressant medication, and reported approximately 90% adherence. She had received a course of CBT in the past and attended a CBT Voices group. She regularly met with her psychiatrist and care coordinator.

Ms Cooper took readily to the techniques. She was particularly enthusiastic about being invited to reflect in detail on a positive experience, remarking that it had been a very long time since she had given herself permission to do so. Over the three sessions, she practised the techniques using the positive experiences of taking a walk by the river, buying a pair of shoes and laughing with an old friend. Ms Cooper then focused on recalling negative experiences of occasions when she had believed that she was being followed or conspired against. These were in the supermarket, on the street and when in her car. Metacognitive insight was promoted by breaking the narrative down into its components in order to identify specific thoughts, feelings, sensations, behaviours and images. For example, when recalling an occasion when she believed she was being followed, she identified thoughts such as 'I think he is in the car behind me', emotions such as fear and anger, physiological sensations such as a racing heart and nausea, behaviours such as walking faster and images such as 'him shouting at me'. The specific words that had salience and caused distress to Ms Cooper were 'humiliate', 'rape' and 'fat'. The therapist used gestalt techniques, describing the colour, weight and shape of these words to alter her relationship with them and their meaning for her. She described the word 'humiliate' as 'hot', 'fiery', 'red', 'heavy' and 'fast moving'. She was able to watch the imagery transform to cool it, make it appear smaller and slower moving. She rated the levels of distress the word caused, until her distress had reduced. She then used defusion techniques, singing the word in different voices and writing it over and over, until she began to laugh and said the word now sounded silly, and that its power had reduced.

At the baseline assessment and pre-EPMA, Ms Cooper rated the intensity of her distress as 'extreme' on the PSYRATS (Haddock *et al.*, 1999). Following therapy, the rating of distress had reduced to 'moderate', and by follow-up this had reduced to 'slight'. Ms Cooper reported a reduction in her use of worry following EPMA. Her score on the PSWQ (Meyer *et al.*, 1990) reduced from 80 to 63, and her score on the measure of rumination reduced from 77 to 57; that is, her worry and rumination had showed large reductions but still remained at high levels. Ms Cooper also reported significant reductions in both anxiety and depression, as measured by the DASS (Lovibond & Lovibond, 1995). She rated her anxiety at 31 (out of a possible 42) pre-intervention; by post-intervention, this had fallen to 4. She rated her depression at 24 (out of a possible 42) pre-intervention and at 4 post-intervention.

3.8   Conclusion

We developed a novel brief intervention for patients with persecutory delusions, drawing upon advances in our understanding of persecutory delusions. It was envisaged that the intervention would be used with other psychological approaches for people with distressing delusions. In our pilot study, EPMA was found to reduce levels of delusion distress. For nine out of the twelve patients, a >25% reduction in distress was achieved. The changes associated with the intervention for these patients were large, clinically important and maintained after 1 month. However, notably, this was a pilot study, with no control group, unblinded assessments and a single therapist. An RCT is needed to more robustly establish the efficacy of the intervention. At this stage, it shows only promise.

There were indications that the EPMA intervention reduced overall levels of the persecutory delusions. However, it is difficult to interpret this finding because there were slight falls in the overall levels of the delusions during the baseline period. Clinically, we observed that many patients readily took to the techniques with little difficulty, expressing that they found the intervention acceptable and accessible. However, others experienced some initial anxiety over directly exposing themselves to their fear experiences, and at times there were initial increases in distress during sessions. A larger trial is needed to test whether this initial level of anxiety predicted outcome. EPMA may not be suitable for all patients with persecutory delusions, or may depend on the stage of a person's illness and their exposure to previous therapeutic approaches. Clearly EPMA, which involves discussion of distressing experiences, has to be carried out gently, with the agreement of patients, and some may not wish to try these techniques at all (and, indeed, the techniques will not be suitable for all). No patient showed a significant increase in distress through participation in EPMA. However, one patient did have an overall increase in their delusion during the period of the study.

EPMA is a simple, brief and highly structured intervention. Following training, this approach could easily be delivered by a range of mental-health professionals. Clearly, however, it does require sensitivity and confidence on the part of therapist to help the patient use the techniques. EPMA provides further support for the idea that direct challenge of delusional content is not required to reduce distress. It may prove to be a useful addition to the early stages of standard CBT for psychosis, in lowering levels of emotional distress before working directly on the content of delusional thinking, or as a booster therapy for clients who have received CBT. It is complementary to mindfulness and acceptance-based approaches, and may be a useful additional approach for clients who require more concrete, tangible exercises.

EPMA as an approach highlights the general issue of how best to help patients talk about their delusional experiences. It might be argued that comprehensive CBT assessments also provide access to this level of exposure, indirectly facilitating emotional processing, as the clinician goes over with the patient their recent instances of paranoid thinking. Encouraging clients to do so in an experiential rather than an evaluative way may enhance this further. EPMA may hold its greatest potential as a complement to other worry intervention approaches being developed for delusions (Foster *et al.*, 2010). This is therefore an approach that shows potential as part of a programme to improve treatment for delusions.

Acknowledgement

This study was supported by a Wellcome Trust Fellowship awarded to Daniel Freeman.

References

Bach, P. & Hayes, S. C. (2002). The use of acceptance and commitment therapy to prevent the rehospitalisation of psychotic patients: a randomised controlled trial. *Journal of Consulting and Clinical Psychology*, 70, 1129–1139.

Bassett, M., Sperlinger, D. & Freeman, D. (2009). Fear of madness and persecutory delusions. *Psychosis*, 1, 39–50.

Becker, C. B. & Zayfert, C. (2001). Integrating DBT-based techniques and concepts to facilitate exposure treatment for PTSD. *Cognitive and Behavioural Practice*, 8(2), 107–122.

Blackledge, J. T. (2007). Disrupting verbal processes: cognitive defusion in acceptance and commitment therapy and other mindfulness-based psychotherapies. *The Psychological Record*, 57(4), 555–577.

Borkovec, T. D., Ray, W. J. & Stober, J. (1998). Worry: a cognitive phenomenon intimately linked to affective, physiological, and interpersonal behavioural processes. *Cognitive Therapy and Research*, 22, 561–576.

Borkovec, T. D. & Costello, E. (1993). Efficacy of applied relaxation and cognitive behavioural therapy in the treatment of generalised anxiety disorder. *Journal of Consulting and Clinical Psychology*, 61, 611–619.

Brown, T. A., Chorpita, B. F., Korotitsch, W. & Barlow, D. H. (1997). Psychometric properties of the Depression Anxiety Stress Scales (DASS) in clinical samples. *Behaviour, Research and Therapy*, 35(1), 79–89.

Chambless, D. L. & Ollendick, T. H. (2001). Empirically supported psychological interventions. *Clinical Psychology Science and Practice*, 3, 685–715.

Ehring, T. & Watkins, E. R. (2008). Repetitive negative thinking as a transdiagnostic process. *International Journal of Cognitive Therapy*, 1(3), 192–205.

Evans, S., Ferrando, S., Findler, M., Stowell, C., Smart, C. & Haglin, D. (2008). Mindfulness-based cognitive therapy for generalized anxiety disorder. *Journal of Anxiety Disorders*, 22(4), 716–721.

Foster, C., Startup, H., Potts, L. & Freeman, D. (2010). A randomised controlled trial of a worry intervention for individuals with persistent persecutory delusions. *Journal of Behavior Therapy and Experimental Psychiatry*, 41(1), 45–51.

Freeman, D. (2007). Suspicious minds: The psychology of persecutory delusions. *Clinical Psychology Review*, 27, 425–457.

Freeman, D. (2011). Improving cognitive treatments for delusions. *Schizophrenia Research*, 132, 135–139.

Freeman, D. & Garety, P. A. (1999) Worry, worry processes and dimensions of delusions: an exploratory investigation of a role for anxiety processes in the maintenance of delusional distress. *Behavioural Cognitive Psychotherapy*, 27, 47–62.

Freeman, D. & Garety, P. A. (2000) Comments on the content of persecutory delusions: does the definition need clarification? *British Journal of Clinical Psychology*, 39, 407–414.

Freeman, D., Garety, P., Kuipers, E., Fowler, D., Bebbington, P. E. & Dunn, G. (2007). Acting on persecutory delusions: the importance of safety seeking. *Behaviour Research and Therapy*, 45, 89 – 99.

Freeman, D., Pugh, K., Antley, A., Slater, M., Bebbington, P., Gittins, M., Dunn, G., Kuipers, E., Fowler, D. & Garety, P. (2008). Virtual reality study of paranoid thinking in the general population. *British Journal of Psychiatry*, 192, 258–263.

Freeman, D., Stahl, D., McManus, S., Meltzer, H., Brugha, T., Wiles, N. & Bebbington, P. (2011). Insomnia, worry, anxiety and depression as predictors of the occurrence and the persistence of persecutory ideation. *Social Psychiatry and Psychiatric Epidemiology*. doi: 10.1007/s00127-011-0433-1.

Foa, E. B. & Kozak, M. J. (1986). Emotional processing of fear: exposure to corrective information. *Psychological Bulletin, 99*, 20–35.

Foster, C., Startup, H., Potts, L. & Freeman, D. (2010b). A randomised controlled trial of a worry intervention for individuals with persistent persecutory delusions. *Journal of Behaviour Therapy and Experimental Psychiatry, 41*, 45–51.

Gortner, E., Rude, S. S. & Pennebaker, J. W. (2006). Benefits of expressive writing in lowering rumination and depressive symptoms. *Behavior Therapy, 37*, 292–303.

Haddock, G., McCarron J., Tarrier, N. & Faragher, E. B. (1999). Scales to measure dimensions of hallucinations and delusions: the psychotic symptom rating scales (PSYRATS). *Psychological Medicine, 29*, 879–889.

Hayes, S. C. & Smith, S. (2005). *Get Out of Your Mind and Into Your Life: The New Acceptance and Commitment Therapy*. Oakland: New Harbinger.

Hayes, S. C., Strosahl, K. & Wilson, K. G. (1999). *Acceptance and Commitment Therapy: An Experiential Approach to Behavior Change*. New York: Guilford Press.

Hepworth, C., Startup, H. & Freeman, D. (2011). Developing treatments for persistent persecutory delusions: the impact of an emotional processing and metacognitive awareness (EPMA) intervention. *Journal of Nervous and Mental Disease, 199*, 653–658.

Levin, M. E., Hildebrandt, M. J., Lillis, J. & Hayes, S. C. (in press). The impact of treatment components suggested by the psychological flexibility model: a meta-analysis of laboratory-based component studies. *Behavior Therapy*, doi: 10.1016/j.beth.2012.05.003.

Lovibond, S. H. & Lovibond, P. F. (1995). *Manual for the Depression Anxiety Stress Scales*. Psychology Foundation of Australia.

Lynch, T.R. (2007). Dialectical behaviour therapy for borderline personality disorder. *Annual Review of Clinical Psychology, 3*, 181–205.

Markowitz, L. (2007). Written emotional disclosure about potential problems. PhD thesis, University of Waterloo.

Masuda, A., Hayes, S. C., Sackett, C. F. & Twohig, M. P. (2004). Cognitive defusion and self-relevant negative thoughts: examining the impact of a ninety year old technique. *Behaviour Research and Therapy, 42*, 477–485.

McLaughlin, K. A., Borkovec, T. D. & Sibrava, N. J. (2007). The effects of worry and rumination on affect states and cognitive activity. *Behavior Therapy, 38*, 23–38.

Meyer, T. J., Miller, M. L., Metzger, R. L. & Borkovec, T. D. (1990). Development and validation of the Penn State Worry Questionnaire. *Behaviour Research and Therapy, 28*, 487–495.

Myers, E., Startup, H. & Freeman, D. (2011). Cognitive behavioural treatment of insomnia in patients with persecutory delusions. *Journal of Behaviour Therapy and Experimental Psychiatry, 42*, 330–336.

National Institute for Health and Clinical Excellence (2009) *Clinical Guideline 1. Schizophrenia: Core Interventions in the Treatment and Management of Schizophrenia in Primary and Secondary Care*. London: National Institute for Health and Clinical Excellence.

Nolen-Hoeksema, S. & Morrow, J. (1991). A prospective study of depression and posttraumatic stress symptoms after a natural disaster: the 1989 Loma Prieta earthquake. *Journal of Personality and Social Psychology, 61*, 115–121.

Pennebaker, J. W. (1989). Confession, inhibition, and disease. In L. Berkowitz (ed.). *Advances in Experimental Social Psychology* (Vol. 22). Orlando: Academic Press, pp. 211–244.

Pennebaker, J. W. & Beall, S. K. (1986). Confronting a traumatic event: toward an understanding of inhibition and disease. *Journal of Abnormal Psychology, 95*, 274–281.

Pennebaker, J. W. & Seagal, J. D. (1999). Forming a story: the health benefits of narrative. *Journal of Clinical Psychology, 55*, 1243–1254.

Pfammater, M., Junghan, U. M. & Brenner, H. D. (2006). Efficacy of psychological therapy in schizophrenia: conclusions from a meta-analysis. *Schizophrenia Bulletin, 32*, s64–s80.

Ross, K., Freeman, D., Dunn, G. & Garety, P. (2011). Can jumping to conclusions be reduced in people with delusions? An experimental investigation of a brief reasoning training module. *Schizophrenia Bulletin, 37*, 324–333.

Sartorius, N., Jablensky, A. & Kortens, A. (1986). Early manifestations and first-contact incidence of schizophrenia in different cultures. *Psychological Medicine, 16*, 909–928.

Segal, Z., Williams, M. & Teasdale, J. (2002). *Mindfulness-based Cognitive Therapy for Depression: A New Approach to Preventing Relapse.* New York: Guilford Press.

Smyth, J. M. (1998). Written emotional expression: effect sizes, outcome types, and moderating variables. *Journal of Consulting and Clinical Psychology, 66*, 174–184.

Startup, H. M. & Erickson, T. M. (2006). The Penn State Worry Questionnaire (PSWQ). In G. C. L. Davey & A. Wells (eds). *Worry and its Psychological Disorders: Theory, Assessment and Treatment.* Chichester: John Wiley & Sons.

Startup, H., Freeman, D. & Garety, P. A. (2007). Persecutory delusions and catastrophic worry in psychosis: developing the understanding of delusional distress and persistence. *Behaviour Research and Therapy, 45*(3), 525–537.

Stober, J. (1998). Worry, problem elaboration and suppression of imagery: the role of concreteness. *Behaviour Research and Therapy, 36*, 751–756.

Stober, J. & Borkovec, T. D. (2002). Reduced concreteness of worry in generalized anxiety disorder: findings from a therapy study. *Cognitive Therapy and Research, 26*, 89–96.

Trower, P., Birchwood, M. et al. (2004) Cognitive therapy for command hallucinations: randomised controlled trial. *British Journal of Psychiatry, 184*, 312–320.

van Os, J., Hanssen, M., Bijl, R. V. and Ravelli, A. (2000). Strauss (1969) revisited: a psychosis continuum in the general population? *Schizophrenia Research, 45*, 11–20.

Vrana, S. R., Cuthbert, B. N., Lang, P. J. (1986). Fear imagery and text processing. *Psychophysiology, 23*(3), 247–253.

Watkins, E. (2004). Adaptive and maladaptive ruminative self-focus during emotional processing. *Behaviour Research and Therapy, 42*(9), 1037–1052.

Wells, A. & King, P. (2006). Metacognitive therapy for generalized anxiety disorder: an open trial. *Journal of Behaviour Therapy and Experimental Psychology, 37*(3), 206–212.

Waller, W., Freeman, D., Jolley, S., Dunn, G. & Garety, P. (2011). Targeting reasoning biases in delusions. *Journal of Behaviour Therapy and Experimental Psychiatry, 42*, 414–421.

Wykes, T. Steel, C. Everitt, B. & Tarrier, N. (2008). Cognitive behavior therapy for schizophrenia: effect sizes, clinical models, and methodological rigor. *Schizophrenia Bulletin, 34*(3), 523–537.

Zimmerman, G., Favrod, J., Trieu, V. H. & Pomini, V. (2005). The effect of cognitive behavioural treatment on the positive symptoms of schizophrenia spectrum disorders: a meta-analysis. *Schizophrenia Research, 77*, 1–9.

4

Clinical Assessment and Assessment Measures

*John Farhall, Fran Shawyer, Neil Thomas
and Eric M. J. Morris*

4.1 Introduction

This chapter introduces both a clinical assessment process and formal measurement instruments for work with people experiencing persisting symptoms and disability associated with psychosis. We first outline the approach to clinical assessment we have developed in our acceptance and commitment therapy (ACT) for psychosis work. Then we outline formal measures of mindfulness and measures designed to tap ACT constructs.

4.2 Clinical Assessment

4.2.1 Overview

4.2.1.1 Aims and Scope

Our approach to clinical assessment in psychosis is designed to support an ongoing formulation of the client's problems within an ACT framework. Much of it mirrors assessment for a nonpsychotic problem. However, people living with psychosis can face challenges that are disorder-specific, such as thinking difficulties that impact on assessment and therapy, and experiences such as voices and delusions that are produced by the mind but are experienced as external rather than internal. In addition, opportunities for valued living may be hampered by multiple domains of disability or impoverished social contexts.

Acceptance and Commitment Therapy and Mindfulness for Psychosis, First Edition.
Edited by Eric M. J. Morris, Louise C. Johns and Joseph E. Oliver.
© 2013 John Wiley & Sons, Ltd. Published 2013 by John Wiley & Sons, Ltd.

The ideal breadth of assessment reflects a conceptualisation of problems into three broad categories: the normal challenges of living; the challenges arising from living with a psychotic disorder; and specific challenges associated with psychotic symptoms. Conceptualising the first two categories is relatively straightforward, but the role of psychotic symptoms may be conceptualised as serving a range of functions – sometimes problematic experiences that are managed by efforts to suppress or avoid them, and sometimes experiences that are preoccupying or valued and serve to separate the person from real-world experiences.

In general, the aims of assessment are to:

(1)   Assess symptoms and identify associated problems, their context and their interactions.
(2)   Assess the client's level of engagement and motivation in order to guide the direction of therapy.
(3)   Generate collaborative goal(s) of therapy and frame these in an ACT-consistent way.
(4)   Develop an ACT formulation as a guide for treatment.

Formulation is covered in Chapter 5, while more detail on the conceptualisation of psychotic symptoms is given in Chapters 2, 7 and 8.

4.2.1.2   *General Principles*
Our experience suggests some general principles for conducting assessments:

- *Engagement is more critical initially than assessment.* Getting bogged down in history or the detail of formal assessment runs the risk of missing opportunities for compassionate connection.
- *Assessment of behaviour in the moment is at least as helpful as reports from outside sessions.* Gently exploring what is happening in the room, such as avoidance or emotion, may demonstrate coping patterns and the nature of internal experiences.
- *Behaviour may be more revealing than words.* ACT is fundamentally interested in behaviour in the outside world; thus, what people do, or fail to do, in relation to valued directions is of greater relevance than what they say.
- *Different ways of working during assessment are to be heralded.* The first two or three contacts typically shape expectations and hope. Assessment tasks serve to 'warm up' the patient to key features of therapy.
- *Assessment never stops.* Initial assessment helps us get going, but a deep under-standing of the individual patient and the phenomena they are struggling with is built up throughout therapy.

4.2.2   Structure and Methods of Assessment

4.2.2.1   *Assessment Interwoven with Interventions*

The initial assessment includes material that will be explored further in core ACT interventions, including the patient's appraisal of how effectively past treatments and their own strategies solved their problems (which may lead later into creative hopelessness or related interventions) and a brief assessment of values/goals in relation to therapy. A mixture of further assessment tasks and initial therapy interventions (e.g. costs of current methods of coping or struggle) may continue over the next couple of sessions. For example, some early exercises, like the 'raisin exercise' (a present-moment awareness experience, Kabat-Zinn, 1990, pp. 27–29), can provide valuable information about habitual reactions to experience, as well as beginning the skill-development process.

As therapy progresses, ongoing assessment can take various forms. Progress may be tracked via monitoring, diaries or reassessment with instruments. Check in with the patient during exercises – how are they going? Are they fusing, avoiding or remaining mindful? Look for clues as to what ACT processes and exercises the client is responding to and not. This gives essential information about strengths in therapy, cognitive deficits and avoidance. Use this understanding to tailor directions. Exercises or metaphors that prompt insight, excitement or laughter (i.e. that clearly connect directly with the client's experience), rather than blankness, indifference or perplexity,[1] can be used as 'Christmas trees' on which other contexts or processes can be 'hung' and appreciated. For example, if the tug-of-war with the monster (see Appendix H) proves to be a powerful experience for the client, later skills such as mindfulness and defusion might be described as ways of 'dropping the rope'.

4.2.2.2   *Use of Assessment Instruments*

Formal assessment instruments can play useful clinical and research roles in assessment, monitoring of change and demonstration of outcomes and processes of therapy. Section 4.3 outlines ACT and mindfulness instruments that might be suitable for each of these purposes. In general, we rely on our clinical assessment for formulation, but test scores can provide a useful context, including scores on positive symptom measures (e.g. the Psychotic Symptoms Ratings Scale, PSYRATS; Haddock *et al.*, 1999), broad assessments of symptoms (Positive and Negative Syndrome Scale, PANSS; Kay *et al.*, 1987) and assessments of cognitive functioning.

4.2.2.3   *Role of Self-monitoring in Assessment*

It is unlikely that all, or even most, psychosis clients will be willing and able to complete monitoring. Nonetheless, where possible, monitoring is encouraged. Monitoring provides useful material with which to work in the session and by which to illustrate key points (e.g. differentiating symptoms from reactions), practice in tuning into experience and observing symptoms and a vehicle for practising ACT strategies and recording homework exercises. It is important to provide a rationale for the client, such as 'Keeping track of your difficult experiences highlights what happens when you are struggling. We can use this diary in sessions to help see what is going on for you when you feel upset.'

If monitoring is proposed, it needs to be adapted to the client's level of functioning, taking sufficient time to explain and practise using the recording form. It should be reviewed as part of the agenda each week. As a general rule, err on the side of simplicity. Having a range of forms with varying levels of complexity available can be useful, but these can also be collaboratively drawn up (and thus tailored) during the session.

For the purposes of assessment, monitoring is directed at simply observing and describing key behaviours and client reactions in context. Depending on the complexity of the form, it may include the date/time, the situation and client reactions, which can range from simply how upset they were, to including specific feelings, thoughts and sensations, to a detailed description of what they did.

4.2.2.4   Goal Setting
Collaboratively work with the client to generate goals for therapy. Writing these down formally, and referring back to and refining them as therapy proceeds, can help both client and therapist remain on track and sustain motivation.

As far as possible, reframe the client's goals in ACT-consistent ways, with a focus on meaningful behavioural outcomes that reflect underlying values (e.g. to meet new people, even if voices don't agree). If the client gives a goal linked to their delusions (e.g. 'To have the CIA stop following me') or a goal of reducing symptoms or distress, seek out the underlying value. For example, if the goal is to be free of voices, ask how being free of voices would affect their lives; if the goal is not remotely realistic, ask what is important about it, in order to access alternative ways of expressing the same value. An example may help: 'I can set a goal of becoming prime minister, but it's unlikely to happen given my circumstances and talents. I can stress myself out and make myself miserable living with this unattainable goal. However, if my underlying value is to contribute meaningfully to society, there are a lot of ways I can do this.' By digging down into values, this is likely to yield immediate possibilities for action: addressing workability will rein in psychotic excess more gently, without causing shame or making the client appear wrong (Luoma *et al.*, 2007). At an appropriate point, it may be helpful to review what aspects of experience can and can't be controlled, in order to help underpin the importance and relevance of values and personal behaviour.

4.2.3   A Guide to Clinical Assessment

4.2.3.1   The Problems Experienced by the Client

Although family members, the treating team and the referrer may have views about what the problem is, it is the client's experience of themselves and the world that is the starting point. We typically do the following:

(1) Obtain an overview of current concerns, whether symptom-related or otherwise.

(2) Assess symptoms the client experiences, with a focus on phenomenology and behavioural analysis. Assessment of symptoms may be cued by the client's reference to them, by their presence in the session or by the referrer's (or another's) mention of them, as appropriate. We first attempt to clarify the experience by asking about:

  (i) *Phenomenology*: Content, frequency, duration and preoccupation.

  (ii) *Subjective experience*: What this experience has been like, including times when it was difficult and times when they managed.

  (iii) *Explanatory model*: How the client understands their psychosis and the experience of their symptoms. Some useful questions here are: 'What do you think caused it?' 'Why did it start when it did?' 'What do your friends/family have to say about it?' 'Why you?'

  (iv) *Contexts*: When symptoms tend to occur and when they are unlikely to occur, particularly with reference to times of the day, the presence of others and stress.

(3) Assess aspects of symptoms that are particularly relevant to the ACT formulation – especially the function of the experiences and their impact on valued behaviour. Fusion and avoidance may arise from voice content, beliefs about voices, delusional ideation, stigma or schemas thought to underlie delusions. Useful questions include:

  (i) How have these symptoms been a problem? Are they getting in the way of living your life? How?

  (ii) What has been the effect on friends/family?

  (iii) What have these problems stopped you doing? If you had a magic wand and could make the symptom/problem disappear, what difference would it make to your life?

  (iv) What thoughts and feelings arise with the symptoms? (Potential sources of fusion.)

  (v) What do you do in response to symptoms? (Explore internally based emotional control strategies, such as negative distraction, and behaviourally focused emotional control strategies, such as smoking, drinking, taking medication 'when required'.)

(4) Clarify attitudes towards psychosis, symptoms and treatment generally (including case management and medication).

(5) Listen to concerns and identify recurring narratives or themes. This can both aid identification and suggest prioritisation of behaviours and contexts.

(6) Clarify the concerns until there is a shared language for understanding and describing them. This serves the dual purpose of helping us be clear about the client's concerns and giving us opportunities to informally introduce the language of ACT ('values', 'struggle' etc.).

4.2.3.2   *Understanding the Client*

Getting to know about the client in their life context provides important information on how symptom-related behaviour fits in with broader behavioural routines and highlights past and ongoing valued activities. A starting point is to gain an appreciation of current daily life, then ask about life before the onset of psychosis. We usually briefly explore the following:

(1) The client's typical day-to-day routines and activities.

(2) The extent and quality of their relationships with others.

(3) The social and daily living context, especially with regard to how rich or impoverished the opportunities for valued action might be.

(4) Pertinent aspects of the client's personal, psychiatric, social and family history. Where time precludes a comprehensive assessment, important things to cover include:

   (i)   duration of the disorder;

   (ii) a brief picture of life before the disorder, so as to assess premorbid functioning and quality of life;

   (iii) anything else in the client's life they think might be of relevance to therapy.

(5) Valued domains of experience over time. This involves asking, 'What wouldn't you want changed in your life?'

4.2.4   Assessing and Addressing Potential Barriers to and Risks Arising from Therapy

In this section we present some of the barriers and risks that might be encountered in working with people living with a psychotic disorder, and some appropriate responses. At first the list may seem daunting, especially for clinicians experienced in using ACT for people who do not have psychosis (watch out for fusion!). However, these are simply pieces of potentially useful assessment information. Some factors to be alert for include:

(1) *Absence of self-referral.* Where the impetus for therapy has come from others rather than the client, greater attention to engagement, desire for change and collaborative goals is needed.

(2) *Chronically low energy and motivation*. These common accompaniments to, and sometimes core symptoms of, psychosis may impact on the pace of therapy, and prompt greater attention to the therapeutic relationship. Finding meaningful goals and introducing simple rewards such as a cup of tea on arrival can help, but for some people changing egosyntonic adaptational habits that have built up over years may be unrealistic.

(3) *Pessimism and anxiety about change*. Awareness of a decline in social and occupational functioning leads some clients to abandon the possibility of a better life. Others feel stuck, fragile and scared of change. These individuals are at risk of dropping out if too much is asked of them, or too much discomfort is exposed, before a hopeful and trusting relationship has developed, or before they have experienced a small change associated with therapy. Therapist responses might include reviewing the pace of sessions and attention to rewards, but also a readiness to back off if the client is becoming overwhelmed and unable to process what is happening. On the positive side, both assessment and therapy can foster a sense of hope, purpose and direction, via the structure of sessions, the identification of treatment goals and the ongoing review of progress. Cultivation of a therapeutic relationship in which the therapist is seen as competent and understanding but also 'a fish swimming in the same sea' can begin at assessment, along with the development of a therapeutic relationship in which the client is not seen as 'broken' and needing to be 'fixed'.

(4) *Absence of struggle in the context of egosyntonic delusions or voices*. Engagement may present challenges if the patient is preoccupied with a delusional world in which psychotic experiences are valued over and dominate others. Assessment might include an exploration of valued directions that are not exercised via delusions, as these may facilitate collaborative engagement around new behaviours.

(5) *Absence of a shared view about the 'reality' of psychotic experiences*. From an ACT perspective, the reality of the experience is not the issue (though its function is!) and need not be debated. A helpful stance is to be 'casually neutral' about the reality of the client's beliefs and – more importantly – to converse and understand from the client's perspective as assessment proceeds. Where the client is sensitive to terminology in discussing psychotic material, it may be possible to link with ACT processes in a natural way, such as by saying, 'When you have the thought that…' without any sense of trying to convince the client that it is a thought (Bach, 2004). If this proves unacceptable, you could use 'concern' or other synonyms. If the reality of their beliefs is directly raised by the client, explain that ACT is not so much concerned about whether beliefs are real or not but with how useful they are in assisting the client to pursue their interests and goals; thus, you might choose to ignore a thought even when you believe it is 'real', because acting on it would interfere with attaining a valued goal. For example, the dieter who really feels hungry

and really wants a piece of cake might choose to disregard the thought in order to attain the goal of losing weight (Bach, 2004).

(6) *Stimulus overload.* This is a risk for some people who are prone to exacerbation of symptoms under even mild stress. Assessment might usefully explore the day-to-day variability of paranoia or voice activity and any apparent association with anxiety or external demands. This might serve as an initial guide to the demands and pace of therapy and its suitability for the client at this point in their life.

(7) *Concentration, abstract thinking and verbal memory.* These may be impaired, so an initial appreciation of the extent to which standard ACT exercises, metaphors and skills development need to be adapted for the client may help ensure positive experiences of therapy.

(8) *Mismatch of goals for therapy.* Clients frequently arrive with avoidance or suppression goals. A useful assessment 'intervention' is to note the client's response to the therapist's translation of their goals into an ACT-consistent form (e.g. translating 'Stop the voices' into 'Find ways to do what is important to you whether the voices stop or not'). Where a referral has been made in order to assist a client adapt to problematic psychotic experiences, the client will not necessarily propose this as a goal. If other issues are raised, the therapist can review with the client the purpose of the referral, and explain that the therapy approach is likely to be useful for these other issues as well. If the client is unable or unwilling to address problems related to the 'symptoms' of psychosis, the assessment and formulation may lead to an initial therapy focus on values and goals, with the expectation that opportunities to engage with problematic symptoms will emerge in this context.

(9) *Thought disorder.* Of the symptoms of psychosis, we have found high levels of thought disorder the most difficult to accommodate, as the delivery of therapy relies so heavily on verbal communication and reflection. Maximising behavioural experience and *in vivo* work seems the best route to minimising their impact.

4.3   Assessment Measures

As with many emerging fields, well-validated instruments measuring processes associated with ACT and mindfulness, particularly those tailored for psychosis, are relatively scarce. Choosing an instrument for clinical or research purposes inevitably involves weighing up competing attributes, such as length, psychometric rigour and clinical utility. This section focuses on measures that have some published psychometric evaluation and that have been used in clinical or research reports about ACT or mindfulness interventions for psychosis, plus a small number of instruments that may also be considered for psychosis clients.

For a wider range of published and unpublished measures relevant to ACT more generally, the ACBS Web site (contextualpsychology.org) is a useful resource, while Baer's (2010) book *Assessing Mindfulness & Acceptance Processes in Clients: Illuminating the Theory & Practice of Change* is an in-depth look at measuring mindfulness.

4.3.1   Issues in the Use of Self-report Measures

Most of the phenomena we wish to assess, such as symptoms or mindfulness, cannot be measured objectively, so interviews or self-report measures are necessary. However, a fundamental challenge in psychosis research and clinical practice is that we are asking people who struggle with cognitive processes to use those cognitive processes to reflect on and report their experiences. Sources of error variance may arise at various levels: the client's awareness of the phenomenon to be reported (awareness of internal experience; concentration; perspective taking/ theory of mind; metacognitive awareness); their difficulties in forming a response to the information sought (concentration; verbal memory; concrete thinking impairing abstract responding; appraisal bias); and how accurately they are able to report the experience (associative thinking; circumstantiality). Valid self-ratings may be particularly difficult for mindfulness processes: not only might it be unrealistic for respondents with little experience of being mindful to validly self-rate aspects of this experience they pay little attention to, but in addition the language of the items may have different meanings for those who have been taught mindfulness and those who have not (Leigh *et al.*, 2005).

The choice of measurement instruments should take into account such difficulties, especially when applying measures that were not specifically designed for psychosis populations. In our experience, cognitive difficulties can be compensated for by a reduction of memory and concentration demands through short scales with briefly worded items, the use of printed as well as verbal questions and friendly environments that minimise distraction and anxiety, and in which assistance is available if required.

4.3.2   Mindfulness Measures

Compared with Buddhist traditions of meditation, mindfulness employed within the pragmatic and time-limited context of psychological therapies has tended to focus more on the cognitive skills of awareness and attention (e.g. Hayes & Plumb, 2007) and relatively less on facets such as the compassionate qualities underpinning a nonjudgemental stance or investigation of ongoing experience in a 'nondiscursive, nonanalytic' way (Grossman & Van Dam, 2011). From the clinician's point of view, pragmatic measures that address these former aspects are of primary interest. Some measures seem to fulfil this brief.

In addition to the reliance of measurement of mindfulness upon a person's metacognitive awareness, some other issues are of note. First, mindfulness measures tend to be self-ratings of perceived competencies, potentially influenced by broader factors affecting self-rated competence. Second, the existing measures differ in scope, addressing from two to five facets of mindfulness. Finally, the questionnaires tend to address mindfulness as a trait, although they do imply that it is modifiable by practice; yet clinical and research applications are often interested in changes in mindfulness following interventions designed to teach it. There is little information available about the sensitivity to change of such measures in psychosis.

There are many mindfulness self-report measures, at least eight of them reporting psychometric evaluation. However, we could find only two that have been applied to psychosis: the Southampton Mindfulness Questionnaire (SMQ), which has a psychosis-specific version, and the Kentucky Inventory of Mindfulness Skills (KIMS).

- *SMQ and SMVQ.* Paul Chadwick and colleagues have produced two related measures, the SMQ and the Southampton Mindfulness of Voices Questionnaire (SMVQ). Each is a self-report questionnaire comprising eight positively- and eight negatively-worded items rated on a 7-point fully-anchored Likert scale. The SMQ directs attention specifically to 'distressing thoughts and images', asking the user to rate statements that address the following: awareness of the present moment; allowing attention to remain on the distressing experience rather than avoiding it; acceptance; and letting go versus struggle (Chadwick *et al.*, 2008). It has been used with clinical and nonclinical populations and seems readily applicable to a range of internal experiences, including delusions. The SMVQ has similarly worded items specifically referring to voices (Chadwick *et al.*, 2007). It has been used with people who have psychosis in two single case reports (Newman-Taylor *et al.*, 2009) and a pilot group programme for the treatment of distressing voices (Ratcliff, 2010).
- *KIMS.* The KIMS (Baer *et al.*, 2004) was designed to measure mindfulness as practised in dialectical behaviour therapy (DBT). The 39 items cover four elements: observation of present-moment experiences; description through verbal labelling; acting with awareness; and accepting present-moment experiences without judgment. There is some evidence for its sensitivity in psychosis: in a pilot RCT of ACT for psychosis (ACTp), the ACT group showed greater change in the KIMS than did the treatment-as-usual (TAU) comparison group (White *et al.*, 2011).

Among other mindfulness measures, the following are of particular note, but we could find no reports of their use in psychosis.

- *Five Facet Mindfulness Questionnaire (FFMQ).* The FFMQ (Baer *et al.*, 2006) may be the best representation of the elements of mindfulness as it is currently conceptualised, given that it was developed from a factor analytic study of five independently developed questionnaires, selecting the best performing items across them (including the SMQ, MAAS and KIMS). It comprises 39 items measuring five facets of mindfulness: observing, describing, acting with aware-ness, nonjudging of inner experience and nonreactivity to inner experience.

- *Mindful Attention Awareness Scale (MAAS).* The difficulty of directly reporting mindfulness is addressed in the MAAS (Brown & Ryan, 2003) by having items covering a range of behaviours that are considered to be inconsistent with mindfulness, rather than attempting to directly describe it. The 15 items encom-pass two aspects of mindfulness: attention and awareness of experience.
- *Toronto Mindfulness Scale (TMS).* The TMS (Lau *et al.*, 2006) was designed to be used after a 15-minute mindfulness exercise to measure the degree of mindful-ness attained via two facets: curiosity and decentring. Its measurement of immediately preceding behaviour makes it attractive as a skills measure.

4.3.3 Measures of ACT Processes and Constructs

The six components of ACT are conceptually distinguishable but are assumed to be synergistic elements contributing to the greater whole of psychological flexibility. In the development of measures for ACT processes, the initial focus has been at this broad level of psychological flexibility. The extent to which 'pure' measures of the component ACT processes are possible remains to be seen. Defusion arguably requires some degree of mindful attention to thoughts, and, conversely, mindfulness of thoughts in itself is a defusing process. Being 'present' may require some level of acceptance of internal experience and so on. Nonetheless, through the development of component scales, it may be possible to disentangle the contributions of such hypothesised components, and initial attempts to provide such measures are considered in this section. As with mindfulness, few scales have been used directly with psychosis: only the Acceptance and Action Questionnaire (AAQ), Voices Acceptance & Action Scale (VAAS) and believability rating scales have been reported to date.

4.3.3.1 Acceptance and Action Questionnaire

The original core construct of ACT was experiential avoidance – an attempt to change or avoid unwanted thoughts, feelings and sensations. The AAQ was devel-oped as a measure of this construct, with the title reflecting the positive expression of the notion; that is, a willingness to have such internal experiences in the course of pursuing valued actions. Although ACT has developed over time, broadening into a six-component hexaflex model and conceptualising the central acceptance/ experiential avoidance construct more broadly as 'psychological flexibility', versions of the AAQ have remained the key measure of theoretically relevant change across many research studies (Hayes *et al.*, 2006) and it has been adapted for specific client groups and translated into various languages. Nonetheless, it has been hampered by uncertainty about its factor structure and by its less than desirable internal consistency. Information about the many variants of the measure can be found on the Contextual Psychology Web site (contextualpsychology.org).

A definitive seven-item revision, the AAQ-II, has now been published, reporting improved internal consistency, a single latent factor structure across clinical and nonclinical populations and evidence of construct and discriminant validity. Although strongly correlated with the Beck Depression Inventory (BDI) and moderately correlated with other measures of depression and anxiety, it nonetheless appears to be tapping a distinguishable construct (Bond *et al.*, 2011).

The AAQ was not reported as a measure in the initial clinical studies of psychosis, but it has been used in research studies on the subject (e.g. Goldstone *et al.*, 2011), contributing to prediction of vulnerability to hallucinatory experiences in both a student and a psychosis sample. White *et al.* (2011) used the AAQ-II in their pilot of ACT for emotional dysfunction in psychosis. Although it did not differentiate ACT and TAU groups, there was evidence of an association between change in AAQ-II scores and change in self-rated depression.

Among alternative measures, the *Avoidance and Fusion Questionnaire for Youth (AFQ-Y)*, developed for children and adolescents, is notable (Greco *et al.*, 2008). It has 8- and 17-item versions, with adequate psychometrics. Initial data suggest it is unidimensional, supporting its claim to measure psychological flexibility. Although originally intended for children, none of the items are age-specific and it has been successfully used with college students (Schmalz & Murrell, 2010). Its simple language and avoidance of ACT-specific terminology suggests that people who have cognitive problems associated with psychosis may find it usable.

4.3.3.2   The Voices Acceptance & Action Scale

Ratcliff *et al.* (2010) reviewed specific assessment instruments for voices using the VAAS, the only published ACT measure specific to psychosis. The VAAS was originally developed for use with people who experience command hallucinations, with its items specifically addressing two constructs: acceptance of the experience of hearing voices and the ability to act independently of them (Shawyer *et al.*, 2007). Section A comprises 12 items designed to be applicable to any voice; the remaining sections are intended for command hallucinations. Further work on the scale using an expanded sample ($n = 103$) has refined Section A, demonstrating improved psychometrics by omitting items (A1, A11, A12), resulting in a standalone scale, the VAAS-9, comprising two factors: acceptance of voices and autonomous action (independence) (Ratcliff, 2010).

4.3.3.3   Believability of Symptoms

'Believability' has been a key measure in case reports and trials of ACT and mindfulness for psychosis. Although it has only been rated with single items, its use in studies provides considerable evidence of its utility. 'Believability' refers to the extent to which one accepts the literal truth of products of the mind, and has long been used as a proxy for defusion (Zettle & Hayes, 1986). Rating the believability of a thought that is, in fact, not literally true makes sense as an indicator of defusion, but such a measure cannot pick up defusion from thoughts that *are* true, such as 'I'm going to die'.

Bach & Hayes (2002) applied believability to positive symptoms of psychosis, asking patients, 'On a scale of zero to 100, to what degree do you believe that it is true [that gang members are stalking you; that the voices are telling you that you are a bad person]?'. A similar scale was also used as an outcome and a process measure in Gaudiano & Herbert's (2006) clinical trial, where it differentiated between groups and mediated change (Gaudiano *et al.*, 2010). On this basis, despite being a simple single-item rating, it is clearly measuring something of interest.

Although this believability rating mediates outcomes, its interpretation – especially its validity as a measure of flexibility of, or fusion with, internal mental activity – is uncertain. The conceptual problem is that from the psychotic person's point of view, delusions and hallucinations may not be recognised as their own cognitive experiences; therefore, being asked about the truth of a delusion operationalises 'believability' as the truth or falsity of the symptom experience itself (i.e. insight) rather than of internally experienced thoughts or beliefs. Thus, two perspectives are possible. First, if believability is intended to measure a dimension of fusion with *thoughts*, asking a question about the 'truth' of *externally* experienced psychotic phenomena might indicate little about the flexibility of thinking, and would traditionally be understood as addressing insight. (Readers familiar with dimensional measurement of psychotic symptoms will note that the wording of the believability question is almost identical to 'conviction' items in measures such as the PSYRATS (Haddock *et al.*, 1999) and Peters *et al.* Delusions Inventory (PDI) (Peters *et al.*, 2004)). The alternative perspective is that because psychotic phenomena are a product of the mind, delusions and hallucinations can be interpreted as the ultimate form of fusion, where even the awareness of their base in one's own thinking is lost. From this perspective, believability could be argued to be a reasonable proxy for such 'fusion'.

The teasing out of ACT change processes, especially for research purposes, would benefit from the development of a measure of believability of *internally attributed* beliefs and appraisal associated with positive symptoms. These might most sensitively identify the ACT construct of 'believability'. For those who interpret psychotic symptoms as fusion, the PDI and PSYRATS are alternatives or additions to the traditional believability rating.

4.3.3.4 Additional Measures

The following measures show promise as supplementary assessments of specific ACT processes.

- *Valued Living Questionnaire (VLQ)*. The VLQ (Wilson *et al.*, 2010) was devised to assess the extent to which respondents are in touch with freely chosen domains of valued living in their everyday life. After rating 10 domains of living for their importance, a rating is made of the consistency over the past week of actions with values within each value domain. The primary measure is a composite score. Limitations of this measure include its use of domains of life as the focus of ratings, rather than individually defined valued directions, and the cognitive demands of rating the 'consistency' of one's actions in relation to valued directions. It seems to be more useful as a clinical tool than a formal assessment measure.

- *The Valuing Questionnaire (VQ).* This new instrument (Smout *et al.*, 2011) aims to measure the extent of valued living in the past week, including in the presence of barriers. Unlike in the VLQ, general domains of life are not rated; rather, the items represent two self-assessed factors: the extent to which values have been 'lived' in the past week ('progress') and the extent to which cognitive and emotional barriers have interfered with enacting values ('obstructed'). There are two versions: 8 and 20 items. Although the clarity of items and scoring on the VQ shows promise, no use in psychosis has been reported.
- *Cognitive Fusion Questionnaire (CFQ13).* Although not yet published, considerable developmental work has gone into this scale, which is publically available, along with psychometric information, at contextualpsychology.org. The scale comprises 13 items, worded in terms of both fusion and defusion. The relatively low reading age of the items augers well for its use with clients who have difficulties in concentration and abstraction.
- *Thought Action Fusion Questionnaire (TAF).* Originally developed to extend the study of obsessive–compulsive disorder (OCD), this 19-item scale assesses beliefs that thinking about an unacceptable thought makes it more likely to occur and that having unacceptable thoughts is as bad as carrying them out (Shafran *et al.*, 1996). There is some evidence that fusion with positive actions is tapped by versions of this measure, not just fusion with avoided actions (Shafran & Rachman, 2004), suggesting it measures the broad relational framing construct of fusion in ACT. In the absence of published fusion measures, this may be a proxy.

4.4 Conclusion

Some useful practice wisdom is now accumulating with which to inform clinical assessment for ACT and mindfulness for psychosis, and the development of specific assessment instruments has begun. In presenting these developments, we are intending to convey the message that the particular needs of people living with psychosis must be considered in assessment as well as in therapy: simply applying assessment approaches and instruments devised for people with nonpsychotic disorders or problems risks engagement failure and a poor understanding of the particular life dilemmas of the people we are endeavouring to assist. However, the challenges of assessment and measurement are not confined to working with psychosis: valid measurement of third-wave constructs is a challenge in itself. With the rapid rise in interest in ACT and mindfulness therapies, measurement research is ripe for development of both general measures of core constructs and specialist measures tuned to the features of specific populations.

Note

1   Confusion or perplexity is often seen as 'good' and expected in ACT, but it appears to be unhelpful in a psychosis population, illustrating an important stylistic difference between general ACT and ACT for psychosis.

References

Bach, P. A. (2004). ACT with the seriously mentally ill. In S. C. Hayes & K. D. Strosahl (eds.). *A Practical Guide to Acceptance and Commitment Therapy*. New York: Springer, pp. 185–208.

Bach, P. & Hayes, S. C. (2002). The use of acceptance and commitment therapy to prevent rehospitalization of psychotic patients: a randomized controlled trial. *Journal of Consulting and Clinical Psychology*, 70(5), 1129–1139.

Baer, R. (2010). *Assessing Mindfulness & Acceptance Processes in Clients: Illuminating the Theory & Practice of Change*. Oakland: Context Press.

Baer, R. A. (2011). Measuring mindfulness. *Contemporary Buddhism*, 12(1), 241–261.

Baer, R., Smith, G. T. & Allen, K. B. (2004). Assessment of mindfulness by self-report: the Kentucky Inventory of Mindfulness Skills. *Assessment*, 11(3), 191–206.

Baer, R., Smith, G. T., Hopkins, J., Krietemeyer, J. & Toney, L. (2006). Using self-report assessment methods to explore facets of mindfulness. *Assessment*, 13(1), 27–45.

Bond, F. W., Hayes, S. C., Baer, R. A., Carpenter, K. M., Guenole, N., Orcutt, H. K., Waltz, T. & Zettle, R. D. (2011). Preliminary psychometric properties of the Acceptance and Action Questionnaire AAQ II: a revised measure of psychological inflexibility and experiential avoidance. *Behavior Therapy*, 42, 676–688.

Brown, K. W. & Ryan, R. M. (2003). The benefits of being present: mindfulness and its role in psychological well-being. *Journal of Personality and Social Psychology*, 84(4), 822–848.

Chadwick, P., Barnbrook, E. & Newman Taylor, K. (2007). Responding mindfully to distressing voices: links with meaning affect and relationship with voice. *Journal of the Norwegian Psychological Association*, 44, 581–588.

Chadwick, P., Hember, M., Symes, J., Peters, E., Kuipers, E. & Dagnan, D. (2008). Responding mindfully to unpleasant thoughts and images: reliability and validity of the Southampton Mindfulness Questionnaire (SMQ). *British Journal of Clinical Psychology*, 47(4), 451–455.

Gaudiano, B. A. & Herbert, J. D. (2006). Acute treatment of inpatients with psychotic symptoms using Acceptance and Commitment Therapy: pilot results. *Behaviour Research and Therapy*, 44(3), 415–437.

Gaudiano, B. A., Herbert, J. D. & Hayes, S. C. (2010). Is it the symptom or the relation to it? Investigating potential mediators of change in acceptance and commitment therapy for psychosis. *Behavior Therapy*, 41(4), 543–554.

Goldstone, E., Farhall, J. & Ong, B. (2011). Synergistic pathways to delusions: enduring vulnerabilities, proximal life stressors and maladaptive psychological coping. *Early Intervention in Psychiatry*, 5(2), 122–131.

Greco, L. A., Lambert, W. & Baer, R. A. (2008). Psychological inflexibility in childhood and adolescence: development and evaluation of the Avoidance and Fusion Questionnaire for Youth. *Psychological Assessment*, 20, 93–102.

Grossman, P. & Van Dam, N. T. (2011). Mindfulness, by any other name: trials and tribulations of *sati* in western psychology and science. *Contemporary Buddhism*, 12(1), 219–239.

Haddock, G., McCarron, J., Tarrier, N. & Faragher, E. B. (1999). Scales to measure dimensions of hallucinations and delusions: the Psychotic Symptom Rating Scales (PSYRATS). *Psychological Medicine*, 29(4), 879–889.

Hayes, S. C., Luoma, J. B., Bond, F. W., Masuda, A. & Lillis, J. (2006). Acceptance and commitment therapy: model, processes and outcomes. *Behaviour Research and Therapy*, 44(1), 1–25.

Hayes, S. C. & Plumb, J. C. (2007). Mindfulness from the bottom up: providing an inductive framework for understanding mindfulness processes and their application to human suffering. *Psychological Inquiry*, 18(4), 242–248.

Kabat-Zinn, J. (1990). *Full Catastrophe Living: How to Cope with Stress, Pain and Illness Using Mindfulness Meditation*. New York: Bantam Dell.

Kay, S. R., Fiszbein, A. & Opler, L. A. (1987). The Positive and Negative Syndrome Scale (PANSS) for schizophrenia. *Schizophrenia Bulletin*, 13, 261–276.

Lau, M. A., Bishop, S. R., Segal, Z. V., Buis, T., Anderson, N. D., Carlson, L. *et al.* (2006). The Toronto Mindfulness Scale: development and validation. *Journal of Clinical Psychology*, 62(12), 1445–1467.

Leigh, J., Bowen, S. & Marlatt, G. A. (2005). Spirituality, mindfulness and substance abuse. *Addictive Behaviors*, 30(7), 1335–1341.

Luoma, J. B., Hayes, S. C & Walser, R. D. (2007). *Learning ACT: An Acceptance & Commitment Therapy Skills-training Manual for Therapists*. Oakland: New Harbinger, pp. vii–304.

Newman-Taylor, K., Harper, S. & Chadwick, P. (2009). Impact of mindfulness on cognition and affect in voice hearing: evidence from two case studies. *Behavioural and Cognitive Psychotherapy*, 37, 397–402.

Peters, E., Joseph, S., Day, S. & Garety, P. (2004). Measuring delusional ideation: the 21-item Peters et al. Delusions Inventory (PDI). *Schizophrenia Bulletin*, 30(4), 1005–1022.

Ratcliff, K. M. (2010). *Acceptance of Experience and Adaptation to Auditory Hallucinations*. PhD thesis, School of Psychological Science, La Trobe University, Australia.

Ratcliff, K., Farhall, J. & Shawyer, F. (2010). Auditory hallucinations: a review of assessment tools. *Clinical Psychology & Psychotherapy*, 18(6), 524–534.

Schmalz, J. E. & Murrell, A. R. (2010). Measuring experiential avoidance in adults: the avoidance and fusion questionnaire. *The International Journal of Behavioral Consultation and Therapy*, 6(3), 198–213.

Shafran, R. & Rachman, S. (2004). Thought-action fusion: a review. *Journal of Behavior Therapy and Experimental Psychiatry*, 35(2), 87–107.

Shafran, R., Thordarson, D. S. & Rachman, S. (1996). Thought–action fusion in obsessive compulsive disorder. *Journal of Anxiety Disorders*, 10(5), 379–391.

Shawyer, F., Ratcliff, K., Mackinnon, A., Farhall, J., Hayes, S. C. & Copolov, D. (2007). The Voices Acceptance and Action Scale (VAAS): pilot data. *Journal of Clinical Psychology*, 63(6), 593–606.

Smout, M. F., Davies, M., Burns, N. & Christie, A. (2011). Development of the Valuing Questionnaire. Presentation at the Association for Contextual Behavioral Science (ACBS) World Conference IX, 13–15 July, Parma, Italy.

Wechsler, D. (2001). *Wechsler Test of Adult Reading*. San Antonio: The Psychological Corporation.

White, R., Gumley, A., McTaggart, J., Rattrie, L., McConville, D., Cleare, S. & Mitchell, G. (2011). A feasibility study of Acceptance and Commitment Therapy for emotional dysfunction following psychosis. *Behaviour Research and Therapy*, 49(12), 901–907.

Wilson, K. G., Sandoz, E. K., Kitchens, J. & Roberts, M. (2010). The valued living questionnaire: defining and measuring valued action within a behavioral framework. *Psychological Record*, 60(2), 249–272.

Yusupoff, L. & Tarrier, N. (1996). Coping strategy enhancement for persistent hallucinations and delusions. In G. Haddock & P. D. Slade (eds). *Cognitive-behavioural Interventions with Psychotic Disorders*. London: Routledge, pp. 86–102.

Zettle, R. D. & Hayes, S. C. (1986). Dysfunctional control by client verbal behavior: the context of reason giving. *The Analysis of Verbal Behavior*, 4, 30–38.

5

Acceptance and Commitment Therapy Case Formulation

Patty Bach

5.1 Introduction

Given recent reports of acceptance and commitment therapy (ACT) in the treatment of psychosis (e.g. see Bach *et al.*, 2012; Gaudiano & Herbert, 2006; Shawyer *et al.*, 2007), there is increasing interest in functional contextual approaches to understanding and conceptualising psychotic disorders. The aim of this chapter is to illustrate the ACT model of psychopathology as it applies to people with psychotic disorders using a lengthy case study. A second case study focuses more on the process rather than the content of case formulation.

5.2 Case Study

Case formulation in ACT for people with psychotic disorders is based on our understanding of a functional contextual account of symptoms of psychosis, ACT in the treatment of psychotic disorders and ACT case formulation more generally. Case formulation in ACT can be carried out using the hexaflex model. That is, client symptoms and target behaviours are considered in terms of core ACT processes. While the Hexaflex model described in Chapter 1 involves six processes associated with psychological flexibility, the ACT model of psychopathology includes processes that lead to inflexible and narrow behavioural repertoires and generally unworkable solutions to client problems. These processes can be characterised in six domains consistent with psychological inflexibility, which Bach & Moran (2008) thus call the 'inflexahex' (see Figure 5.1).

Acceptance and Commitment Therapy and Mindfulness for Psychosis, First Edition.
Edited by Eric M. J. Morris, Louise C. Johns and Joseph E. Oliver.
© 2013 John Wiley & Sons, Ltd. Published 2013 by John Wiley & Sons, Ltd.

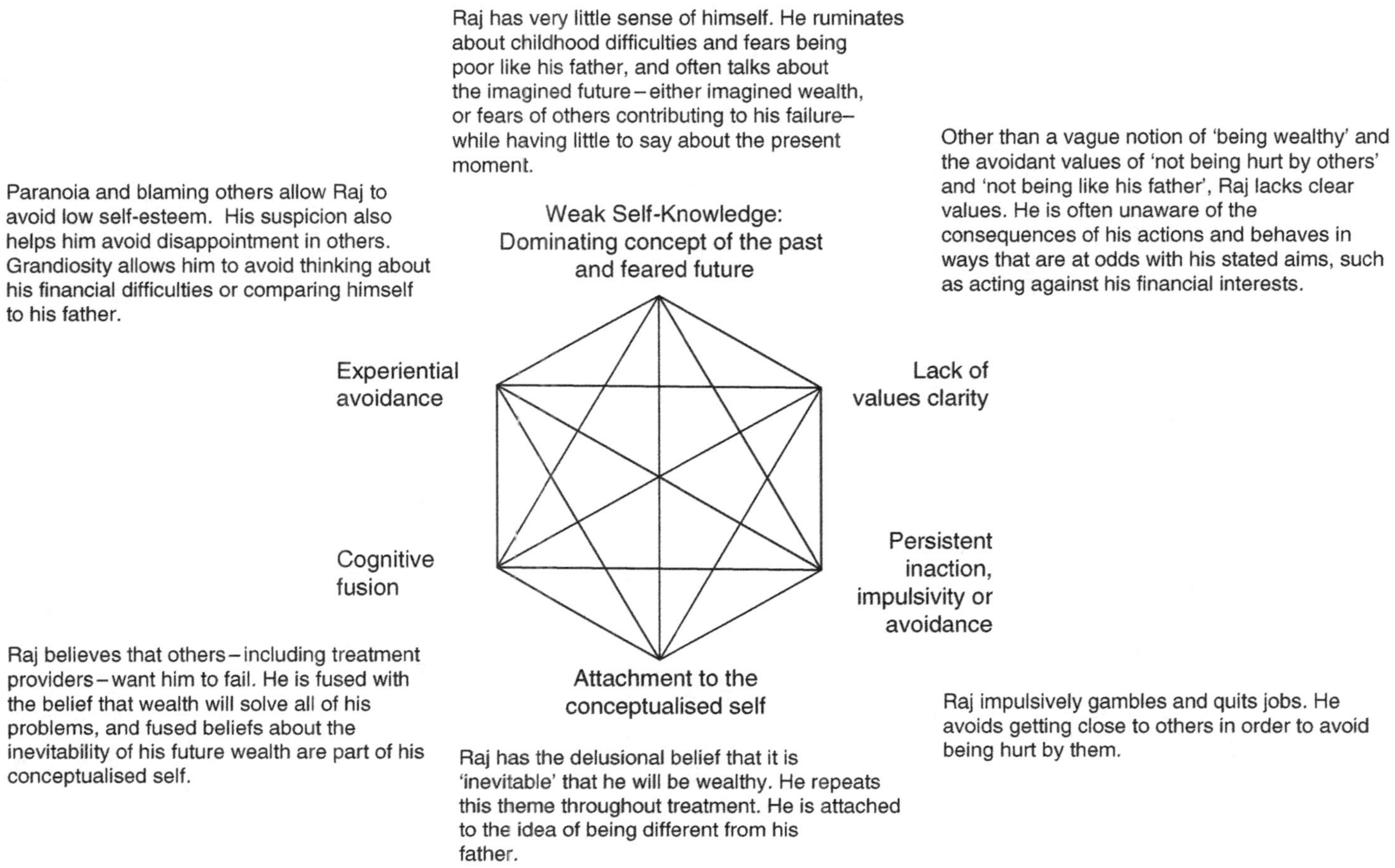

Raj has very little sense of himself. He ruminates about childhood difficulties and fears being poor like his father, and often talks about the imagined future – either imagined wealth, or fears of others contributing to his failure – while having little to say about the present moment.

Other than a vague notion of 'being wealthy' and the avoidant values of 'not being hurt by others' and 'not being like his father', Raj lacks clear values. He is often unaware of the consequences of his actions and behaves in ways that are at odds with his stated aims, such as acting against his financial interests.

Weak Self-Knowledge: Dominating concept of the past and feared future

Lack of values clarity

Persistent inaction, impulsivity or avoidance

Raj impulsively gambles and quits jobs. He avoids getting close to others in order to avoid being hurt by them.

Paranoia and blaming others allow Raj to avoid low self-esteem. His suspicion also helps him avoid disappointment in others. Grandiosity allows him to avoid thinking about his financial difficulties or comparing himself to his father.

Experiential avoidance

Cognitive fusion

Attachment to the conceptualised self

Raj has the delusional belief that it is 'inevitable' that he will be wealthy. He repeats this theme throughout treatment. He is attached to the idea of being different from his father.

Raj believes that others – including treatment providers – want him to fail. He is fused with the belief that wealth will solve all of his problems, and fused beliefs about the inevitability of his future wealth are part of his conceptualised self.

Figure 5.1 An ACT model of psychopathology (adapted from Hayes *et al.*, 2006)

Symptoms of psychosis and target behaviours common in people with psychotic disorders can be conceptualised in an ACT-consistent manner using such a model. Consider the case of Raj. Raj was a 27-year-old Indian immigrant who left Mumbai with his family when he was six years old. He dropped out of college and travelled across the country at the age of 20, cutting off all contact with his family. He was first hospitalised at age 24 after he threatened to kill himself by jumping off a building following a confrontation with a casino manager. He was unemployed, homeless, earned money by begging, and at the time of his hospitalisation he hadn't eaten in 2 days. He denied delusions and hallucinations, though both paranoia and grandiosity were evident. He was assigned a diagnosis of paranoid schizophrenia.

Raj began treatment, including medication, participation in skills training groups and ACT therapy, while in the hospital, and continued treatment as an outpatient. The ACT model was useful in developing a treatment plan for Raj. Formulation of his case will be considered in order to illustrate ACT case conceptualisation using the ACT model of psychopathology and is illustrated in Figure 5.1.

5.2.1   Avoidance

Experiential avoidance occurs when one attempts to avoid unwanted inner experience, or private events, such as thoughts, feelings and sensations. Avoidance often fails, and can even increases unwanted private events. For instance, trying to suppress a thought may work in the very short term, but has been shown to be followed by an increase in the suppressed thought (Wegner *et al.*, 1987). Even when avoidance appears successful, there is often a cost in diminished vitality and life opportunities, such as when a person with panic disorder or paranoid thoughts avoids leaving their home. Attempts to avoid private events can also lead to more and bigger problems, as when an individual uses alcohol to avoid sad feelings or auditory hallucinations, or leaves a job or relationship in order to avoid anxiety. During case formulation the clinician should note when the client engages in experiential avoidance.

In Raj's case, it was clear that his paranoia and grandiosity allowed him to avoid confronting his rather dire circumstances, to blame others for his perceived failures and to avoid comparing himself to his father. For instance, he viewed his homelessness as 'a lifestyle choice' that would allow him to save money in order to start up a business that would surely make him a millionaire. His lack of business success was attributed to unnamed others who wanted him to fail. When he did accumulate any money, he usually went to a casino in the hopes of making more, only to leave with nothing. He was most afraid of 'being poor like my mother and father'. Raj's behaviour nicely illustrates the ACT slogan that 'if you aren't willing to have it, you've got it' (Hayes *et al.*, 1999, p. 122). That is, Raj's attempts to avoid being poor involved him in homelessness and begging! He quit jobs because they didn't pay enough, and gave up an apartment so he could save the rent money 'for bigger and better things'. He gambled away the little money he did save, then railed against the 'cheating casinos' and 'people that want to see me fail like my father'. Recent research suggests that symptoms of paranoia may have the function of avoiding low self-esteem even while paradoxically serving to increase it (Udachina *et al.*, 2009). Raj's grandiose dreams of future wealth also allowed him to avoid confronting fears about his precarious financial situation.

5.2.2   Cognitive Fusion

When behaviour is influenced more by thoughts than by actual experience and evaluations, and beliefs such as 'I am bad' or 'I will certainly fail' are regarded as if they correspond with literal truth, a person is said to be fused with their thoughts. Fusion can affect a person's mood and behaviour, for instance making them feel afraid and stay home from work when they have the thought, 'They are out to get me'. Fusion is often related to avoidance when an individual tries to avoid an unwanted thought they are fused with. In contrast, an individual who can defuse from a thought might simply notice that thought when going about their planned activities. It matters little whether we regard the thought as a 'true' thought, an irrational belief or a delusion: it is one's relationship to the thought rather than its content that is targeted in ACT. In the case of symptoms of psychosis, hallucinatory and delusional content is targeted in ACT by altering how the client relates to it, rather than by trying to eliminate it or replace it with 'more accurate' content.

Raj was fused with thoughts that others wanted him to fail. These thoughts led him to behave inappropriately in many situations, such as when he confronted employers or casino workers. In the context of treatment, he was mistrustful of most treatment providers. He was also fused with the thought that wealth was the solution to all of his problems and that it was inevitable that he would be wealthy. While Raj's fused thoughts became apparent during his initial evaluation, fusion is a common verbal process that a clinician might observe at any phase of treatment.

5.2.3   Attachment to Content

The conceptualised self consists of all the verbal content an individual might use to describe and evaluate themselves (Hayes *et al.*, 1999). Much verbal content is benign, and even useful. For instance, 'My name is Raj and I was born in India' is content. 'I enjoy football' is content. 'I am good at math' and 'I feel anxious' are more content. A conceptualised self allows us to interact in a verbal social community. However, when an individual rigidly holds descriptions and evaluations that increase their suffering, or that lead to ineffective behaviour, they may be attached to their verbal content. When content is rigidly held, rather than being useful it becomes problematic.

Raj was also rigidly fused with the notion that it was 'bad' to be like his father, and avoided both his father (by leaving home) and taking responsibility for any action that might be associated with a comparison with his father. A conceptualised self depends on perspective-taking skills; that is, the ability to interact with the self in relation to others, 'here' in relation to 'there', and with the present in relation to the past and future. People with schizophrenia appear to have more limited perspective-taking skill than is normal (Vilatte, *et al.*, 2010), and Raj showed limited perspective-taking in his very limited conceptualised self: beyond rather vague descriptions, he had little to say about himself that was unrelated to delusional content or fused thoughts.

5.2.4   Weak Self-knowledge, Dominating Concept of the Past or Feared Future

The ability to know and describe one's self is useful when self-descriptions are not held to rigidly. Weak self-knowledge shows up when an individual can say very little about themselves or when the conceptualised self is dominated by one or a few notions of the self (e.g. 'I am a failure' or 'I lost my job'). Weak self-knowledge may manifest as a general lack of verbal content pertaining to the self and little sense of direction and purposeful goal setting. These processes may be especially evident in negative symptoms of schizophrenia (Bach, 2007). Like his self-descriptions, Raj's goals were vague and did little to contribute to purposeful actions.

Clients may also be out of touch with the present moment when they are fused with the verbally constructed past or future. Raj tended to lack contact with the present moment. Though Raj was very bright, quite good looking and had many skills, he seemed unaware of or unmoved by this, with a narrow focus on being wealthy 'some day'. His speech was always about the imagined future – whether visions of wealth or of the unnamed others preventing his success. He was also embroiled in the past, and the fear he would end up like his unsuccessful father. Raj's fears of being poor or 'like his father' in the future led to bad choices in the present, such as quitting jobs and gambling. Raj also failed to connect with others in the present because he was focused on paranoid and grandiose content that was neither 'here' nor 'now'.

5.2.5   Lack of Values Clarity

In case formulation it is helpful to enquire about client goals and values. Clients who are unclear about their values are likely to behave ineffectively and/or have little sense of purpose and direction in their lives. Identifying values is important to both case formulation and treatment planning, because values can be useful in building willingness for treatment, and behaviour change in the service of valued action is a key part of most treatments (Bach & Moran, 2008). The primary value Raj reported was becoming wealthy, which he elaborated upon with notions of wealth being associated with his being important and unlike his father. He did not know how he might become wealthy or what he would do with the money once he earned it. Given his lack of values clarity, he did not carry out many activities beyond those that met his immediate physical needs, or which he perceived would gain him money quickly.

Values may also be problematic when they are excessively aimed at experiential avoidance and / or at pleasing others at the expense of other valued outcomes. Like many people with prominent negative symptoms, Raj showed little interest in pleasing others. He did however show much avoidance in his values statements, such as wanting to avoid anxiety by avoiding others whom he feared might harm him and focusing on the future at the expense of the present moment, such as when he abruptly quit jobs. Even his professed value of accumulating wealth appeared more in the service of avoiding comparison with his father rather than being associated with a real interest in wealth itself.

A lack of awareness of the consequences of one's behaviour can lead to problems with valued action, in that an individual may take actions that are inconsistent with their values or which otherwise fail to move them in the direction of their values. Raj clearly articulated a value of accumulating wealth, yet he behaved in a manner inconsistent with this when he quit his jobs or lost his money gambling.

5.2.6   Persistent Inaction, Impulsivity or Avoidance

This domain usually includes the most obvious problems a client presents with, such as substance abuse, compulsions, staying in bed, responding to hallucinations or delusions and medication nonadherence. Ideally, committed actions move people in the direction of their values. Inaction, impulsivity and avoidance are associated with more limited values-directed actions; that is, with rigid and inflexible behavioural repertoires. Raj showed behaviour aimed at avoiding paranoid content. He impulsively gambled and quit jobs. In other ways he was very inactive, in that he was unable to describe a recent history of behaviour aimed at anything other than meeting his most basic needs. His description was of a rather empty life devoid of all but the most superficial human relationships, and limited primarily to activities aimed at avoiding feared persecution or (mostly ineffective strategies for) making money.

The overall ACT case formulation for Raj was that he was fused with paranoid and grandiose thoughts. He avoided or quit activities that made him feel like a failure. He had weak self-knowledge and a limited sense of direction in his life. These features led to inaction on many behavioural fronts and to making impulsive choices with respect to work and gambling behaviour. Raj's treatment focused on skills training, so that he might develop his social, vocational and independent living skills, and on therapy, so that he could improve his contact with the present moment, clarify his values and commit to actions that better served his interests. Raj made steady progress, and after 2 years he was employed and contemplating going back to college; he was living in his own apartment; and he had reconnected with one of his sisters. Towards the end of treatment, for the first time ever, Raj expressed interest in friendships and romantic relationships.

5.3 Case Formulation using the Inflexahex Model

While Raj's case provides a detailed description of the ACT model of psychopathology, the case of Sarah will be used to illustrate the process of case formulation using the inflexahex model. Sarah was a 32-year-old woman with a diagnosis of schizoaffective disorder. She was referred to a day-treatment pro-gramme after she was briefly hospitalised following a transition in her living arrangement from a group home to a shared apartment. Sarah had stopped taking her medications, which exacerbated her auditory hallucinations. She was depressed and reported that while she enjoyed 'being more independent', she was bored and lonely in her new home.

While Bach (2005) has recommended that case conceptualisation might begin with values clarification when clients show little treatment motivation, Sarah was highly motivated for treatment, so her case formulation began with acceptance/ avoidance. Sarah reported that 'the voices are louder' when she was alone, so she would spend much of her time at the apartment complex seeking out two on-site social workers. She did not inform them of her distress because she 'didn't want to be a bother' and instead engaged them in idle conversation, which led them to minimise her problems and focus their attention on seemingly more needy clients. Sarah felt rejected and would return to her room and cry. She would often decide not to take her medication so that she might 'get worse and be sent back to the group home'. At the same time, Sarah 'wanted to be living like a real grown up and even have a job' and was reluctant to risk failure. Sarah appeared to be both avoiding her symptoms and avoiding fear of failure. Avoidance of symptoms led her to seek help excessively and avoidance of perceived failure led her to minimise her symptoms so that she did not appear to be seeking help. Symptom underre-porting, because of its negative treatment implications, is common in people with psychotic disorders (Waters, 2010) and can have disastrous consequences. Bach & Hayes (2002) found that reporting symptoms of psychosis was more common in inpatients who received treatment with ACT, who stayed out of the hospital longer than those who persisted in denying symptoms.

Sarah's self-report also led the clinician to probe for signs of cognitive fusion. She was asked about thoughts she wished to avoid, or which troubled her, includ-ing auditory hallucinations. She reported that 'the voices tell me I'm a bad person and I can't bear it', suggesting fusion with thought content. She was also fused with thoughts that others did not like her, that she would not make friends in her new home and that she would ultimately fail to attain what she wanted. She acknowledged that she felt ambivalent at times about leaving the group home and that she feared that these thoughts, rather than being a fairly normal part of making a transition, meant that she wanted to return to the group home and would ultimately fail at her opportunity to live more independently.

Sarah's expression of fears about the future led the clinician to further explore her sense of self and her orientation to the present moment. Sarah reported that she had 'a hard time being in the here and now because that's when I feel lonely and the voices start up'. When she thought about the future, she felt afraid, seeing only visions of failure. Sarah was able to describe several interests, including her relationship with her family, friendships, animals, going for walks and eating ice cream. While she liked other people, she was not sure that they liked her. She may have had underdeveloped perspective-taking or theory-of-mind skills that impaired her ability to understand what others were thinking (Corcoran, 2001). Her orientation to the future rather than the present moment led her to feel ungrounded and fearful.

Values clarification was easier with Sarah than with some clients with schizophrenia-spectrum disorders, because she was able to articulate some goals and interests. Though her values were not clearly articulated, Bach (2005) has suggested that questions about goals can lead to identification of values. For instance, it was clear that Sarah wanted to live independently; when probed further about this goal, she responded that she wanted to be self-sufficient and not to be a financial burden. Her response here led to questions about her vocational goals. She initially reported a goal of becoming a veterinarian. This appeared rather unrealistic given her limited educational background, but further questioning led her to express a value of 'caring for animals'. She also described valuing her friendships, taking care of her health and 'being a good sister and daughter' to her family.

In the domain of committed action, Sarah reported that 'I have failed. I don't have a job and I was just hospitalised.' While she did not note it, Sarah agreed when the clinician pointed out that she did not appear to seek social support when she was distressed, even while she valued friends and family. She also acknowledged that when she felt overwhelmed she tended to 'give up and stop taking medication'.

This case formulation allowed for a treatment plan that included ACT and participation in skills-training groups. In ACT, Sarah learned to defuse from thoughts of failure and to relate to her voices differently. When more defused, she was less likely to engage in avoidant behaviours. Mindfulness training facilitated defusion and she found that when she was less focused on the future she was more able to engage in goal-directed actions. Values-clarification work combined with skills training led her to set vocational goals and to work on developing her social skills. Sarah participated in skills-training groups on social skills, coping with symptoms, independent-living skills and vocational skills. In time, Sarah obtained first a volunteer position and then a paying job at an animal shelter. She was able to better cope with her voices because she was more defused, and when distressed she was able to seek appropriate social support from friends and staff. This ultimately successful treatment plan was developed directly from the ACT case formulation.

Sarah's experience illustrates both the functional nature of ACT and its orientation towards capitalising on strengths through values clarification. The functional nature of ACT is what most distinguishes it from many other cognitive-behavioural approaches to psychotherapy for psychosis. The ultimate aim of ACT is to increase psychological flexibility. With this aim, it is important to understand how avoidance, fusion and other processes limit the behavioural repertoire of the client. Thus, it is more important to understand how the individual's behaviours and symptoms function in their environment than to merely note the presence or absence of symptoms (Bach & Moran, 2008). This is in contrast to approaches that emphasise changing the content of symptoms such as hallucinations, which are not always effective (Tarrier & Wykes, 2004). In ACT there is no aim of reducing symptoms; nor is there an assumption that the presence of symptoms *per se* is problematic. Individuals such as Raj and Sarah can function in the presence of symptoms if they can learn to relate differently to them.

Cognitive reappraisal is a common technique in many cognitive approaches to psychotherapy for psychosis (Kuipers *et al.*, 2006). Defusion differs somewhat from reappraisal, though both approaches may have the shared outcome of reducing the believability of thoughts. The primary distinction is that defusion techniques aim to alter how one relates to private events: to make one see thoughts as thoughts and not as events that should be taken literally. Reappraisal techniques, in contrast, aim to alter the *content* rather than the *function* of thoughts. Bach *et al.* (in press) have suggested that one might contrast reappraisal and defusion thus: the aim of reappraisal is to decrease the believability of problematic thoughts, while the aim of defusion is to decrease the believability of all thoughts.

Because defusion leads to reduced believability of thoughts, the client may be less inclined to engage in avoidance behaviours. For instance, the client who is troubled by the content of hallucinations may be less likely to act out impulsively in order to reduce them if they can see hallucinations as mere verbal content rather than as statements to be taken as literally true.

As the publication of this volume attests, work on contact with the present moment has recently gained traction as a viable approach to the treatment of psychosis. Contact with the present moment and defusion are intertwined, as one can only defuse in the present moment. Identifying where the client is fused with thoughts about the past and future can facilitate work on both defusion and mindfulness.

The conceptualised self is also related to fusion and contact with the present moment. Many clients with psychotic disorders have limited and negative self-conceptualisations. This may be due to deficits in perspective-taking skill (Vilatte *et al.*, 2010) and/or an effect of institutionalisation (Bach, 2005). In ACT case formulation, the clinician must take care to note both where the client has a deficient sense of self and where the client is fused with negative or delusional content about the self. For instance, Raj had a limited conceptualised self in that he had very little self-description or interests, and the content that was apparent was largely delusional. Defusion, values clarification and committed action can aid in work on the conceptualised self.

The committed action domain of ACT is where important treatment outcomes can most often be found. Bach & Hayes (2002) and Gaudiano & Herbert (2006) used days to rehospitalisation as the primary outcome measure and found that those treated with ACT were far less likely than treatment-as-usual (TAU) controls to be rehospitalised at follow-up ranging from 4 months to 1 year. Hospitalisation accounts for one of the greatest financial costs of schizophrenia to society (Knapp, 2005). It is also costly to the individual, because the hospitalised individual is most likely removed from opportunities to engage in valued action. Medication adherence is similar and may also be a committed action for many people with psychotic disorders. While medication nonadherence is common in people with psychotic disorders (Bellack, 2006) and its improvement is a common treatment outcome goal, failure to take medication is a common reason for rehospitalisation. The emphasis in ACT on values clarification provides an incentive for improved medication adherence. Only a functional account of behaviour can provide the therapist with an understanding of why the client may fail to take medication as prescribed and, more importantly, provide the client with reasons to adhere to treatment. That is, when taking medication is linked to valued goals and outcomes, it may become more important to take it. Individualised treatment outcomes will vary as much as individuals themselves, and the outcomes will tend to be behavioural; for example, get a job, smoke less, attend a social-skills training group, attend meetings with the case manager, improve hygiene and grooming, get out of the house more and soon. The exact nature of the outcomes or committed actions is less important than that they are clearly linked to client values.

5.4   Conclusion

It should be clear that the core processes involved in both the ACT model of psychopathology and the ACT model of treatment are intertwined. While it is useful to talk about them separately, ultimately behaviour linked to any one process is likely to be linked to other processes as well. As treatment unfolds, it is likely that the initial case formulation will be modified and elaborated upon. However, a thorough initial case formulation made with regard to the core ACT processes and the ACT model of psychopathology will enhance the clinician's ability to develop a treatment plan that can, if followed, increase the psychological flexibility and vitality of even the most severely ill.

References

Bach, P. (2005). ACT with the seriously mentally ill. In S. C. Hayes & K. Strosahl (es). *Acceptance and Commitment Therapy: A Practical Guide*. New York: Plenum Press.

Bach, P. (2007). Psychotic disorders. In D. W. Woods & J. Kanter (eds). *Understanding Behavior Disorders: A Contemporary Behavioral Perspective*. Reno: Context Press.

Bach, P. A. & Hayes, S. C. (2002). The use of Acceptance and Commitment Therapy to prevent the rehospitalization of psychotic patients: a randomized controlled trial. *Journal of Consulting and Clinical Psychology*, 70, 1129–1139.

Bach, P. A. & Moran, D. J. (2008). ACT in Practice: Case Conceptualization in Acceptance and Commitment Therapy. Oakland: New Harbinger.

Bach, P., Hayes, S. C. & Gallop, R. (2012). Long term effects of brief Acceptance and Commitment Therapy for psychosis. *Behavior Modification*, 36, 167–183.

Bach, P., Gaudiano, B. A., Hayes, S. C. & Herbert, J. D. (in press). Acceptance and Commitment Therapy for psychosis: intent to treat, hospitalization outcome, and mediation by symptom believability. *Psychosis: Psychological, Social, and Integrative Approaches*. doi: 10.1080/17522439.2012.671349.

Bellack, A. S. (2006). Scientific and consumer models of recovery in schizophrenia: concordance, contrasts, and implications. *Schizophrenia Bulletin*, 32, 432–442.

Corcoran, R. (2001). Theory of mind in schizophrenia. In D. Penn & P. Corrigan (eds). Social cognition in schizophrenia. Washington, DC: American Psychiatric Association, pp. 149–174.

Gaudiano, B. A. & Herbert, J. D. (2006). Acute treatment of inpatients with psychotic symptoms using acceptance and commitment therapy: pilot results. *Behaviour Research and Therapy*, 44, 415–437.

Hayes, S. C., Luoma, J., Bond, F., Masuda, A. & Lillis, J. (2006). Acceptance and Commitment Therapy: model, processes, and outcomes. *Behaviour Research and Therapy*, 44, 1–25.

Hayes, S. C., Strosahl, K. D. & Wilson, K. G. (1999). *Acceptance and Commitment Therapy: An Experiential Approach to Behavior Change*. New York: Guilford Press.

Knapp, M. (2005). Costs of schizophrenia. *Psychiatry*, 4, 33–35.

Kuipers, E., Garety, P., Fowler, D., Freeman, D., Dunn, G. & Bebbington, P. (2006). Cognitive, emotional, and social processes in psychosis: refining cognitive behavioral therapy for persistent positive symptoms. *Schizophrenia Bulletin*, 32, S24–S31.

Shawyer, F., Ratcliff, K., Mackinnon, A., Farhall, J., Hayes, S.C. & Copolov, D. (2007). The Voices Acceptance and Action Scale: pilot data. *Journal of Clinical Psychology*, 63, 593–606.

Tarrier, N. & Wykes, T. (2004). Is there evidence that cognitive behaviour therapy is an effective treatment for schizophrenia? A cautious or cautionary tale? *Behaviour Research and Therapy*, 42, 1377–1401.

Udachina, A., Thewissen, V., Myin-Germeys, I., Fitzpatrick, S., O'Kane, A. & Bentall, R. P. (2009). Understanding the relationships between self-esteem, experiential avoidance, and paranoia: structural equation modeling and experience sampling studies. *Journal of Nervous and Mental Disease*, 197, 661–668.

Villatte, M., Monestes, J. L., McHugh, L., Esteve, F. B. & Loas, G. (2010). Adopting the perspective of another in belief attribution: contribution of Relational Frame

Theory to the understanding of impairments in schizophrenia. *Journal of Behavior Therapy and Experimental Psychiatry*, 41, 125–134.

Waters, F. (2010). Auditory hallucinations in psychiatric illness. *Psychiatric Times*, 27, 54–58.

Wegner, D. M., Schneider, D. J., Carter, S. R. & White, T. L. (1987). Paradoxical effects of thought suppression. *Journal of Personality and Social Psychology*, 53(1), 5–13.

6

Engaging People with Psychosis in Acceptance and Commitment Therapy and Mindfulness

Brandon A. Gaudiano and Andrew M. Busch

6.1 Introduction

Treating patients with psychotic disorders such as schizophrenia is a challenging endeavour for many therapists. Even though practice guidelines recommend the provision of adjunctive psychosocial interventions in the treatment of psychosis (Dixon *et al.*, 2010; National Institute for Health and Clinical Excellence, 2009), most patients are not being offered such interventions (Moran, 2003). Part of the problem is that many therapists are intimidated by the prospect of treating severe mental illness and have not obtained the training or experience required to deliver newer psychosis interventions (Berry & Haddock, 2008). Furthermore, patients with psychosis can be more difficult to engage and retain in therapy, and treatment nonadherence is a frequent clinical problem that requires attention (Kreyenbuhl *et al.*, 2009). In this chapter, we will examine issues related to engagement in treatment and present techniques and strategies designed to improve the implementation of acceptance/mindfulness interventions for psychosis.

6.1.1 Treatment Adherence and Engagement in Psychosis

Treatment adherence is defined as 'The extent to which a person's behaviour – taking medication, following a diet, and/or executing lifestyle changes, corresponds with agreed recommendations from a healthcare provider' (World Health

Acceptance and Commitment Therapy and Mindfulness for Psychosis, First Edition.
Edited by Eric M. J. Morris, Louise C. Johns and Joseph E. Oliver.
© *2013 John Wiley & Sons, Ltd. Published 2013 by John Wiley & Sons, Ltd.*

Organization, 2003). Nonadherence is a frequent problem in patients with psychotic disorders, with research indicating that approximately 50% of patients with schizophrenia are nonadherent to medications (Lacro *et al.*, 2002). Abrupt medication discontinuation is associated with a three-times increased risk for relapse in schizophrenia (Weiden *et al.*, 2004). Furthermore, behavioural nonadherence is equally problematic and includes attendance at scheduled appointments and the implementation of recommended lifestyle changes (e.g. diet/exercise plans, behavioural strategies, social activities) (Colom *et al.*, 2005). Studies in samples with severe mental illness demonstrate high rates of community treatment attrition (Bergen *et al.*, 1998; Kreyenbuhl *et al.*, 2009; Nuttbrock *et al.*, 1997).

Furthermore, it can be difficult to engage patients with psychosis in psychosocial treatments because the neuroleptic medications prescribed for these conditions provide benefits in some areas (reducing positive symptoms) at the cost of drawbacks in others (oversedation, muscle rigidity, memory impairment) (Moncrieff *et al.*, 2009; Reilly *et al.*, 2006). The negative symptoms (avolition, blunted affect, anhedonia, alogia) commonly associated with psychotic disorders can inhibit efforts at behaviour change, and the effects of neuroleptics on the brain may further contribute to these symptoms by impairing cognitive functioning and decreasing motivation and interest (Artaloytia *et al.*, 2006; Ho *et al.*, 2011). In addition, abrupt discontinuation from neuroleptics can produce impairing withdrawal symptoms and rebound psychosis, which dramatically increase the risk for relapse (Chouinard & Chouinard, 2008; Margolese *et al.*, 2002; Moncrieff, 2006). Thus, therapists treating patients with psychosis must deal with multiple challenges, including behavioural and medication nonadherence, negative symptoms and the disadvantages of concurrent pharmacological treatment, all of which may make behaviour change more difficult to achieve.

6.2   Acceptance and Commitment Therapy

Acceptance and commitment therapy (ACT) (Hayes *et al.*, 2012) has demonstrated efficacy in three randomised trials for treating patients with psychosis, two with inpatients (Bach & Hayes, 2002; Gaudiano & Herbert, 2006) and one with outpatients (White *et al.*, 2011). For example, Gaudiano & Herbert (2006) conducted a randomised trial testing a brief ACT intervention for inpatients with psychosis. A total of 40 inpatients with current psychotic symptoms (58% with a primary psychotic disorder such as schizophrenia) were randomly assigned to treatment as usual (TAU) alone or TAU augmented by individual sessions of ACT. The number of sessions received varied based on the patient's length of stay, with an average of three. Patients found the treatment acceptable, and one patient withdrew from each condition during hospitalisation. Intent-to-treat analyses demonstrated that ACT produced significant advantages over TAU alone at discharge in terms of self-rated distress about psychotic symptoms, interviewer-rated mood symptoms, self-rated social disability related to illness and clinically significant improvement in symptoms (50 versus 7%). The ACT group demonstrated a significantly longer time to rehospitalisation (based on insurance records) over a 4-month follow-up period after controlling for baseline severity compared with TAU (Bach *et al.*, in press). Consistent with the proposed mechanisms of ACT, improvements in the believability of psychotic symptoms statistically mediated the effects of treatment condition on distress related to psychotic symptoms at discharge (Gaudiano *et al.*, 2010) and rehospitalisation rates at 4-month follow-up (Bach *et al.*, in press).

Hayes *et al.* (2011) have proposed several distinctive elements of contextual approaches such as ACT compared with traditional cognitive and behavioural approaches, including a focus on the function more than the content of psychological events, the use of similar principles and techniques across diagnostic groups, an emphasis on improving functioning and quality of life rather than symptom elimination alone, relevance and application to the clinician's behaviour and not just the patient's, and an interest in addressing more complex problems, including values, relationships and existential issues. These characteristics may be particularly useful for engaging and retaining patients in treatment (Bach, 2004; Levitt & Karekla, 2005). ACT emphasises acceptance rather than change of internal events while pursing goals, focuses on the process of change rather than the outcomes achieved and places behaviour change efforts in the service of the patient's deeply held values, all of which can increase motivation and promote persistence in the face of challenges and setbacks.

There is emerging evidence that acceptance-related processes and strategies can improve persistence in distressing behavioural tasks and promote treatment adherence. Tait *et al.* (2003) found that a 'sealing-over' or avoidant post-psychosis recovery style predicted decreased service engagement at 6-month follow-up beyond the effects of insight or symptoms. In addition, experimental studies demonstrate that values and acceptance interventions consistent with ACT improve distress tolerance related to anxiety and pain (Branstetter-Rost *et al.*, 2009; Levitt *et al.*, 2004; Marcks & Woods, 2007; Masedo & Rosa Esteve, 2007; McMullen *et al.*, 2008; Paez-Blarrina *et al.*, 2008). A recent randomised trial of individuals in an inpatient substance-use programme demonstrated that those assigned to a brief ACT intervention demonstrated higher rates of treatment attendance and more days abstinent following discharge compared to those receiving TAU (Luoma *et al.*, 2011). In addition, White *et al.* (2011) conducted a randomised trial in outpatients of the treatment of emotional dysfunction following a psychotic episode and found lower rates of attrition and greater improvements in mood symptoms in ACT compared with TAU.

6.3   Functional Analytic Psychotherapy

Functional analytic psychotherapy (FAP) (Kohlenberg & Tsai, 1991; Tsai *et al.*, 2009) is another third-wave behavioural treatment of relevance to the engagement of patients with psychosis in psychotherapy. FAP assumes that out-of-session client problems (e.g. paranoid behaviour in interpersonal relationships) will manifest themselves in the therapeutic relationship (e.g. paranoid behaviour in session) and that the therapist can shape this behaviour '*in vivo*', meaning live, in session. Out-of-session problems that manifest during the therapy session are referred to as CRB1s ('clinically relevant behaviours') and in-session improvements in these problems are referred to as CRB2s. Using a functional case conceptualisation, the FAP therapist will be mindful of CRBs and will purposefully elicit them. This provides the therapist the opportunity to contingently respond to them as they occur. Specifically, CRB2s are followed by natural positive reinforcement, although the therapist may exaggerate a natural response. CRB1s are extinguished, (mildly) punished or blocked, after which the therapist will attempt to elicit a CRB2. Over the course of treatment, a decrease in CRB1s should occur, as they are shaped into increasingly skilled CRB2s. These skills shaped in session can then be assigned as out-of-session homework (interacting with with peers in a nonparanoid manner). In order for this process to unfold, the therapist must first establish him or herself as a potent social reinforcer.

FAP and ACT have been compared and contrasted in detail elsewhere (Kohlenberg & Callaghan, 2010). The treatments are theoretically consistent, but there are differences in emphasis (i.e. FAP focuses on interpersonal processes whereas ACT focuses on intrapersonal processes); thus integration may be particularly fruitful. Several authors have provided guidance on how to combine ACT and FAP techniques (Baruch *et al.*, 2009; Callaghan *et al.*, 2004; Kohlenberg & Callaghan, 2010) and recent FAP texts have more clearly integrated mindfulness, acceptance and valuing into a FAP context (Tsai *et al.*, 2009). Further, a large randomised trial of smoking cessation has demonstrated the efficacy of an integrated ACT and FAP treatment (Gifford *et al.*, 2011).

6.4   Acceptance-based Methods and Techniques for Improving Engagement

Several components of ACT and FAP are particularly relevant when it comes to promoting treatment engagement and adherence: using workability as a guide to coping, placing goals in the service of the patient's deeply held values, bringing acceptance and nonjudgmental awareness to distressing experiences, promoting committed action and utilising the therapeutic relationship. In this section, we review each of these components in turn, focusing on how they can be used to promote treatment engagement and how they can be delivered in ways that make them more acceptable and understandable to patients with psychosis (Table 6.1).

Table 6.1 Methods for promoting engagement and adherence with treatment

Component	Description	Techniques and methods
Workability	• Review past attempts to cope unsuccessfully with symptoms, especially those related to excessive struggle/avoidance and nonadherence • Emphasise 'workability' when choosing coping strategies and encourage exploration of new approaches such as acceptance • Explore the workability of taking medications and attending appointments	• Chinese fingercuffs exercise • Person-in-the-hole metaphor
Valuing	• Explore client's deeply held values and examine the distress associated with actions that are inconsistent with these values • Examine values in relation to adherence/nonadherence behaviours • Place treatment in the service of specific values	• Compass metaphor • Skiing metaphor • Valued Living Questionnaire
Acceptance and mindfulness	• Increase willingness to experience unwanted private events and persistence in the face of adversity in the service of chosen values • Practise bringing nonjudgmental awareness in the present moment to nonadherence beliefs, instead of evaluating them as true or false • Apply this to medication side effects and lack of motivation as well	• Leaves-on-the-stream exercise • Tug-of-war-with-the-monster metaphor
Committed action	• Develop a behavioural activation plan • Focus on engagement in the process as the goal, instead of a specific outcome • Emphasise patient choice in changing behaviours	• Break complex goals into manageable steps that can be started in session • Provide support for client's completion of steps • Replace avoidance with acceptance-based coping responses • Use failed assignments as illustrations of experiential avoidance
Therapist factors	• Model acceptance • Shape client's behaviour '*in vivo*'	• Show acceptance of client's and your own content in actions and discussion • Reinforce client acceptance that occurs during session • Reinforce improvements in client's interpersonal behaviour in session

6.4.1   Workability

Often, patients with psychosis excessively struggle with or attempt to avoid their experiences, which can paradoxically lead to more persistent symptoms and increased distress and impairment (Farhall *et al.*, 2007; Romme & Escher, 1993; Shawyer *et al.*, 2007; Tait *et al.*, 2003). Instead of reinforcing counterproductive attempts to control internal experiences, the ACT therapist emphasises 'workability' as a guide to how to choose responses to psychosis or other symptoms. The emphasis is not on whether or not patients' coping attempts are 'right' or 'wrong', but whether they are helpful in achieving their goals. Workability can be applied to nonadherence behaviours (e.g. refusal to take medications or failure to attend treatment sessions), which can be conceptualised as further maladaptive attempts to avoid or control distress. Use of Chinese fingercuffs, a simple children's toy, is one method by which to highlight problems with a reliance on avoidant coping (Hayes *et al.*, 2012). A patient will quickly learn that when she tries to pull her index fingers out of the paper fingercuffs, the device only further tightens its grip. The therapist can draw parallels between this experience and the patient's history of attempting to escape or avoid the aspects of treatment that she finds difficult, such as dealing with medication side effects or lacking motivation to attend appointments.

In addition, the person-in-the-hole metaphor (see Appendix D) is a useful story by which to demonstrate the unworkability of a patient's control strategies (Hayes *et al.*, 2012). In this scenario, the patient is asked to imagine herself blindfolded and using a shovel in an attempt to 'dig out' of the hole she has fallen into, simply because she has no other tool to use. The therapist encourages the patient to consider putting down the shovel and exploring other ways of escaping the hole that she may have missed. Examination of unsuccessful past coping attempts and a focus on workability when exploring new strategies fosters creativity and hope that a different way is possible, setting the stage for the development of more functional responses to symptoms.

6.4.2   Values Clarification

Exploration of the (un)workability of a patient's coping attempts leads to the question of what the patient is actually working to achieve. In ACT, values are described as what gives a person's life meaning and purpose (Wilson & Murrell, 2004). The therapist starts by exploring values that may be relevant to the patient (e.g. family, romantic relationships, work, health). If a patient has difficulty generating ideas, the therapist can suggest some based on the values that implicitly showed up during the discussion of past coping attempts. To keep the values discussion from becoming too abstract or unfocused, the therapist can ask the patient to complete the Valued Living Questionnaire (VLQ) (Wilson *et al.*, 2010), which records ratings of perceived importance and behavioural consistency across 10 commonly valued domains. Discrepancies between a person's valued area and her daily actions are highlighted, along with the distress this tends to cause. The therapist suggests that being more consistent with values can lead to a more fulfilling and healthy life. Specific behavioural goals consistent with these values are then elicited and a plan for implementing them after the session is developed. In addition, the therapist can use a real compass as a model to explain the idea of values as an individual's personal life guide, which helps to determine the direction to move in when things are uncertain. Many of the goals associated with values can be difficult to achieve or require patience on the part of the patient (e.g. reconnecting with an estranged son or daughter). The skiing metaphor (see Appendix G) is a useful story by which to highlight how the ongoing process of working towards values is important and meaningful in and of itself, regardless of the specific outcome obtained (Hayes *et al.*, 2012).

Several characteristics of values clarification make it relevant for engaging patients in treatment. The focus on the process of 'valuing' in one's actions, instead of achieving a particular and narrow outcome, can help patients persist when making positive behavioural changes, even if they are not immediately rewarded for doing so. For example, starting a new medication involves a time of increased side effects, which can lead to premature termination. If taking medication is placed in the service of an important value (e.g. getting back to work), the patient will be better able to tolerate any discomfort. Also, the emphasis on choice when identifying and defining values places the motivation within the patient instead of some external source. Highlighting choice also strengthens the patient's commitment to change.

6.4.3   Acceptance and Mindfulness

Implementing values-consistent actions can be challenging for patients because of the emotional reactions that this process can evoke. Various experiential exercises are conducted to help patients work on ACT concepts in the present moment with the help of the therapist. For example, the experience of mindfulness can be introduced using various meditation practices. To make mindfulness exercises more tolerable for patients with psychosis, they can be limited to 5 minutes' duration at first. In one form of meditation practice, patients are instructed to visualise leaves falling into a stream (Hayes *et al.*, 2012) (see Appendix B). They are told to place any thoughts, feelings or symptoms (hallucinations and delusions) that arise on these leaves and watch them flow down the stream without trying to control them. Other activities can be substituted for patients who have difficulty concentrating, including mindful eating or walking exercises (Kabat-Zinn, 1994). At first, patients often struggle and have difficulty letting go of their internal experiences when attempting to place them on their mental 'leaves'. The therapist emphasises that the aim of the exercise is not to produce any particular outcome (e.g. to achieve relaxation or have less thoughts) and that simply doing the exercise itself is the 'success'. In addition, there are numerous metaphors and stories that also communicate these concepts. For example, in the tug-of-war metaphor (see Appendix H) the patient is asked to imagine being in a tug-of-war with a monster, with a bottomless abyss separating them (Hayes *et al.*, 2012). The option of dropping the rope is explored, and represents the idea of acceptance as an alternative to continued struggle with symptoms. The patient is encouraged to practise 'dropping the rope' in order to cope with troublesome experiences such as voices in between sessions.

Acceptance and mindfulness exercises build patients' resilience and provide skills to promote persistence even in the face of increased distress or discomfort during goal-directed activities. However, it is important to simplify acceptance and mindfulness exercises for patients with psychosis so that they are more understandable and easier to practise, including limiting the duration of practice or making it more concrete (e.g. mindful eating or walking). The practice of bringing nonjudgmental awareness to internal experiences can be applied to potential treatment barriers as well, including stigma about illness, negative beliefs about treatment, fatigue and lack of motivation. The ACT therapist stresses that the patient does not need to eliminate these negative feelings or thoughts in order to choose to remain consistent with a treatment regimen that supports a valued domain.

6.4.4   Committed Action

Committed action, or encouragement of values-based changes in out-of-session behaviour, is a major component of all ACT manuals. However, in our clinical experience we have found that adaptations are often necessary for patients with psychosis. For example, it is often helpful to introduce small committed action assignments very early in treatment. When patients with psychosis start with a new therapist they are often reluctant to share the content of their thoughts, feelings and hallucinations, and may not do so until later in treatment. This makes ACT techniques that are dependent on this content, such as acceptance and mindfulness, difficult early in treatment. However, patients are often willing to discuss their values and accept assignments to take small steps towards these values early in treatment. Successful completion of such assignments can improve mood, but unsuccessful completion is often just as useful. A functional analysis of noncompletion often indicates that failure was due to experiential avoidance, and this can prompt a useful discussion of acceptance and workability.

In addition, we have found that patients with psychosis need more support in the out-of-session assignment process than is included in most ACT manuals. Behavioural activation provides suitable intensive supportive techniques (for a full review, see Kanter *et al.*, 2009). In particular, gently graded task assignment (starting small and raising the complexity and difficulty slowly), preassignment basic problem solving (e.g. if the assignment is to get a library card, the therapist may need to first help problem solve transportation to the library), intensive stimulus control (e.g. having the patient write down the assignment in multiple locations and call her own voicemail during the session to leave a reminder message) and assignment-specific skills training (e.g. if the assignment is to plan a social outing with a peer, the therapist might first roleplay this specific interaction several times) are often useful.

6.4.5   The Therapeutic Relationship

The therapeutic relationship provides an opportunity for the therapist to model acceptance and shape improved client behaviour during a session. Therapist modelling of acceptance of the patient's experience may be particularly important when working with patients with psychotic symptoms. These patients sometimes report hallucinations or delusions with content that is uncomfortable for the therapist to hear (e.g. violence, sexual acts). The therapist should be mindful of their own (understandable) temptation to avoid this content (e.g. change the topic, end the session early), and instead approach the content as the patient is asked to deal with it (i.e. as what it is and not what they say it is). Therapists can also model acceptance by describing their own acceptance behaviour both in session ('I am feeling tired today as well, but am going to do my best to have a productive session with you anyway. Are you willing to try that with me?') and out of session ('I hate getting the flu shot. It makes me very anxious. However, I do it anyway because it is important for me to stay healthy to take care of my kids').

Dykstra *et al.* (2010) provide recommendations for applying FAP with people with psychosis. Common CRB1s (real-world patient problems that occur in the therapeutic relationship) in this population include odd behaviours, expression of delusional thoughts, obvious ongoing symptoms that are not reported or are denied (e.g. the patient is responding to auditory hallucinations in session, but denying them to the therapist), lack of goal-directed behaviour, lack of expression of wants and needs and lack of basic social skills (e.g. eye contact). In many patients with psychosis, these behaviours are long-standing and have been reinforced by others. Thus, with this population, it is particularly important to notice and reinforce subtle improvements in in-session behaviour. For example, for a patient who very rarely expresses any needs, even a very unclear and passive request could be considered an improvement (i.e. a CRB2) and be reinforced (by granting the request). Given this low threshold for reinforcement and the likelihood that this population will not attend to subtle social reinforcement, it is often necessary for the therapist to amplify their natural reaction to a level that is salient to the patient and make functional relationships concrete. For example, a therapist might choose to reinforce a patient for very brief periods of eye contact by saying, 'You are looking at me much more today than usual. This makes me feel like you are engaged and really working with me.'

When FAP and ACT are integrated, acceptance and mindfulness can also be shaped in session (Kohlenberg & Callaghan, 2010). For example, auditory hallucinations occurring during a session provide an opportunity to shape acceptance in the moment. Sitting with but not responding to these experiences can be prompted ('I know you are experiencing a lot right now. I wonder if you can notice those voices and still work with me today?') and reinforced ('I am so proud of how you dealt with your voices today. To me, it shows that you are making great progress'). Successive approximations of mindfulness can be similarly shaped. For example, all patient 'I feel...' statements could be considered improvements (CRB2s) and reinforced.

Regardless of the target behaviour, it is always important for therapists to observe the effects of their attempts at contingent responding by noting the frequency of the patient's behaviour or by discussing the shaping process with the patient (Dykstra *et al.*, 2010; Kohlenberg & Tsai, 1991). It is important to remember that FAP techniques are functional; a therapist may intend to reinforce a patient behaviour by saying 'I am proud of you', but that statement could also be punishing for a particular patient. Observing the effects of attempts at shaping allow the therapist to adjust contingent responding ideographically.

6.5   Special Contexts and Issues

6.5.1   ACT Made Even Simpler

In the Gaudiano & Herbert (2006) study of ACT for psychosis, patients received a variable and flexible number of sessions based on their length of stay on the hospital unit. Each session was 'self-contained', with all the core elements of ACT presented briefly, including the treatment rationale, acceptance and mindfulness strategies for coping with hallucinations and delusions, and values-clarification work (Bach *et al.*, 2006). In addition to these core elements, various themes were rotated over sessions. One session format examined unsuccessful past attempts to cope with psychotic symptoms by highlighting those focused on struggle and control in order to motivate exploration of new coping strategies. Acceptance and willingness were then introduced as alternative approaches to psychotic symptoms. Other sessions expanded upon this theme, and introduced new concepts consistent with the ACT rationale, including workability as a guide to coping and perspective-taking in order to develop a more stable sense of self (Gaudiano, in press). The therapist can promote treatment engagement and increase the patient's adherence to ACT for psychosis by simplifying the

Table 6.2 ACT to improve treatment engagement made even simpler

Brief session format

1. Explore the patient's history, highlighting the unworkability of control-orientated strategies applied to psychotic symptoms and nonadherence behaviours.
2. Introduce and practise acceptance and mindfulness towards experiences as alternative coping strategies.
3. Place acceptance and mindfulness in the service of a valued life domain.
4. Identify a value-consistent goal and formulate a specific action plan that supports treatment and can be implemented between sessions.

intervention using this basic format: accept and stay present when experiencing psychotic symptoms, choose a value and take action. A brief ACT session format is presented in Table 6.2.

6.5.2   Involuntary Admission and Lack of Insight

Working with hospitalised patients with psychosis who are involuntarily committed can pose significant challenges (Fiorillo *et al.*, 2011). Many patients with psychosis lack insight into their psychotic symptoms at various times and thus may not view them as requiring change or treatment (Trauer & Sacks, 2000). These patients in particular can benefit from the values–goals clarification strategies used in ACT. Values work helps the therapist develop an alliance with the patient and identify potential treatment goals. ACT's deemphasis on symptom elimination and on judging whether or not a hallucination or delusion is 'true' or 'false' sidesteps many of the typical pitfalls when working with these patients. The goal of the ACT therapist is not to convince the patient that treatment *per se* is necessary, nor is it to treat a particular 'disease'. Instead, the therapist explores the patient's values system and the workability of her actions in helping her move closer in line with it. Discrepancies between values and actions can be explored to build motivation for change. Such work can permit the ACT therapist and patient to find common ground, develop a working alliance and explore other clinical issues, based on the patient's level of willingness.

6.5.3   Other Cognitive Behavioural Approaches for Psychosis

6.5.3.1   Traditional CBT

The methods used to engage patients and increase adherence in traditional CBT for psychosis (CBTp) include an emphasis on building a strong therapeutic alliance, providing psychoeducation, setting individualised goals and applying techniques to nonpsychotic symptoms before hallucinations or delusions (Kingdon & Turkington, 2005). For example, there is an emphasis at the start of traditional CBTp on building rapport with the patient so that cognitive strategies (e.g. Socratic questioning) can be employed without rupturing the therapeutic relationship. Also, the therapist normalises psychotic experiences by explaining that these symptoms are more prevalent in the general population than is commonly believed and that they can be produced in a number of different situations, including drug use and sleep deprivation. Goal setting in CBTp focuses on eliciting definable and measurable behavioural achievements that are desired by the patient. Typically, the therapist works with the patient to apply cognitive and behavioural strategies to nonpsychotic symptoms first. This allows time for the therapist to strengthen the therapeutic alliance and permits the patient to experience the potential benefits of these techniques. Also, in traditional CBTp, the therapist uses problem-solving and cognitive techniques for nonadherence behaviours (Wright *et al.*, 2009). For example, the therapist might encourage the patient to use written/electronic reminders and pill organisers to promote medication adherence or treatment appointment attendance. Also, cognitive-restructuring techniques are applied to dysfunctional thoughts about illness and treatment in order to encourage adherence.

ACT and traditional CBTp share a focus on normalising psychotic experiences so as to promote engagement with treatment. The ACT therapist can also use practical strategies to help patients remember to take their medications more consistently if forgetfulness is producing nonadherence. However, goal-setting and problem-solving activities in ACT are placed in the context of the patient's personally held values in order to foster change and increase persistence during difficult behaviour-change efforts. The dual themes of patient choice and workability as a guide to action are emphasised when discussing adherence issues. In addition, ACT does not focus on directly changing patients' beliefs about treatment or on judging whether they are incorrect or inaccurate; rather, the ACT therapist encourages the patient to bring nonjudgmental awareness to nonadherence beliefs while choosing to engage in values-consistent actions.

6.5.3.2 Motivational Interviewing

Motivational interviewing (MI) (Miller & Rollnick, 2002) is a person-centred approach to assisting patients in resolving ambivalence about behaviour change and increasing motivation to make that behaviour change, including attending treatment or taking medication. MI seeks to elicit and reinforce 'change talk' (e.g. statements of desire, ability, reason, need or commitment to behaviour change). In order to accomplish these goals, MI relies heavily on open-ended questioning, affirmation of patient effort and struggles, and reflections. Given that the standard pharmacological treatments for psychosis often help some symptoms but have aversive side effects (Artaloytia *et al.*, 2006), it is not surprising that many patients are ambivalent regarding acceptance of and engagement in treatment. Research supports the use of MI in patients with psychosis (Barrowclough *et al.*, 2001).

Interestingly, at the technique level, MI and ACT have significant overlap. For example, both treatments do a careful assessment of patient values and link them to behaviour change (Wagner & Sanchez, 2002). The MI technique of 'rolling with resistance' leads MI therapists to avoid directly challenging the content or factuality of a patient's statements. For example, like an ACT therapist, an MI therapist would not directly confront a patient statement that 'I do not need any treatment' or judge a particular delusion as true or false. Theoretically, however, MI and ACT are inconsistent. MI's posited mechanism is a cognitive shift (e.g. ambivalence to commitment to change), while ACT posits that cognitive content change is not required for behaviour change.

6.6   Case Study

The following case is a blend of several patients, so as to protect their confidentiality, and illustrates how to integrate ACT and FAP approaches when working with patients with psychosis. John presented for treatment days after being discharged from an inpatient unit, where he was treated for a depressed mood and psychosis (auditory hallucinations, suspiciousness regarding the motives of his family and treatment providers). John had had several therapists in the past, but reported that he never attended sessions for long as all of his therapists eventually 'betrayed' him. In the first session, John stated that he would not talk about his hallucinations because when he did, he ended up in the hospital.

6.6.1   Early Sessions (1–5)

Early sessions focused on values clarification, committed action and building an open and honest therapeutic relationship through the therapist modelling acceptance. When first asked about his values, John reported several goals (e.g. 'Stay out of the hospital'), including some related to his delusions ('Get better at knowing good people from evil people'). However, after further exploration using the compass metaphor, it became clear that John deeply valued independence and relationships with his family. John agreed to simple, graded behavioural activation assignments in the service of these goals, such as going on outings with his family and attending classes at a vocational centre. The therapist provided intensive support for assignment completion (e.g. filling out the class-sign up form collaboratively in session).

Given John's history of interpersonal paranoia and treatment nonadherence, the therapist was careful to build a therapeutic relationship that would support session attendance and treatment engagement. For example, the therapist made it explicit that feelings of paranoia might come up in the therapeutic relationship and that expressing these thoughts and feelings to the therapist would be helpful, even if the content were negative (e.g. 'I feel betrayed by you'). This is an example of modelling acceptance (the therapist is willing to sit with this content nonjudgmentally) and sets up later opportunities to shape improved in-session behaviour.

6.6.2   Mid-treatment Sessions (6–15)

Mid-treatment sessions focused on the unworkability of the experiential avoidance agenda and the alternative of acceptance and mindfulness. By this point in treatment, John was willing to share more about his hallucinations and other upsetting thoughts and feelings. Metaphors, including person-in-the-hole and tug-of-war-with-the-monster, were presented. In addition, many opportunities for natural discussions of acceptance were provided by successful and failed behavioural activation assignments. Successful completion often included some degree of acceptance ('I was anxious, but I went to my class anyway'), and failure was often due to experiential avoidance ('Even thinking about doing X increased the voices, so I did not do it').

At this point in treatment, John and the therapist had a positive therapeutic relationship that was conducive to *in vivo* shaping. Collaboratively, John and the therapist discussed ways that his interpersonal challenges outside of treatment came up in the therapy relationship. They agreed that cutting people out when he felt betrayed and not expressing his needs clearly were such challenges (i.e. CRB1s). It was agreed that the therapist would point out these behaviours when they occurred in session and encourage John to engage in more effective behaviour (i.e. CBR2s). The therapist shaped successive approximations of these behaviours. For example, initially the therapist fulfilled (i.e. reinforced) John's requests even if they were poorly presented (e.g. 'I know you will say "no", but will you…), while later in treatment the therapist followed these types of request with prompts for more skilled and socially effective ones.

6.6.3   Late-treatment Sessions (16–20)

Later treatment sessions focused on applying skills shaped and practised *in vivo* in real relationships and pursuing long-term, value-linked goals. For example, John could now express his needs clearly to the therapist, but still did so infrequently with peers and family because it made him anxious. Thus, John was asked to do so repeatedly as homework. These assignments were presented both as a generalisation of skills practised in session and as values-based experiential approach assignments (e.g. 'We know you will be anxious when you are asking your sister for help, but does the possibility of it increasing the intimacy of your relationship make it worth it to try anyway?').

6.7   Conclusion

Engaging and retaining patients with psychosis in treatment can be challenging at times. ACT and FAP can be combined in ways that complement and strengthen the therapist's ability to promote treatment adherence. However, certain modifications can be helpful. Adherence can best be targeted by focusing on themes of workability, valuing, acceptance/mindfulness applied to treatment-related distress/lack of motivation, committed actions and relationship factors. The ACT therapist needs to attend to the potential complexity or difficulty of skills training or behavioural assignments, and help the patient to break them down into manageable steps or simpler exercises (e.g. mindful walking or eating) in order to improve success. Abstract concepts in ACT can be communicated using visual aids (e.g. cartoons, illustrations) or stories that can improve comprehension and retention of therapy content. In addition, FAP strategies can help the therapist attend to interpersonal relationships in and out of session and successively shape more effective social behaviours in the patient. This is particularly important for patients who exhibit paranoia or confusion due to hallucinations, which can disrupt the therapeutic alliance. Although ACT and FAP overlap in some ways with traditional CBT and MI, they differ in their approach to case conceptualisation (i.e. functional analysis) and offer a variety of novel strategies that can be useful for helping patients in the pursuit of their valued behavioural goals.

References

Artaloytia, J. F., Arango, C., Lahti, A., Sanz, J., Pascual, A., Cubero, P. *et al.* (2006). Negative signs and symptoms secondary to antipsychotics: a double-blind, randomized trial of a single dose of placebo, haloperidol, and risperidone in healthy volunteers. *American Journal of Psychiatry*, 163, 488–493.

Bach, P. (2004). ACT with the seriously mentally ill. In S. C. Hayes & K. D. Strosahl (eds). *A Practical Guide to Acceptance and Commitment Therapy*. New York: Springer, pp. 185–208.

Bach, P., Gaudiano, B., Pankey, J., Herbert, J. D. & Hayes, S. C. (2006). Acceptance, mindfulness, values, and psychosis: applying Acceptance and Commitment Therapy (ACT) to the chronically mentally ill. In R. A. Baer (ed.). *Mindfulness-based Treatment Approaches: Clinician's Guide to Evidence Base and Applications*. San Diego: Academic Press, pp. 93–116.

Bach, P., Gaudiano, B. A., Hayes, S. C. & Herbert, J. D. (in press). Acceptance and Commitment Therapy for psychosis: intent to treat hospitalization outcome and mediation by believability. *Psychosis*, doi: 10.1080/17522439.2012.671349.

Bach, P. & Hayes, S. C. (2002). The use of acceptance and commitment therapy to prevent the rehospitalization of psychotic patients: a randomized controlled trial. *Journal of Consulting and Clinical Psychology*, 70, 1129–1139.

Barrowclough, C., Haddock, G., Tarrier, N., Lewis, S. W., Moring, J., O'Brien, R. *et al.* (2001). Randomized controlled trial of motivational interviewing, cognitive behavior therapy, and family intervention for patients with comorbid schizophrenia and substance use disorders. *American Journal of Psychiatry,* 158, 1706–1713.

Baruch, D. E., Kanter, J. W., Busch, A. B. & Juskiewicz, K. (2009). Enhancing the therapy relationship in Acceptance and Commitment Therapy for psychotic symptoms. *Clinical Case Studies,* 8, 241–257.

Bergen, J., Hunt, G., Armitage, P. & Bashir, M. (1998). Six-month outcome following a relapse of schizophrenia. *Australian and New Zealand Journal of Psychiatry,* 32, 815–822.

Berry, K. & Haddock, G. (2008). The implementation of the NICE guidelines for schizophrenia: barriers to the implementation of psychological interventions and recommendations for the future. *Psychol. Psychother.,* 81, 419–436.

Branstetter-Rost, A., Cushing, C. & Douleh, T. (2009). Personal values and pain tolerance: does a values intervention add to acceptance? *Journal of Pain,* 10, 887–892.

Callaghan, G. M., Gregg, J. A., Marx, B., Kohlenberg, B. S. & Gifford, E. (2004). FACT: the utility of an integration of Functional Analytic Psychotherapy and Acceptance and Commitment Therapy to alleviate human suffering. *Psychotherapy: Theory, Research, Practice, Training,* 41, 195–207.

Chouinard, G. & Chouinard, V. A. (2008). Atypical antipsychotics: CATIE study, drug-induced movement disorder and resulting iatrogenic psychiatric-like symptoms, supersensitivity rebound psychosis and withdrawal discontinuation syndromes. *Psychotherapy and Psychosomatics,* 77, 69–77.

Colom, F., Vieta, E., Tacchi, M. J., Sanchez-Moreno, J. & Scott, J. (2005). Identifying and improving non-adherence in bipolar disorders. *Bipolar Disorder,* 7(Suppl. 5), 24–31.

Dixon, L. B., Dickerson, F., Bellack, A. S., Bennett, M., Dickinson, D., Goldberg, R. W. *et al.* (2010). The 2009 schizophrenia PORT psychosocial treatment recommendations and summary statements. *Schizophrenia Bulletin,* 36, 48–70.

Dykstra, T. A., Shontz, K. A., Indovina, C. V. & Moran, D. J. (2010). The application of FAP to persons with serious mental illness. In J. W. Kanter, R. J. Kohlenberg & M. Tsai (eds). *The Practice of Functional Analytic Psychotherapy.* New York: Plenum.

Farhall, J., Greenwood, K. M. & Jackson, H. J. (2007). Coping with hallucinated voices in schizophrenia: a review of self-initiated strategies and therapeutic interventions. *Clinical Psychology Review,* 27, 476–493.

Fiorillo, A., De Rosa, C., Del Vecchio, V., Jurjanz, L., Schnall, K., Onchev, G. *et al.* (2011). How to improve clinical practice on involuntary hospital admissions of psychiatric patients: suggestions from the EUNOMIA study. *European Psychiatry,* 26, 201–207.

Gaudiano, B. A. (in press). Brief acceptance and commitment therapy for the acute treamtent of hospitalized patients with psychosis. In C. Steel (ed.). *CBT for Schizophrenia: Evidence-based Interventions and Future Directions.* Hoboken: John Wiley & Sons.

Gaudiano, B. A. & Herbert, J. D. (2006). Acute treatment of inpatients with psychotic symptoms using Acceptance and Commitment Therapy: pilot results. *Behaviour Research and Therapy,* 44, 415–437.

Gaudiano, B. A., Herbert, J. D. & Hayes, S. C. (2010). Is it the symptom or the relation to it? Investigating potential mediators of change in acceptance and commitment therapy for psychosis. *Behavior Therapy,* 41, 543–554.

Gifford, E. V., Kohlenberg, B., Hayes, S. C., Pierson, H., Piasecki, M., Antonuccio, O., Palm, K. (2011). Does acceptance and relationship focused behavior therapy contribute to bupropion outcomes? A randomized controlled trial of functional analytic psychotherapy and acceptance and commitment therapy for smoking cessation. *Behavior Therapy*, 42, 700–715.

Hayes, S. C., Strosahl, K. D. & Wilson, K. G. (2012). *Acceptance and Commitment Therapy: The Process and Practice of Mindful Change* (2nd edn). New York: Guilford Press.

Hayes, S. C., Villatte, M., Levin, M. & Hildebrandt, M. (2011). Open, aware, and active: contextual approaches as an emerging trend in the behavioral and cognitive therapies. *Annual Review of Clinical Psychology*, 7, 141–168.

Ho, B. C., Andreasen, N. C., Ziebell, S., Pierson, R. & Magnotta, V. (2011). Long-term antipsychotic treatment and brain volumes: a longitudinal study of first-episode schizophrenia. *Archives of General Psychiatry*, 68, 128–137.

Kabat-Zinn, J. (1994). *Wherever You Go, There You Are: Mindfulness Medication in Everyday Life*. New York: Hyperion.

Kanter, J. W., Busch, A. M. & Rusch, L. C. (2009). *Behavioral Activation: Distinctive Features*. London: Routledge.

Kingdon, D. G. & Turkington, D. (2005). *Cognitive Therapy of Schizophrenia*. New York: Guilford Press.

Kohlenberg, B. & Callaghan, G. M. (2010). FAP and Acceptance Commitment Therapy: similarities, divergence, and integration. In J. W. Kanter, R. J. Kohlenberg & M. Tsai (eds). *The Practice of Functional Analytic Psychotherapy*. New York: Plenum.

Kohlenberg, R. J. & Tsai, M. (1991). *Functional Analytic Psychotherapy: A Guide for Creating Intense and Curative Therapeutic Relationships*. New York: Plenum.

Kreyenbuhl, J., Nossel, I. R. & Dixon, L. B. (2009). Disengagement from mental health treatment among individuals with schizophrenia and strategies for facilitating connections to care: a review of the literature. *Schizophrenia Bulletin*, 35, 696–703.

Lacro, J. P., Dunn, L. B., Dolder, C. R., Leckband, S. G. & Jeste, D. V. (2002). Prevalence of and risk factors for medication nonadherence in patients with schizophrenia: a comprehensive review of recent literature. *Journal of Clinical Psychiatry*, 63, 892–909.

Levitt, J. T., Brown, T. A., Orsillo, S. M. & Barlow, D. H. (2004). The effects of acceptance versus suppression of emotion on subjective and psychophysiological response to carbon dioxide challenge in patients with panic disorder. *Behavior Therapy*, 35, 747–766.

Levitt, J. T. & Karekla, M. (2005). Integrating acceptance and mindfulness with cognitive behavioral treatment for panic disorder. In S. M. Orsillo & L. Roemer (eds). *Acceptance and Mindfulness-based Approaches to Anxiety*. New York: Springer, pp. 165–188.

Luoma, J. B., Kohlenberg, B. S., Hayes, S. C. & Fletcher, L. (2011). Slow and steady wins the race: a randomized clinical trial of acceptance and commitment therapy targeting shame in substance use disorders. *Journal of Consulting and Clinical Psychology*, 80, 43–51.

Marcks, B. A. & Woods, D. W. (2007). Role of thought-related beliefs and coping strategies in the escalation of intrusive thoughts: an analog to obsessive-compulsive disorder. *Behavior Research and Therapy*, 45, 2640–2651.

Margolese, H. C., Chouinard, G., Beauclair, L. & Belanger, M. C. (2002). Therapeutic tolerance and rebound psychosis during quetiapine maintenance monotherapy in patients with schizophrenia and schizoaffective disorder. *Journal of Clinical Psychopharmacology*, 22, 347–352.

Masedo, A. I. & Rosa Esteve, M. (2007). Effects of suppression, acceptance and spontaneous coping on pain tolerance, pain intensity and distress. *Behav. Res. Ther.*, 45, 199–209.

McMullen, J., Barnes-Holmes, D., Barnes-Holmes, Y., Stewart, I., Luciano, C. & Cochrane, A. (2008). Acceptance versus distraction: brief instructions, metaphors and exercises in increasing tolerance for self-delivered electric shocks. *Behavior Research and Therapy*, 46, 122–129.

Miller, W. R. & Rollnick, S. (2002). *Motivational Interviewing: Preparing People for Change* (2nd edn). New York: Guilford.

Moncrieff, J. (2006). Why is it so difficult to stop psychiatric drug treatment? It may be nothing to do with the original problem. *Medical Hypotheses*, 67, 517–523.

Moncrieff, J., Cohen, D. & Mason, J. P. (2009). The subjective experience of taking antipsychotic medication: a content analysis of Internet data. *Acta Psychiatrica Scandinavica*, 120, 102–111.

Moran, M. (2003). Psychosocial treatment rates for schizophrenia patients. *Psychiatric News*, 38, 12.

National Institute for Health and Clinical Excellence (2009). *Core Interventions in the Treatment and Management of Schizophrenia in Primary and Secondary Care*. UK: National Institute for Health and Clinical Excellence.

Nuttbrock, L. H., Ng-Mak, D. S., Rahav, M. & Rivera, J. J. (1997). Pre- and post-admission attrition of homeless, mentally ill chemical abusers referred to residential treatment programs. *Addiction*, 92, 1305–1315.

Paez-Blarrina, M., Luciano, C., Gutierrez-Martinez, O., Valdivia, S., Ortega, J. & Rodriguez-Valverde, M. (2008). The role of values with personal examples in altering the functions of pain: comparison between acceptance-based and cognitive-control-based protocols. *Behavior Research and Therapy*, 46, 84–97.

Reilly, J. L., Harris, M. S., Keshavan, M. S. & Sweeney, J. A. (2006). Adverse effects of risperidone on spatial working memory in first-episode schizophrenia. *Archives of General Psychiatry*, 63, 1189–1197.

Romme, E. & Escher, S. (1993). *Accepting Voices*. London: MIND Publications.

Shawyer, F., Ratcliff, K., Mackinnon, A., Farhall, J., Hayes, S. C. & Copolov, D. (2007). The voices acceptance and action scale (VAAS): pilot data. *Journal of Clinical Psychology*, 63, 593–606.

Tait, L., Birchwood, M. & Trower, P. (2003). Predicting engagement with services for psychosis: insight, symptoms and recovery style. *British Journal of Psychiatry*, 182, 123–128.

Trauer, T. & Sacks, T. (2000). The relationship between insight and medication adherence in severely mentally ill clients treated in the community. *Acta Psychiatrica Scandinavica*, 102, 211–216.

Tsai, M., Kohlenberg, R. J., Kanter, J. W., Kohlenberg, B., Follette, W. C. & Callaghan, G. M. (2009). *Functional Analytic Psychotherapy: A Therapist's Guide to Using Awareness, Courage, Love, and Behaviorism*. New York: Springer.

Wagner, C. C. & Sanchez, F. P. (2002). The role of values in motivational interviewing. In W. R. Miller & S. Rollnick (eds). *Motivational Interviewing: Preparing People for Change* (2nd edn). New York: Guilford.

Weiden, P. J., Kozma, C., Grogg, A. & Locklear, J. (2004). Partial compliance and risk of rehospitalization among California Medicaid patients with schizophrenia. *Psychiatric Services*, 55, 886–891.

White, R., Gumley, A., McTaggart, J., Rattrie, L., McConville, D., Cleare, S. *et al.* (2011). A feasibility study of Acceptance and Commitment Therapy for emotional dysfunction following psychosis. *Behavior Research and Therapy*, 49, 901–907.

Wilson, K. G. & Murrell, A. R. (2004). Values work in acceptance and comitment therapy: setting a course for behavioral treatment. In S. C. Hayes, V. M. Follette & M. M. Linehan (eds). *Mindfulness and Acceptance: Expanding the Cognitive-behavioral Tradition*. New York: Guilford.

Wilson, K. G., Sandoz, E. K., Kitchens, J. & Roberts, M. E. (2010). The Valued Living Questionnaire: defining and measuring valued action within a behavioral framework. *The Psychological Record*, 60, 249–272.

World Health Organization (2003). *Adherence to Long-term Therapies: Evidence for Action*. Geneva: World Health Organization.

Wright, J. H., Turkington, D., Kingdon, D. G. & Basco, M. R. (2009). *Cognitive-behavior Therapy for Severe Mental Illness: An Illustrated Guide*. Washington, DC: American Psychiatric Publishing.

7

Acceptance and Commitment Therapy for Voices

Neil Thomas, Eric M. J. Morris, Fran Shawyer
and John Farhall

7.1 Introduction

Auditory hallucinations are one of the most common symptoms of schizophrenia, frequently persisting despite treatment with antipsychotic medication, resulting in ongoing distress and functional disability. Consequently, they have become a common target for psychological interventions (Chadwick & Birchwood, 1994; Farhall *et al.*, 2007; Haddock *et al.*, 1998; Thomas *et al.*, 2010; Trower *et al.*, 2004), and have been one of the main treatment targets in early applications of acceptance and commitment therapy (ACT) to psychosis (Bach & Hayes, 2002; Gaudiano & Herbert, 2006; Shawyer *et al.*, 2012). ACT has particular synergies with intervention for auditory hallucinations, a phenomenon characterised by verbal content, which may be a source of fusion (see Chapter 2) and for which acceptance has already been heralded as important in promoting adaptation (Romme & Escher, 1989). In this chapter we consider the specific ways in which we have applied ACT to the experience of hearing voices in our work with medication-resistant psychosis in Melbourne and with early psychosis in London.

7.2 Formulating how Voices are a Problem

ACT is primarily concerned with assisting people to disengage more effectively from unproductive struggle with uncontrollable experiences and to promote fuller engagement in life. There are at least three layers of the experience of hearing voices that may contribute to client struggle and interference with valued living:

Acceptance and Commitment Therapy and Mindfulness for Psychosis, First Edition.
Edited by Eric M. J. Morris, Louise C. Johns and Joseph E. Oliver.
© 2013 John Wiley & Sons, Ltd. Published 2013 by John Wiley & Sons, Ltd.

(1) *Intrusiveness and salience of experience.* Voices are attention-capturing. They are an intrusive and hard-to-escape auditory experience and, in the context of psychosis, one which may be experienced as particularly personally meaningful and salient (Kapur, 2003). The capture of attention by hallucinatory experience can divert a person from valued living, and when regarded as unwelcome, this can become a source of frustration, demoralisation or anxiety, often generating attempts to suppress or control it.

(2) *Verbal content.* Voices are a verbal phenomenon, providing potential material for cognitive fusion. In particular, voices frequently include emotive material such as criticism, threats, warnings and harmful commands.

(3) *Interpersonal qualities of voice experience.* People are frequently drawn into reacting to hallucinatory experience as if being addressed by another person. Patients often ascribe their voices' identities and intentions, see them as sentient others existing in external reality and view them as possessing great power (Chadwick & Birchwood, 1994). Meanwhile, behaviourally, people are commonly drawn into verbal responses to their hallucinations (either aloud or in thought), generating a dialogue. Common responses include arguing with voices, telling them to go away and trying to engage, persuade or appease them. These responses are unhelpful because they maintain attention on the voice experience, possibly also maintaining activation of neural networks involved in the generation of voices, reinforcing the phenomenon itself. In addition, the resistant responses to voices that are particularly common seem to be associated with distress (Romme & Escher, 1989; Farhall & Gherke, 1997).

Hence, ACT for voices most often has the primary aim of helping a patient more effectively disengage attention from these salient aspects of hallucinatory experience and break associated habitual behavioural responses. In line with the standard ACT model, this involves promoting a process of letting go of resistance to (or unworkable engagement with) voices (*acceptance*) when such resistance interferes with living a valued life. This process can be supported by *cognitive defusion*, by adopting the stance of a mindful observer of voice experience (*present moment, self-as-context*) and by fostering an attitude of willingness to experience voices while pursuing valued action (*values, committed action*).

7.3   Overall Considerations in Conducting ACT with Voices

The application of ACT to psychotic phenomena such as voices requires some modification of its application to nonpsychotic disorders:

(1) *Gentle rate of progress.* Applying ACT to people with psychotic disorders necessitates a greater degree of gentleness and caution than when applying it

to anxiety or depressive disorders. Compared with other psychological therapies, ACT is quite a confronting intervention. It contains elements which aim to shake up the patient's view of reality, and to disrupt an established equilibrium of avoiding distressing experiences as a primary means of coping. Psychotic patients, who may have considerable existing difficulties in making sense of the world, may become overwhelmed relatively easily, and stepping outside of their usual avoidant repertoire might elicit significant anxiety and arousal. Each of these responses has the potential not only to threaten engagement in therapy but also to increase psychotic symptomatology. Hence we carefully track a patient's responses to therapy activities, through observation and by asking for feedback, in order to inform the pace and direction of therapy. With individual exercises, we typically seek permission from the patient each time an exercise is conducted and make it clear that they can stop at any time.

(2) *Experience of voices as external.* Unlike thoughts, the content of verbal material generated from voices is not usually experienced as originating from the self. In addition, the patient may have delusional beliefs about the existence of their voices in external reality, often held with a level of conviction that leads to reactance when threatened. In this context, therapists need to exercise caution around referring to voices as 'internal' experiences, or differentiating voice content from external reality. Therefore, we tend not to utilise the common ACT differentiation between 'internal' and 'external' experiences in considering their controllability in work with voices. Instead, we help people to consider the extent to which experiences such as voices are 'controllable' versus 'uncontrollable', without special reference to their location or origins. This allows us to maintain a central focus upon the workability of different ways of dealing with psychotic experience, joining with the patient in developing the most workable ways of living with such experiences while pursuing a meaningful life. When there is some existing flexibility present, we might help the patient recognise that voice content, as with any speech or thought content, is not 'real' in the same sense as objects in the external world – but only with care. If there is a danger of inadvertently eliciting reactance or becoming drawn into a debate about whether or not voices are real, we would steer the focus away from these issues on to the basic agenda of considering what works in dealing with such experiences.

(3) *Use of metaphor.* Given the difficulties in abstract thinking, metacognition and memory that can be present in psychotic disorders, people with psychosis may have difficulties understanding standard ACT metaphors. We use metaphors and exercises quite selectively, preferring those that are most easily understood, especially those which provide vivid illustrations of experience or demonstrate more workable ways to respond to voices (e.g. the tug-of-war-with–the-monster (see Appendix H) and swamp metaphors

(see Hayes *et al.*, 1999)), rather than those that are more abstract. To make metaphors more memorable, we often act them out physically, use illustrations or draw things out with the patient, and seek opportunities to practise or roleplay their application to voices when we can.

7.3.1   Sequence of Therapy

In general, therapy will proceed by addressing each of the ACT processes in parallel, with each therapy session incorporating a number of elements of the ACT model, and helping the patient to make links between them. For example, one might introduce a defusion exercise, discuss how this could be applied to letting go of struggle with voices and then consider how the patient might use it in the context of engaging in a valued activity. Nonetheless, a natural starting point is often formed by noting the costs of struggle with voices and introducing the patient to the idea of acceptance as an alternative response, with an increasing focus on values, willingness and action as therapy progresses.

7.3.2   Acceptance: Letting Go of Struggle with Voices

In promoting acceptance, the main therapeutic aims are to:

(1) Help the client see ways in which they become caught up in struggle or engagement of attention with voices.
(2) Help the client recognise habitual responses to voices that are ineffective or counterproductive, in light of valued directions.
(3) Introduce an alternative attitude of letting go of voices: abandoning attempts to control the experience and instead disengaging attention from it.

A range of ACT methods can be applied to this, as described in detail elsewhere (e.g. Hayes *et al.*, 1999). The following are specific methods which we have found particularly helpful.

7.3.2.1   *Discussing Responses to Voices*
A useful starting point is to develop a detailed understanding of voice experience, including basic information on voice phenomenology: number of voices, gender, loudness, frequency, duration, content and so on (see Chapter 2). This can then lead to a more focused discussion of responses to voices. The aim here is to identify both helpful and unhelpful responses in order to begin establishing which appear to be workable and which appear not to work and/or to be increasing the problem. For example, what are some of the different things the client finds themselves doing in response to voices? How have they attempted to cope with this experience? How

helpful have these responses been in the short term? What have been their effects in the long term? Are there any costs associated with using them?

In doing this, coping strategies may be identified that appear to be effective, such as keeping oneself occupied or listening to music. While these do not represent acceptance of the phenomenon, we would encourage the use of them within an ACT framework – effective strategies for the relief of distress, even if only of short-term benefit, may be a 'workable' way to get on with valued living. Meanwhile, we would be alert to any attempts to suppress or change the voices, which will either restrict the patient's life or draw the patient into more engagement with the voices. Hence the therapist's role is to help the patient make a distinction between responses that do work and those that are engaged in habitually but seem to be ineffective or counterproductive. This has much in common with conducting an assessment of responses to voices for coping strategy enhancement (Tarrier, 1992). However, with an ACT approach the main thing that one should be drawing out is a recognition that while there are some things that can be done to minimise the impact of voices, ultimately it is hard to either directly suppress them or to modify them by interacting with them. This puts the issue of workability on the agenda, setting the scene for the promotion of acceptance and willingness as an alternative to elimination or control.

7.3.2.2   Letting Go of Struggle

A number of metaphors and exercises exist for highlighting the fact that struggle can be counterproductive (e.g. 'quicksand', 'Chinese fingertrap'), including attempts to suppress thoughts (e.g. white bear-type exercises) or emotions (e.g. the polygraph metaphor; see Appendix E) (Hayes *et al.*, 1999). However, probably the most important message to convey in work with voices is to let go of struggle, which we have found most usefully illustrated by tug-of-war with the monster (Appendix H). We implement this metaphor with the therapist and client physically enacting a tug-of-war: the therapist plays an unbeatable monster pulling the patient towards an imaginary abyss (if patients are reluctant, we might do this while sitting down, or the therapist might act out the exercise by themselves). The therapist then guides the patient in noticing how all-consuming the struggle is and prompts them to consider alternative ways of responding (noting that the monster is infinitely strong and unbeatable), eliciting the response that dropping the rope is more workable than trying to win the battle. This exercise can then be discussed in relation to the experience of hearing voices ('With the voices, what can you do to drop the rope?'). This exercise can also be adapted to incorporate other aspects of the ACT model, such as values ('If your son were sitting in the corner of the room while you were doing this, how easy would it be to talk with him?'), defusion (e.g. the 'monster' verbalising voice content) and committed action ('What would dropping the rope to focus on this value look like?').

Struggle is not always evident. In some people, it may be minimal, and they simply wish to live with their voices more effectively, and in this case they might be directly introduced to the defusion, mindfulness and values methods in order to facilitate this. In others, however, voices may be seen as benevolent and actively engaged with, often at the cost of engagement in life in the nonpsychotic world (and possibly functioning to avoid it). In such situations, it may be more helpful to start with an initial focus on clarifying values, which might lead on to exploration of what gets in the way of the person acting in line with valued activity, and in turn a consideration of the effects of engaging with voices.

7.3.3   Defusion

As voices are a verbal phenomenon, fusion may be particularly applicable in understanding how the patient can become drawn into them. In some ways, voices can be similar to negative thoughts, often having emotive aspects which may be related to the patient's self-concept. However, given that the content of voices is not owned as internally generated, the most important source of fusion may alternatively be the meaning imposed upon the experience of hearing them. In line with the three-layer model, fusion may relate to:

(1)   The intrusiveness and salience of the experience, e.g. 'I can't do anything because of the voices', 'I can't get away from the voices', 'It's essential I listen', 'This is a punishment'.
(2)   The verbal content of the voices, e.g. specific criticism, threats, warnings.
(3)   Interpersonal meaning imposed upon the voices, e.g. 'They are trying to wind me up', 'They'll harm me', 'They won't like it if I go out', 'I have to stop them getting the better of me'.

There is, nonetheless, typically overlap between voice content and the patient's thoughts, so in practice defusion directed at voice content can often incorporate related thoughts and vice versa.

Following on from promoting the idea of letting go of voices, defusion can often be introduced by discussion of the ways in which the patient can find themselves automatically responding to particular voice or thought content. For example:

> So it seems that at times you can dismiss what the voices are saying, not get caught up with it, you can get on with doing stuff and let them 'mumble away' in the background. And at other times you find yourself getting hooked in. They say something and then you're having the thought, 'What if that's true?' or 'I can't let them say that', and before you know it you're arguing with them and they're getting more and more persistent... So it sounds like one of the key things that can help is finding ways not to get hooked in.

This can lead on to basic manoeuvres which encourage distancing, such as writing down particular voice or thought content on paper, explicitly referring to voice or thought content as 'words' or using basic distancing metaphors such as referring to content as being like a radio station that plays nothing but bad news.

Irrespective of whether or not voices are seen as existing in external reality, voice (and thought) content can also be highlighted as comprising ideas which are sometimes useful and sometimes not useful. We have found the monkey metaphor (e.g. Bowden & Bowden, 2010) to be a helpful illustration of workability. Here, the patient imagines themselves shipwrecked on a desert island. While trying to prepare shelter, they notice a little monkey who seems intent on getting their attention by bringing them things: sometimes useful (firewood, bananas), sometime less useful (damp leaves, rancid coconuts) and sometimes unpleasant (handfuls of poo).

While exercising some caution around the more abstract metaphors, further defusion methods can be used to highlight the effects of distancing on the impact of verbal content and reinforce that (1) thought/voice content is distinct from literal reality (e.g. 'finding a place to sit', Hayes *et al.*, 1999, pp. 152–153), (2) opinions are different from facts (e.g. 'bad cup', Hayes *et al.*, 1999, p. 169) and (3) thought/voice content does not lead to action. Differentiating thoughts from action is often particularly important, both in undermining the effect of voices in limiting behaviour and in reducing the influence of command hallucinations. For example, the patient might be instructed to pick up a pen while repeating the words 'I can't pick up the pen' (Bach, 2005). With care, this exercise can be elaborated to incorporate fused voice content (e.g. 'If you pick up the pen, we'll get you') or thought content relating to voices (e.g. 'I can't pick up the pen while I'm hearing voices', 'The voices won't let me pick up the pen', 'If I pick up the pen, the voices will win'), as well as to replace picking up pens with behaviours analogous to those which the voices might be seen as interfering with.

7.3.4   Mindfulness: Present Moment and Self as Observer

The ACT processes of getting in touch with the present moment and taking the perspective of an observer ('self-as-context') are mainly conveyed through the use of mindfulness exercises. We have tended to introduce mindfulness exercises into sessions as early as we are able to, usually presenting them to the patient as a general skill and applying them to the experience of voices once the patient has gained some familiarity with them. We tend to use mindfulness practices which involve focusing one's attention on a particular anchor, such as one's breath or an external object, rather than exercises involving opening up awareness without focus. We start carefully, first giving a brief description of the process in order to reduce uncertainty ('For a couple of minutes, notice your breathing, and notice when your mind gets hooked on to other things') and beginning with a brief exercise to check for aversive reactions and build trust. Although the duration is gradually increased, it is usually unrealistic to expect clients to be willing to commit to the

45-minute meditations used in mindfulness-based stress reduction. Instead we have usually used mindfulness exercises of up to 20 minutes' duration, plus 10- or 15-minute CD-guided practices for home use, which we actively encourage. Most often, we have used versions of the 'raisin exercise' (Kabat-Zinn, 1990, pp. 27–29; Segal *et al.*, 2002, pp. 101–110), 'mindfulness of the breath' (Kabat-Zinn, 1990, pp. 47–58) and the 'body scan meditation' (Kabat-Zinn, 1990, pp. 75–93; Segal *et al.*, 2002, pp. 110–120) used in mindfulness-based cognitive therapy. We also often incorporate the brief '5-5-5' (Harris, 2008, p. 156) or 'centring' (Eifert & Forsyth, 2005, p. 125) exercises at the beginnings of sessions.

When the patient is experiencing voices, we use two types of mindfulness instruction, which we incorporate into standard mindfulness exercises:

(1) *Focus away from voices.* Here mindfulness is used to help the patient develop the response of disengaging from attentional focus on voices and from automatic responses to them. For example, 'Whenever you find yourself distracted by sounds or voices, bring your attention back as best you can... allow those sounds and voices to remain there as part of your awareness, while turning the focus of your attention back to the breath...'

(2) *Focus towards voices.* The other use of mindfulness is to turn attention towards voices and to explore them from an observer stance, without responding to them. In conjunction with focusing away from voices, this may be useful in promoting acceptance of the phenomenon. For example, 'If voices are present, you might wish to experiment with directing your attention towards them, exploring them as another element of your experience... bringing a curiosity to observe what these experiences are like as sounds... observing their qualities as sounds, their location, their volume, patterns of pitch and rhythm... simply observing them, not trying to push them away, not engaging with them, just noticing them as part of your current experience... and just allowing these and other sounds be there, just as they are, while remaining present and focused on each passing moment.'

If voices do not arise within a session, we may play quiet recorded speech to provide an analogous stimulus from which to disengage. This might initially be done with neutral prerecorded material (e.g. podcasts), building up to more emotionally salient material that corresponds more closely to voice content. Voice-like material can be created by using a voice recorder to record examples of voice content and playing them back on a loop (this has practical advantages over the therapist role-playing voice content themselves, freeing them up to provide the client with instructions). The process of recording this material may itself be useful in promoting distancing from the content.

In promoting self-as-context, we discuss the idea of an 'observer self' as distinct from a 'thinking self' with clients. This can be combined with instruction during mindfulness exercises, such as, 'Notice as you sit here that part of you is simply an observer of these thoughts and experiences as they pass by… Recognise that this part of you is always there, constant, able to stand back and observe these passing experiences, moment by moment'. Depending upon the patient's cognitive capacity, we may also utilise metaphors emphasising the constancy of the observer self, such as in the mountain-meditation (Kabat-Zinn, 1994, p. 135), chessboard (see Appendix A) (Hayes *et al.*, 1999, p. 190) and sky-and-weather (Harris, 2009) metaphors.

7.3.5   Willingness: Values and Committed Action

Clarification and consolidation of personal values and promotion of commitment to action in spite of the presence of aversive symptoms complete the range of ACT interventions. The patient is supported in identifying things in life which are personally important to them and which provide a more important guide to behaviour than habitually falling into behavioural patterns dominated by engagement with or avoidance of voice activity. Alongside this, there is promotion of the principle of being willing to experience discomfort related to voice activity or fears related to voices, in order to live a more fulfilling life. The idea of willingness is well described by the swamp metaphor (Hayes *et al.*, 1999), which illustrates that one may be willing to tolerate wading through unpleasantness in order to get to a valued destination.

Values themselves can be clarified using a range of activities, including card sorts (e.g. Ciarrochi & Bailey, 2008), identification of values in specific domains (e.g. relationships, leisure, work/education and health/well-being; Harris, 2007) and imagining looking back on one's life from one's 80th birthday (Hayes *et al.*, 1999). In addition, the therapist is attentive to value-related themes that may arise during the course of therapy. Such exercises can be conducted without specific reference or adaptation to voices, although the therapist may need to steer the patient into identifying real-world values if the values and goals which are elicited are delusion-based. It should also be borne in mind that, while the process of identifying personal values can be quite motivating in people with nonpsychotic disorders, who can draw on their resources to reorient their lives, people with psychotic disorders often have significant social problems which present barriers to valued action (e.g. lack of friends, poverty, unemployment). Hence, in working with values, our usual aims for behaviour change are not so much based around major and long-term life goals, but rather involve fostering a stance towards life that embodies approach rather than avoidance. Hence we would encourage patients to identify small, achievable, value-congruent activities that can be carried out over the next day or two, or simply to experiment with doing things outside of their usual comfort zone, in order to learn what they find vital and meaningful. If identified goals end up reflecting further engagement with voices or delusions, one might return to drawing out the underlying broader values in order to identify expression of them in the nondelusional world.

In providing a metaphor for committed action in the face of voice activity, a useful exercise is taking your voices for a walk (adapted from Hayes *et al.*, 1999, p. 163), in which the therapist walks alongside the patient while the patient walks a particular route, and the patient's task is not to get caught up with or buy into things that the therapist says as they do so. In this way the therapist can roleplay the patient's voice or thoughts. This can begin with neutral material (e.g. 'What's that over there?') and move on to include imperatives which encourage the patient to act independently of voice content (e.g. 'Turn left!') and finally examples of common voice content. The exercise can be readily translated to other activities, such as playing music. This can be a very powerful exercise, but caution is required as the patient may readily become overwhelmed if they strongly fuse with distressing content. It is important to prepare well by setting clear parameters with the patient (e.g. agree on voice content to be roleplayed), emphasising that the therapist is just playing a role and debriefing frequently during the exercise (don't wait till the end). This exercise can then lead on to discussion of the patient's commitment to engage in identified valued activities.

7.4   Case Study

In this section we outline the case example of Hazel, a 33-year-old white British woman who had been persistently hearing voices and was referred for psychological therapy in a recovery-orientated mental-health team following a period of increased anxiety, worry and social isolation. Hazel had a history of experiencing command hallucinations and deliberate self-harm. She was unemployed and single, on a disability allowance and living in supported accommodation.

Hazel described her therapy goal as follows: 'Basically, I am trying to take charge of my life, and not let the voices dictate what I can and can't do.'

7.4.1   Current Mental-health Problems

Hazel reported ongoing experiences of hearing voices, which frequently criticise her and give her advice about what to do. She described the voices as 'evil' and said they were trying to make her 'do bad things' in order to destroy her. She stated that the voices did not want her to experience happiness and interfered with her having trusting relationships.

Hazel expressed a fear of hearing the voices' commands and feeling compelled to act, despite not hearing compelling commands to harm others/herself for 2 years. She worried about physically hurting others as a result of commands, so tried not to get close to people. She felt very ashamed of acting on the voices' commands; she ruminated about this when going to sleep at night. She also worried about embarrassing herself by talking out loud to the voices when in public, which sometimes stopped her from going out.

Hazel reported frequently having intrusive thoughts about shameful memories, and about losing control by acting on command hallucinations. She coped by using distraction and trying to block the thoughts.

Hazel reported a depressed mood and anxiety, with diminished enjoyment, pessimism, poor sleep, reduced motivation and fearful feelings on leaving home.

7.4.2   Mental-health History

Hazel said she had been hearing commanding voices for 9 years, following the birth of her first child, when she was diagnosed with schizophrenia (ICD 10, F20.0). She also described past problems with engaging in deliberate self-harm (cutting herself). Hazel had been prescribed a stable dose of clozapine, and felt that it reduced the voices' intensity.

7.4.3   Relevant Background

Hazel was brought up by her maternal grandparents, and had little contact with her parents. She was placed into care when she was 9 years old, after her grandmother passed away. This lasted until she was 14 years old, when she lived with her mother for a year. At 15, Hazel returned to care, following allegations that her mother sexually abused her. Hazel lived in a variety of foster homes until 18, when she lived with her father; she describes this as a stable period.

Hazel became homeless at 23 years old, following her father's death. She moved in with a man, and discovered after a short period that she was pregnant. Hazel gave birth to her son and three weeks after the birth was admitted to a psychiatric unit, with a first episode of psychosis. Hazel had two sons to her partner. The relationship broke down after the birth of their second boy, when her partner physically assaulted her. Hazel decided to give her infant children up for adoption after hurting her youngest child, while acting on command hallucinations; she no longer has contact with her children.

She described having no friends and said that the closest people in her life were her father and her two sons. Hazel felt she had a responsibility to stay alive for her sons, hoping to rekindle their relationship when they are older. She reported that she tends to keep to herself and not initiate friendships as she felt it was 'safer this way'.

7.4.4   Assessment and Formulation

Hazel reported hearing many voices, which she described as 'like a crowd at a football pitch', occurring three to five times a day and lasting up to an hour. They were as loud as her own voice. These were second- and third-person hallucinations heard outside of the head, male and female, and unidentified. Hazel described the content as 90% unpleasant and negative. She stated that the voices call her names, comment on her choices and actions, but there have been no recent threats or commands. She described the voices controlling her by causing physical pain if she did things they disapprove of, rather than giving direct commands. She believed she would feel compelled to act if given commands, and was fearful of this happening.

Hazel stated that she did not know what caused the voices, but believed the voices were real people contacting her in some way (80% conviction); she also reported that perhaps her voices were created by her mind (50% conviction). She perceived her voices as powerful and knowledgeable. Hazel denied trying to get in contact with the voices, or finding them helpful. She did not believe that she had any control over when the voices occurred.

Hazel described attempting to suppress the voices through distraction (listening to music), trying to think of other things and keeping busy. She also reported trying not to upset the voices, by avoiding social contact, particularly situations involving a degree of vulnerability.

7.4.5   ACT Case Formulation

The therapist focused on assessing the workability of Hazel's experiential avoidance of voices, and how this was supported by fusion with beliefs about the power and threatening nature of the voices. This perpetuated avoidance and escape in contexts that could provide opportunities for valued action, and rumination about the consequences of disobeying the voices. They considered how fusion between the voice-hearing experience and elicited feelings of shame, memories of voice compliance leading to unwanted outcomes and Hazel's history of unfulfilling relationships had become reasons for avoiding social interactions that could build friendships and any intimate relationship.

7.4.6   The ACT Approach

Hazel participated in 10 ACT sessions, initially focused on values clarification and then moving on to developing willingness by building the skills of defusion and acceptance (mindfulness). Each session started with a present-moment exercise, promoting active noticing for Hazel and the therapist, and then moved on to a discussion of valued actions taken and the practice of acceptance/defusion towards barriers. Sessions ended with planning of valued actions and a review of the main points (written on a summary sheet).

7.4.6.1   Initial Phase (Sessions 1–3)

Introducing defusion and acceptance through metaphor and mindfulness   In the first session, the rationale for mindfulness was introduced as a means of noticing experiences and the tendency to get caught up in them, and of practising 'just observing'. The therapist introduced the idea of 'you and your mind' as a way of talking about the process. Hazel appeared both intrigued and amused, finding it funny to hear the therapist talk this way: 'You are crazier than I am'.

The workability of coping with voices by struggling or obeying was explored through the tug-of-war-with-the-monster metaphor (Appendix H), which became the scaffolding story for the sessions.

Hazel was given a mindfulness CD for home practice. In the second session, she reported using the CD 'even though the voices don't like it' and attributed a shoulder pain to their displeasure. Hazel described persisting despite the pain, in order to exercise freedom from the voices. She reported some benefit from the CD as a means of shifting her attention, rather than being 'locked' on the voices.

During the sessions, the therapist modelled acceptance and defusion towards his own mental experiences through using self-disclosure about in-session experiences, as well as past occasions of fusion and experiential avoidance. Hazel responded positively to these discussions, and expressed surprise that the therapist struggled with intrusive thoughts.

Clarification of values and fostering committed action   The therapist used the lifetime achievement award exercise (a variant of the 'what do you want your life to stand for?' exercise, Hayes *et al.*, 1999, 215–218) to explore what Hazel would want to be doing in valued life domains, if she had a free choice. This exercise appeared to touch upon the sacrifices Hazel had made in order to cope with the voices: she recounted tearfully wanting to be able to have friends, an intimate relationship and a family. Hazel stated she would like to act in a 'loving and kind' way towards people in her life. She indicated that changing her behaviour to act more consistently with her values would involve experiencing fear and the possibility of the voices causing her pain, expressing disagreement and giving her commands. The therapist linked these actions with using mindfulness and letting go as possible ways of enabling her to do these things.

7.4.6.2   Mid-therapy (Sessions 4 – 7)

Use of imagery   Hazel engaged in several imagery exercises in order to develop defusion and acceptance. Some were variants of the physicalising exercise (Hayes *et al.*, 1999, pp. 170–171), in which the client imagines experiences as physical objects with properties such as size, shape and so on; this was done with the voices, intrusive thoughts and self-harm urges in turn.

The leaves-on-the-stream exercise (Appendix B) was introduced as both a mindfulness exercise and a written task. In the latter case, the therapist drew out the stream and used a set of Post-it notes as leaves, and encouraged Hazel to notice current experiences, placing them on the stream.

Finally, Hazel and the therapist acted out the taking-your-voices-for-a-walk exercise (Hayes *et al.*, 1999, p. 163). This involved imagining walking in a valued direction, while the therapist played 'the voices', saying the types of thing that Hazel usually heard. Three stances towards the voices were practised: one of struggling with them, another of obeying them and finally one of 'dropping the rope'/showing willingness. They reflected on the experience of each during the exercise and considered their workability in terms of valued action.

7.4.6.3   *End Sessions (Sessions 8 − 10)*

Towards the end of therapy, Hazel reported that she had been 'dropping the rope' more and engaging in conversations with others at her accommodation, as well as sharing more, despite the voices' comments. At times this resulted in enjoyable interactions, though they were disappointing on other occasions. Hazel stated that she was able to practise being mindful towards this, with a greater sense of meaning in what she was doing.

The last session reviewed the work done, reinforcing the actions that Hazel had taken through mindfulness and acceptance, and linking them with valued directions. Hazel reported benefiting from ACT, particularly in discovering that she did not need to obey the voices' commands. She and the therapist summarised this in her own words in a 'Learning from ACT' handout:

(1)   I know now that I can operate without having to listen to everything that the voices are saying. Just because the voices are there, doesn't mean I need to do what they are saying. I can do what I want to do, not what the voices want.

(2)   In friendships I am more willing to get closer to people, and to keep trying with sharing.

7.4.7   Outcomes

The outcome measures for the therapy are listed in Table 7.1. As can be observed, Hazel reported improvements across a range of areas at the close of therapy.

7.4.7.1   *Psychotic Symptoms*

Hazel reported hearing voices at the end of therapy, although there were changes, with the voices being less frequent (occurring two to three times a week) and perceived as less disruptive to her life. Hazel also reported believing that the voices were coming from her own mind (70% conviction), rather than being real people talking to her (30% conviction). She stated that her voices were not powerful, compared to her; she was also less fearful of them, although she was still slightly apprehensive about the pain she perceived as occurring because of her disobedience.

Table 7.1   Hazel's scores on therapy measures

Measure	Pretherapy	Post-therapy	Outcome
Beck Depression Inventory	51	9	Improvement
Beck Anxiety Inventory	24	8	Improvement
MANSA (Quality of Life)	43	71	Improvement
Social Functioning Scale	93.5	100	–
Voices Acceptance and Action Scale			Improvement
Acceptance	46	63	
Action	30	50	
KIMS Acceptance without Judgement	14	41	Improvement

7.4.7.2   *Depression and Anxiety*

Hazel's responses on the Beck Depression Inventory-II and the Beck Anxiety Inventory demonstrated clinically significant improvements in the levels of depressive and anxiety symptoms at the end of therapy.

7.4.7.3   *Valued Action, Quality of Life and Social Functioning*

Hazel reported increased levels of activity at the end of therapy, particularly related to her valued directions of friendships and relating to others in an open and caring manner. Her responses on the Manchester Short Assessment of Quality of Life (MANSA) (Priebe *et al.*, 1999) suggested clinically significant improvement, with gains made in the areas of friendship (she reported having a friend, post-therapy), accommodation, satisfaction with people she was living with and leisure activities.

Similarly, on the Social Functioning Scale (Birchwood *et al.*, 1990), there were improvements in Hazel's reported levels of interaction with others, particularly in describing approaching others post-therapy, rather than fearing and avoiding them, as well as a reduction in levels of social withdrawal.

7.4.7.4   *Changes in Mindfulness towards Voices and Thoughts*

On the Voices Acceptance and Action Scale (VAAS) (Shawyer *et al.*, 2007), at the start of therapy Hazel endorsed items suggesting that she had a low degree of *autonomy* in terms of her actions from the voices, and low *acceptance* of this as an experience. At the end of therapy her responses suggested a greater sense of autonomy and acceptance (both significant changes).

On the acceptance without judgement subscale of the Kentucky Inventory of Mindfulness Skills (KIMS) (Baer *et al.*, 2004), Hazel reported low acceptance of her experiences, with frequent judgements about whether they were good/bad, healthy and so on. Following therapy, Hazel's responses suggested that she had greater nonjudgement towards her experiences.

7.4.8   Discussion

This case description provides an example of how ACT may be helpful for those who are distressed and disabled by auditory hallucinations, particularly those experiencing command hallucinations.

The use of acceptance and defusion builds mindfulness skills, pragmatic means by which to enable engagement in valued actions, which can provide greater contact with potentially reinforcing contexts, and the shaping of approach behaviours to feared situations.

The therapeutic relationship models a compassionate and validating stance towards how the client copes with voices – in this case, this was particularly helpful, as it helped to build engagement: Hazel reported feeling understood, and not criticised by the therapist for past actions that were attached to a sense of shame. Of note also was that the *experiential* nature of ACT seemed like a novel context for Hazel, as she reported thinking that the therapist was 'crazier' than her and that the exercises had encouraged her to consider fundamentally what was important to her, the costs of coping in the usual way and an alternative approach that she could use. Hazel continued to experience auditory hallucinations, but she now had a few more options available in terms of how she could respond to these experiences, and the means to potentially improve her quality of life and engage in recovery-orientated goals.

References

Bach, P. (2005). ACT with the seriously mentally ill. In S. C. Hayes & K. D. Strohsal (eds). *A Practical Guide to Acceptance and Commitment Therapy.* New York: Springer.

Bach, P. & Hayes, S. C. (2002). The use of acceptance and commitment therapy to prevent the rehospitalization of psychotic patients: a randomized controlled trial. *Journal of Consulting and Clinical Psychology,* 70, 1129–1139.

Baer, R. A., Smith, G. T. & Allen, K. B. (2004). Assessment of mindfulness by self-report. *Assessment,* 11(3), 191–206.

Birchwood, M., Smith, J., Cochrane, R., Wetton, S. & Copestake, S. (1990). The Social Functioning Scale. The development and validation of a new scale of social adjustment for use in family intervention programmes with schizophrenic patients. *The British Journal of Psychiatry,* 157(6), 853–859.

Bowden, T. & Bowden, S. (2010). Thought cards. Retrieved from http://actonpurpose. com.au/Thought%20Cards.pdf, last accessed 16/11/2012.

Chadwick, P. D. J. & Birchwood, M. (1994). The omnipotence of voices: a cognitive approach to auditory hallucinations. *British Journal of Psychiatry,* 164, 190–201.

Ciarrochi, J. & Bailey, A. (2008). *A CBT-practitioner's Guide to ACT: How to Bridge the Gap between Cognitive Behavioral Therapy and Acceptance and Commitment Therapy.* Oakland: New Harbinger.

Eifert, G. H. & Forsyth, J. P. (2005). *Acceptance and Commitment Therapy for Anxiety Disorders*. Oakland: New Harbinger.

Farhall, J., Greenwood, K. M. & Jackson, H. J. (2007). Coping with hallucinated voices in schizophrenia: a review of self-initiated strategies and therapeutic interventions. *Clinical Psychology Review, 27,* 476–493.

Farhall, J. & Gehrke, M. (1997). Coping with hallucinations: exploring stress and coping framework. *British Journal of Clinical Psychology, 36,* 259–261.

Gaudiano, B. A. & Herbert, J. D. (2006). Acute treatment of inpatients with psychotic symptoms using Acceptance and Commitment Therapy: pilot results. *Behaviour Research and Therapy, 44,* 415–437.

Haddock, G., Slade, P. D., Bentall, R. P., Reid, D. & Faragher, E. B. (1998). A comparison of the long-term effectiveness of distraction and focusing in the treatment of auditory hallucinations. *British Journal of Medical Psychology, 71,* 339–349.

Harris, R. (2007). Lungdren's bull's eye exercise (revised by Russ Harris). Retrieved from http://www.actmindfully.com.au/articles_&_papers, last accessed 16/11/2012.

Harris, R. (2008). *The Happiness Trap: How to Stop Struggling and Start Living*. Boston: Trumpeter Books.

Harris, R. (2009). *ACT Made Simple: An Easy to Read Primer on Acceptance and Commitment Therapy*. Oakland: New Harbinger.

Hayes, S. C., Strosahl, K. D. & Wilson, K. G. (1999). *Acceptance and Commitment Therapy: An Experiential Approach to Behavior Change*. New York: Guilford Press.

Kabat-Zinn, J. (1994). *Wherever You Go, There You Are: Mindfulness Meditation in Everyday Life*. New York: Hyperion.

Kapur, S. (2003). Psychosis as a state of aberrant salience: a framework linking biology, phenomenology, and pharmacology in schizophrenia. *American Journal of Psychiatry, 160,* 13–23.

Priebe, S., Huxley, P., Knight, S. & Evans, S. (1999). Application and results of the Manchester Short Assessment of Quality of Life (Mansa). *International Journal of Social Psychiatry, 45*(1), 7–12.

Romme, M. & Escher, S. (1989). Hearing voices. *Schizophrenia Bulletin, 15,* 209–216.

Segal, Z. V., Williams, J. M. G. & Teasdale, J. D. (2002). *Mindfulness-based Cognitive Therapy for Depression: A New Approach to Preventing Relapse*. New York: Guilford.

Shawyer, F., Farhall, J., Mackinnon, A., Trauer, T., Sims, E., Ratcliffe, K., Larner, C., Thomas, N., Castle, D., Mullen, P. & Copolov, D. (2012). A randomised controlled trial of acceptance-based cognitive behavioural therapy for command hallucinations in psychotic disorders. *Behaviour Research and Therapy, 50,* 110–121.

Tarrier, N. (1992). Management and modification of residual positive psychotic symptoms. In M. Birchwood & N. Tarrier (eds). *Innovations in the Psychological Management of Schizophrenia*. Chichester: John Wiley & Sons.

Thomas, N., Rossell, S., Farhall, J., Shawyer, F. & Castle, D. (2010). Cognitive behavioural therapy for auditory hallucinations: effectiveness and predictors of outcome in a specialist clinic. *Behavioural and Cognitive Psychotherapy, 39,* 129–138.

Trower, P., Birchwood, M., Meaden, A., Byrne, S., Nelson, A. & Ross, K. (2004). Cognitive therapy for command hallucinations: randomised controlled trial. *British Journal of Psychiatry, 184,* 312–320.

8

Acceptance and Commitment Therapy for Delusions

*José Manuel García Montes, Marino Pérez Álvarez
and Salvador Perona Garcelán*

8.1   Introduction

This chapter describes the psychological treatment of delusions based on
acceptance and commitment therapy (ACT) (Hayes *et al.*, 1999). ACT is one of the
most recent developments in functional contextualism for the treatment of a
diversity of problems in outpatients (Dougher & Hayes, 1999; Kohlenberg *et al.*,
1993). Although it was first developed for the treatment of emotional problems
(Zettle & Hayes, 1986), it did not take long for it to spread to the field of psychotic
symptoms (Bach & Hayes, 2002; García-Montes & Pérez-Álvarez, 2001; Pankey &
Hayes, 2003), and there are conceptual, clinical and empirical reasons for its
application in patients with psychosis (García-Montes & Pérez-Álvarez, 2005;
García-Montes *et al.*, 2006).

8.2   Delusions as Ways of Making Contact with Experience

According to the DSM-IV-TR (American Psychiatric Association, 2000), delusions
are 'erroneous beliefs that usually involve a misinterpretation of perceptions or
experiences' (p. 299). Having listed the most frequent types of delusion, the manual
admits that the distinction between a delusion and a strongly held idea is sometimes difficult to make and depends in part on the degree of conviction with

Acceptance and Commitment Therapy and Mindfulness for Psychosis, First Edition.
Edited by Eric M. J. Morris, Louise C. Johns and Joseph E. Oliver.
© 2013 John Wiley & Sons, Ltd. Published 2013 by John Wiley & Sons, Ltd.

which the idea is held despite clear contradictory evidence regarding its veracity (American Psychiatric Association, 2000).

This definition has the advantage of acknowledging that the delusional experience makes a certain sense. When it says that the delusion is 'a misinterpretation of perceptions or experiences', it is offering a sort of functional explanation of the delusion. Some time ago, Maher (1974, 1988, 1999) presented a similar understanding of delusions when he asserted that they are false beliefs that arise as normal responses to anomalous experiences. However, it seems that this type of 'anomalous' experience is present in the general population (Bradbury *et al.*, 2009; Shevlin *et al.*, 2007) and that delusional patients are not characterised by having more anomalous experiences than other groups in the nonclinical population (Bell *et al.*, 2007).

Why then do some people react to certain anomalous experiences by developing delusions and others not? One line of research addresses how patients with delusions arrive at conclusions. Huq *et al.* (1988), using a probabilistic reasoning task, found that patients with delusions need less information for decision-making and that, furthermore, they appear to be more confident that their decision is right. This has been called the 'jumping-to-conclusions' bias, and has been replicated a number of times in this client group (Dudley *et al.*, 1997; Moritz & Woodward, 2005). It has also been observed that this bias is related to intolerance of uncertainty (Bentall & Swarbrick, 2003).

Even though this analysis is interesting in terms of psychological processes, other contextual factors influencing the delusional experience cannot be overlooked. According to Myin-Germeys *et al.* (2001), the presence of family members or acquaintances lowers the probability of a person having delusions, while if a person stops their activities, the probability of the symptom appearing is higher. Moreover, the occasions when psychotic patients have delusions are marked by a negative affective state. It has also been highlighted that there is a correspondence between delusions and worrying and the motivations important to the patient at the current point in their lives (Jakes *et al.*, 2004; Rhodes & Jakes, 2000, 2004). So, some delusions can be considered symbolic expressions that employ a different type of metaphor or metonym to refer to a patient's current life experiences.

8.2.1   Delusions as Active Forms of Experiential Avoidance

In view of all this, we think delusions are not just metaphorical understandings of anomalous experiences or complex life situations. Freud (1924) said that delusions are like a patch on a tear in the relationship between the self and the outside world. More recently, Bentall *et al.* (1994) proposed a model of delusions of persecution in which their function is to reduce any discrepancies between the 'real self' and the 'ideal self'. This model has been supported by several empirical studies

(Bowins & Shugar, 1998; Kinderman & Bentall, 1996, 2000; Kinderman *et al.*, 2003; McKay *et al.*, 2007).

Based on Bentall *et al.*'s model, García-Montes *et al.* (2004) proposed that delusions are *'active' forms* of experiential avoidance.[1] According to the canonical definition, experiential avoidance (which we call *'passive' forms* of experiential avoidance here) takes place when a person is not willing to make contact with their private experiences and behaves in a way that attempts to change both the form and frequency of those experiences and the conditions that generate them (Hayes *et al.*, 1996). In passive experiential avoidance, what the patient tries to avoid is the symptom itself (obsessions, anxiety, etc.). In delusions, on the other hand, experiential avoidance, in our opinion, is more elaborate, such that the symptom itself becomes a form of avoidance of some other matter. Delusions are ways of elaborating a reality that does not exist, while at the same time escaping from the one that does. This is especially clear in delusions of grandeur, in which the patient shows themselves and others an image and a social position that are not real and that they are unlikely ever to have. In persecutory delusions there may also be active forms of experiential avoidance related to, for example, guilt the patient feels over certain past behaviour, reversing their position as the author of something reprehensible and making them the victim. All of this, obviously, occurs without affecting passive forms of experiential avoidance that are just as important in maintaining the delusional symptomology, so that avoiding certain thoughts or ideas which the verbal community considers inappropriate may make them appear even more intensely.

The authors of ACT have at least partly picked up on this conception of delusion when they say that, in therapy, delusions are seen 'not so much as a *target* of avoidance, but as *means* of avoidance' (Bach *et al.*, 2006, p. 96, their emphasis). However, as we understand it, the 'active' aspect of delusions must still be stressed: that is, how they serve to not only escape or avoid but at the same time verbally *construct* an alternate reality or world. We think that this distinction between 'active' and 'passive' forms of experiential avoidance is not merely academic. In principle, it aligns with conceptions of psychopathology of diverse origins that underline the distinction between 'neurotic' or 'emotional' disorders and 'psychotic' ones (e.g. Freud, 1924/1993; Jaspers, 1963/1996; Wolpe, 1970). Furthermore, it agrees with research on the role of language in human behaviour developed in the Relational Frame Theory (RFT) paradigm (Hayes *et al.*, 2001). Thus, this differentiation between active and passive forms of experiential avoidance highlights how a person can lose contact with things by pursuing only verbal success (e.g. someone who interprets a fond greeting as a sexual proposition in order to keep up his 'seductive' self-concept). When most severe, these active forms of experiential avoidance can even create insensitivity to the practical consequences of one's behaviour, leading to one becoming installed in a sort of 'private world' where the only thing that is important is to be in agreement with oneself (e.g. if after repeatedly being clearly rejected by someone who does not want to have an intimate relationship, the person believes they were really rejected because the other party is afraid to have such a wonderful lover). Finally, the active forms of experiential avoidance emphasise the importance of a psycho-pathological model that situates the patient's symptoms in their biographical context with regard to their personal aspirations (Chadwick, 2006; Chadwick *et al.*, 1997; García-Montes & Pérez-Álvarez, 2003).

8.3   Intervention with ACT

In this section, the six core goals of ACT (Hayes *et al.*, 1999) are briefly described in relation to working with delusions. It should be kept in mind that in our explanations, the order is more logical than chronological, and that in clinical practice, several different aspects can be worked on in the same session, always paying attention to the subjects that are relevant to the patient at any given time. Several clinical dialogues taken from an intervention with a 19-year-old patient we call Luis are given as examples of the techniques. Luis was diagnosed with 'delusional disorder' 1 year before he came to the office for the first time. He is the younger son in a family that currently consists of his mother and older brother, living in the south of Spain. Luis's father died suddenly 8 months before his psychological problems appeared, while on vacation in the Canary Islands. During the time between his father's death and the onset of his psychological problems, Luis was fired from his job, which he had held while studying, because of staff cuts. Also during that time, his girlfriend broke off their relationship of over 2 years. At the time we saw Luis, he showed paranoid ideation related to his persecution by the secret service, which also involved several celebrities (mainly famous musicians).

8.3.1   Create a State of Creative Hopelessness

This goal attempts to help the patient establish contact with the strategies that they have been using to escape from the situation they are in, but which in the end have proven fruitless.

One way to start could be to ask the patient to think about everything they have done to try and live a better life. It is important for the therapist to recognise both the sense that these attempted solutions make to the patient and their desire to carry them out (Bloy *et al.*, 2011). The following dialogue illustrates this validation and provides a metaphor that can be used to help the patient realise the results of the strategies they have put into practice:

THERAPIST: I've taken note of everything you have done to get out of your situation. It all sounds rather logical to me. For example, you've tried to look for proof that the secret service is after you. Surely anyone who believed that would also try to find proof to find out for sure whether they are really looking for him. And I don't doubt that you want to get out of this situation. However, something doesn't make sense to me.

LUIS: What?

THERAPIST: You see, what you have done is quite logical and I am sure that you have tried hard, but what doesn't make sense is that, even though they are logical decisions made with good intentions, you are not getting good results. You are getting more and more closed in, more afraid... Your situation reminds me of a friend I had at school who was afraid of dogs. One day when she was going to school with her lunch in her bag, a dog started following her as soon as she left the house. My friend was so afraid that, to keep the dog away, she gave it a piece of her lunch. The dog stopped to eat it and my friend went on her way to school. But do you know what happened the next day when she went to school?

LUIS: The dog was there again?

THERAPIST: That's right! The dog was there again! And do you know what my friend did?

LUIS: She gave him some of her lunch again.

THERAPIST: Almost! She had to give it *two* pieces, and, of course, it kept on following her. Do you know what happened the next day?

LUIS: The dog was there again?

THERAPIST: That's right. The dog was there again. My friend was having more and more trouble with the dog and finally she stopped going to school. Do you see what I am trying to tell you?

As suggested by Hayes *et al.* (1999), it can be hard for patients to 'understand' things. Their 'understanding' usually translates into what has been said being incorporated into the control strategies they are already using and which have led them to the situation they are in. So it might be advisable to highlight paradoxes that keep rules from being followed. The clinical dialogue would be something like this:

THERAPIST: A serious problem we have is that, to begin with, you've come here to get something to feed the dog...

LUIS: Well... I came because I can't stand this situation anymore...

THERAPIST: That's right... and, in the past, every time you've felt like you couldn't stand it anymore you've done something to calm yourself down... Given the dog some lunch...

LUIS: Yes...

THERAPIST: So, anything that I told you now, any clue that I gave you, might be used to feed the dog...

LUIS: I don't understand exactly what you are trying to tell me.

THERAPIST: Perfect! Maybe the fact that 'you don't understand' might be something different from feeding the dog... Let's see what happens...

This is intended to make the patient come into emotional contact with uncertainty. Patients with delusions, as we have mentioned, are characterised by very low tolerance to uncertainty (Bentall & Swarbrick, 2003), so this stage of therapy would work equally well as exposure therapy. Additionally, as Baruch *et al.* (2009) said so well, 'the therapeutic relationship also provides a context in which *in vivo* interpersonal behaviors may be evoked and addressed' (p. 243). Such techniques should always be used within a safe therapeutic relationship. The bottom line is that the patient has to find out that there are different ways of reacting to uncertainty and that the therapist is not going to require them to do anything in particular in situations or experiences that are difficult for them to understand or which do not lend themselves to rational analysis.

8.3.2   Clarify and Strengthen the Patient's Values

When this point is undertaken, it should be kept in mind how the psychotic patient's values may be characterised by what Stanghellini (2001) has called '*antagonomy*'; that is, by a:

> … refusal to conceptualize the world through the simplifying views given by common sense. Since conventional knowledge is experienced as a dangerous source of loss of individuality, their rejection manifests itself as the deliberate attempt to disconnect oneself from the others in which conventionality is embodied (p. 214).

Due, then, to this desire for 'specialness' and 'individuality', it could be said that individuals with delusions, and patients with psychosis in general, are the opposite of patients with emotional disorders. If they have not found anything worth resisting their discomfort for, they maintain a 'hard core of values' which lead them to rectify their own reality to accommodate the ideals that provide them with a sense of identity. Therefore, in the case of patients with delusions, the difficulty is not so much that they lack values as that these values are disconnected from their practical realisation in the world. Thus, in this field of values, the basic goal with this client group should be to seek ways in which they can convert their ideal values into pragmatic matters. A metaphor which might illustrate the implementation of this in therapy would be the following:

THERAPIST: Since you like Arabian architecture, can you tell me about a building or monument you especially value?
LUIS: I like the Alhambra in Granada a lot.
THERAPIST: Good. Then imagine that you are one of the architects put in charge of building the Alhambra in Granada. You and your fellow architects have drawn the plans. It is a monumental design. Perfect. But how do you go about it making it? What elements do you need to build it?

LUIS:	Stones, no?
THERAPIST:	Exactly, but stones are not beautiful, are they? Do you think stones are as beautiful as the Alhambra?
LUIS:	No, of course not.
THERAPIST:	Imagine that a fellow architect suddenly told you that stones are not sufficiently beautiful and noble to be used in such a majestic building. What would happen?
LUIS:	I suppose we would argue.
THERAPIST:	What would you tell him?
LUIS:	That stones are the only material there is to build the Alhambra with and that if we don't use them we won't be able to build it at all.
THERAPIST:	Good, that's right. Although it is true that stones in themselves are not beautiful. What is beautiful is the form the stones take on when they *make* the Alhambra, no? Does this remind you somehow of your ideal of having an intimate relationship with someone? What are the elements you could use to build intimate relationships with others?

ACT has a values assessment form (Hayes *et al.*, 1999, pp. 224–228) with which a patient can decide the guiding values in their life in a series of areas (intimate relationships, family relations, social relations, etc.), set concrete goals linked to them and finally determine the actions that will enable each of these goals to be met. Any barriers in their achievement will also be identified. Although this specification may have certain advantages, it is also true that it could lead to a certain rigidity in a person's behaviour and keep them from a more dynamic and sensitive adaptation to circumstances that come up. An alternative way of helping a patient come into contact with their values might be the therapeutic dialogue itself, where daily situations in which emotional reactions arise can be discussed. The following clinical dialogue with Luis illustrates how a person can be made more aware of their values:

THERAPIST:	So, you were upset because the lady cut in line in front of you at the supermarket?
LUIS:	Yes, I was really angry. I started to think that she was a secret service agent… and that made me even more nervous. And I started to make a fuss right then and there…
THERAPIST:	Can you tell me about a similar situation in which you felt angry or annoyed, even if it didn't happen this week?
LUIS:	Yes, something similar happened when I was going to take my driving test a few months after my father died. They were calling people out and they didn't call me. I thought the secret service was there again, trying to annoy me, and I started to argue with the examiner…
THERAPIST:	And, for example, when you were a child, were you that upset when someone cut in line?
LUIS:	Yes! A lot! I used to get into a lot of trouble for that!

THERAPIST: It seems like respect for order is very important to you. It also seems like you sometimes get into trouble by trying to make people stay in line. What could you do if someone didn't go to the end of the line and tried to cut in?

It would also be pertinent to emphasise that there are certain behaviours that may not be consistent with one's own values but which nonetheless have to be followed. These are called 'social practices'. These practices, according to the Spanish philosopher José Ortega y Gasset (1883–1955):

> … are human forms of behavior the individual assumes and complies with because, in one way or another, to some extent or other, he has no other choice. They are imposed on him by living together in his surroundings, by 'others', by 'people', by … society (Ortega y Gasset, 1957, p. 76)

A person's values can only be realised in a social medium that is made up of practices. The following clinical dialogue can illustrate the point we want to make:

LUIS: I hate saying hello to people. Friends of my mother come to our house and I have to say 'hello', I have to pretend that I care about them… I feel so false. I'd rather stay in my room.

THERAPIST: Well, imagine that you are out driving on your way to meet a girl you are head over heels in love with. You are a few miles from her house and, suddenly, the police stop you. What would you do?

LUIS: Stop, of course…

THERAPIST: And you wouldn't feel 'false'? Aren't you just doing the opposite of what you feel like doing?

LUIS: But if I didn't stop the car, I would probably end up in jail and it would take even longer to get to see my girlfriend.

THERAPIST: Exactly! Sometimes you have to do things you don't feel like doing and that could, at first, seem to be the opposite of what you want. We've talked about how important your mother is and how important it is to you that she knows and loves you as you really are. It is not a matter of you greeting your mothers' friends because you like to, just as it is not a matter of whether you feel like stopping your car when the police order you to do it… It is enough just to respect the social norms.

Finally, the goals or targets related to the patient's values need to be kept in mind, in that they must be coordinated with the patient's 'real possibilities' and be kept continually present so that the patient does not lose sight of the 'contingencies of life'. This is especially important in the case of patients with delusions (Veiga-Martínez *et al.*, 2004). It is therefore a matter of matching up the person's life goals and the real circumstances of their life. Instead of asking a patient with delusions about their general 'values', use the concrete situations they bring up in sessions to determine their goals. The following dialogue with Luis illustrates how this might be done:

LUIS: I don't know if the teachers or other students are spying on me. When I go to the university some people stare at me for a long time. They could in the secret service, I don't know.

THERAPIST: By the way, how are you doing at the university? Do the classes interest you? Do you like your subjects this year? How's it going?

LUIS: I'm really bored in class and with the other students.

THERAPIST: Do you like any one subject more than the rest? Is there anything that makes you want to go to class? Did they recommend a good book to you? Have you heard an idea that interested you? Did you have subjects in high school that were more interesting than your classes at the university now? When did you enjoy studying most? Did you feel better in summer when you were working at your aunt and uncle's bar?

From here on, the therapist, again using therapeutic dialogue, should discuss possible life goals with the patient, always openly, and keeping in mind that it is the capacity for enthusiasm perceived in the client's behaviour that will make later goals clear.

8.3.3   Suggest the Possibility that the Problem is Control

Now it is time for the patient to realise that there are certain aspects of their experience that it is impossible for them to control. This is done under the premise that 'the cost associated with putting these experiences "in the closet" (emotional avoidance, escape, and numbing) is greater than the damage the original experiences would have done if they were allowed in without defense' (Hayes *et al.*, 1999, p. 115).

One way of presenting the impossibility of controlling certain aspects of life would be to use the polygraph metaphor (see Appendix E) (Hayes *et al.*, 1999, pp. 123–124). The therapist describes the metaphor and the patient is asked to identify situations in their life that are like the polygraph. The therapist could also highlight examples of different emotional problems in other patients in which control strategies have proven counterproductive. The idea would be to take away the specialness of the psychotic symptoms and liken them to emotional problems that are traditionally considered less severe or disabling (Bach, 2004; Pankey & Hayes, 2003). In the case of patients with paranoid delusions, like Luis, it might be worth stressing this metaphor, especially with regard to possible attempts to control fear when paranoid ideas or feelings of failure appear, in which delusions might be a form of avoidance or justification. Patients with delusions of grandeur could especially benefit if the therapy successfully links the metaphor to their feelings of inferiority in certain social situations. In short, it is a matter of establishing the appropriate equivalencies between the polygraph described in the metaphor and active or passive attempts at avoidance of certain experiences, which as discussed, explain the delusional symptomatology as active forms of experiential avoidance.

It would also be fundamental for the therapist to play down the importance of certain private experiences that people usually attribute importance to in order to achieve the kind of life they want. The importance usually given to thoughts as immediate precursors of behaviour could lead patients with delusions to react to the appearance of bizarre ideas with alarm and worry; escape / avoidance behaviour might begin, which would increase the probability of the patient having the same kinds of idea or thought in the future. It would therefore be of use to dedramatise certain bizarre ideas the patient has with an exercise based on self-irreverence. In this respect, García Montes & Pérez Álvarez (2001) have suggested that during sessions, the client be requested to vocalise any strange, wild or out-of-place idea that occurs to them. Luis, for example, was told to say any strange idea that occurred to him. The therapist reacted by encouraging him to intentionally look for other ideas that were even more threatening to him, and in which his safety was more compromised. When Luis said, for example, that not only was the Spanish secret service after him, but that there was a connection with all the European services, this idea was recognised as being much more threatening than the other, but still capable of being surpassed – it was agreed that other, still more intimidating and distressing ideas might occur to him. It might also be beneficial to the patient to write down ideas that occur to them in their daily life and bring them to the next session. The therapist should remind them to bring as many as they can and that the ideas should be very strange. This would favour a 'proximal development zone' between the therapist and the patient (Chapter 10 of Chadwick (2006) for a long discussion of the 'proximal development zone'). It will make it more likely that the patient will limit themselves to making contact with the bizarre ideas they have and will not try to control them, if they see a distant and irreverent attitude in the clinician. While doing this exercise, the therapist should act with respect, avoiding at all times what Bach (2004) calls 'a patronizing position'.

Finally, a metaphor that might be especially useful with patients with delusions is the one known as the 'passengers on the bus' (see Appendix C) (Hayes *et al.*, 1999, p. 157–158). It should be emphasised how easily parallels can be drawn between the person's delusions and the annoyed passengers on the bus. The metaphor also emphasises how important it is to stay in control of the bus (steer towards matters of personal value) even when the passengers are bothering the driver (that is, even with delusions or other bizarre ideas in the way). Once this metaphor has been presented, the client should be asked what they can do. As a general rule, people answer metaphorically with solutions they have used in real life. At this point, it is important for the clinician to try to make the client think about the results of the strategy that they used in practice and whether it was able to 'throw the passengers off the bus'. It is a matter of establishing equivalencies between any solutions the patient might have for the presence of the annoying passengers on one hand and those they puts into practice in their life to try and fight against their delusions or any other type of thought on the other. One solution, for example, that occurred to Luis was to stop the bus until the annoying passengers got off. He was asked whether he had ever put that solution into practice in his life, whether he had somehow stopped his activities until the delusional ideas stopped appearing, and whether in the end he had been able to make the passengers get off the bus. Since the strategies that he had implemented had not had good results, his attention was called to something more important than the passengers: the direction in which the bus was going. Where does the patient want to take the bus? Are they driving it in the direction they want? The therapist can assure them of one thing: if they drive the bus in the direction they want, the passengers will annoy them even more, especially at the beginning. However, if the client decides to steer the bus in a certain direction, it will go in that direction, even if the passengers shout and threaten them the whole time.

8.3.4   Create a Distance from Language

When approaching delusions as active forms of experiential avoidance, we mentioned that the patient places themselves in an alternate or private reality through language. This new reality, which is the delusion, begins to influence the person's behaviour, although to different degrees depending on the case.

In this respect, an exercise that has often been found to be useful in the treatment of psychotic patients (Bach, 2004; García-Montes & Pérez-Álvarez, 2001) is the one known as 'taking your mind for a walk' (Hayes *et al.*, 1999, pp. 162–163). This is a dramatisation exercise in which the patient is separated from their mind. The patient is usually first asked how many people are in the room, to which the patient usually answers two: the therapist and the patient themselves. The therapist comments that there are really four people: the patient, their mind, the therapist and the therapist's mind. The exercise consists of the patient playing themselves and the therapist playing the patient's mind, as they take a walk for about 10 minutes. Afterwards, the therapist plays themselves and the patient plays the therapist's mind, again for 10 minutes. Finally, for another 10 minutes, the patient and the therapist split up and walk alone, and the patient is made to realise that, although no one is representing their mind, it is still functioning: evaluating, warning, criticising, commenting, relating, remembering, interpreting and so on. The purpose of this exercise is to teach the patient to act independently of their mind. In this respect, it is worth mentioning that the exercise involves a certain amount of evaluation of the extent to which the patient is controlled by their delusions. It would be indicative of a high degree of fusion with thoughts if the patient always did what their mind said, or if they always did the opposite. In either case, the patient's behaviour is controlled directly or inversely by the 'mind'. We found with Luis that when the therapist played his mind, he did exactly the opposite of what was suggested to him. If the mind told him not to go to a café because secret service agents were usually there, Luis went to that café; if he was told to cross the street because the person coming towards him was a spy, Luis stayed on the same side of the street and passed by that person. When he came back to the office after the exercise was over, it was explained to him that doing the opposite of what his mind said was still being controlled by it. In the following session, work on creative hopelessness was continued, in an attempt to get Luis to understand that the intervention being proposed was not based on his symptoms, but on the values and goals he pursued in life.

In the same way, it can be helpful for the clinician to give examples of common cases in which a person has a certain thought but does not act accordingly (Bach, 2004). For example, someone who is on a diet may think about eating a piece of chocolate cake and not do it.

8.3.5   Help Create a Transcendental Sense of Self

ACT distinguishes three senses of the self: the conceptualised self, ongoing self-awareness and the observing self (Hayes *et al.*, 1999; Wilson & Luciano, 2002).

It has been mentioned that delusions, especially of persecution, partly compensate for the discrepancy between the 'real self' and the 'ideal self' (Bentall *et al.*, 1994). This is because the delusional person has established an ideal self – a 'conceptualised self' – which is in constant conflict with experience. It is important to develop a sense of the self as an 'observing self', detached from a concrete self-conception, which gives the person a margin for making contact with the varied experiences of life.

A metaphor commonly used for this is the 'chessboard metaphor' (Appendix A) (Hayes *et al.*, 1999, pp. 190–192):

THERAPIST: According to what you've told me, your chessboard does not seem be in the right place. It seems like you are playing the game in an annoying and unpleasant position. In the distance you can see a place where you would like to be playing. But for now you are concentrating more on the game than on where you are playing it. Would you like to change places? Would you like to change your life?

LUIS: Yes. I don't like the way my life is going. I should move, or move the chessboard. What do I have to do to go from being the one who should win the game and move the board?

THERAPIST: Mmmm... I see that you are waiting for me to tell you what the next move the white pieces have to make is.

LUIS: What?

THERAPIST: Could you change without knowing how to do it? Could you move the chessboard when the black pieces are winning?

Another exercise that can be used is the 'observer self' (Hayes *et al.*, 1999, pp. 193–196). This basically involves setting the conditions for the client to make contact with the variety of thoughts, emotions, feelings, roles, appearances and so on that they have had during their life. All this variety has not caused a certain aspect of their identity as a person to be diminished. In spite of such varied states, behaviours and roles, there is something that has remained constant in any experience the client has had: the 'self' that observes the experience. The purpose of this exercise is for the patient to make contact with that experience of personal continuity. To do this, they are asked to sit in a comfortable chair and close their eyes. They are told to make contact with the situation at the present moment. They should note the contact of their body with the chair and with their clothes, with the floor, their breathing, the noises in the room and so on. When they have done this, different situations present themselves. For example, they are asked to remember a moment when they were a child a few years old, and another when they were older; or a time when they were happy and another when they were sad. The important thing is that as the exercise goes on, the client notes that there is something in all of the situations, no matter how contradictory they are, that has remained constant. That 'something' is 'the observer self'. It should be pointed out that the client is not dealing with an 'idea', but an experience.

8.3.6   Developing Willingness

As shown by Bach & Moran (2008), defining willingness is extremely difficult. For a start, according to Hayes *et al.* (1999), willingness is not the same as what one wants. Indeed, a person may not feel like suffering and nevertheless be willing to do so if they thereby achieve something they particularly value. In this sense, willingness assumes a hierarchical order of purposes and confronts a person with the conflictual nature of life. In other words, one's will is always exerted when there are several possibilities for acting, each with certain inevitable costs.

Bach (2004) has stressed the therapeutic possibilities that the 'swamp metaphor' (Hayes *et al.*, 1999, p. 248) and the 'looking for Mr Discomfort' exercise (Hayes *et al.*, 1999, p. 247) have with the seriously mentally ill. The swamp metaphor suggests that the patient has decided to go on a trip somewhere they can see quite clearly, such as a mountain peak that can be seen from the valley where they are now. Sometime after the journey has begun, an enormous foul-smelling swamp comes into sight which will make the journey hard to finish without difficulty, such as getting wet, having to move slowly through the water and so on. However, there is no other choice; if the patient wants to get to the peak, they have to cross the swamp. Obviously, they can also decide not to go on. It could be suggested that life is something like this. We do not go into the swamp because we want to, but rather because we want to get to the peak.

Looking for Mr Discomfort is an exposure exercise recommended for contexts in which problems appear (a walk down the street, going into a shopping mall, etc.). The patient has to look back on their experiences to see what they have been avoiding, so that they can come into contact with the experiences as they are, and even welcome them. When the patient begins to feel these experiences, the therapist should advise them to pay attention to the atmosphere they are in. It is intended that the client learn to exist in the world with the experiences that were blocking them and causing them to retreat to their private world.

It may be easily understood that developing willingness situates therapy in life and incorporates relapses as just one more aspect of it. In fact, it could be said that relapses constitute an essential component of this goal, in as much as they offer an opportunity for willingness to be developed in its own setting: the patient's life. Thus, at the end of the clinical sessions, it was suggested to Luis that the therapy had not really yet begun, and that the true therapy would come from what he did from that time forward in his life. The basic thing is not whether he begins to believe in his delusional ideas again, or whether he tries to control his symptoms; what is really important is whether, when he makes a mistake, he is willing to continue on towards the peak, knowing that there will be another swamp ahead that may also be hard to cross.

8.4　Conclusion

As we have attempted to show, treatment of delusions using ACT is nowhere near simple. It requires the creation of situations in which the client is exposed to experiences that they have been actively avoiding, while keeping up a warm, secure therapeutic relationship. It is a good idea to normalise the delusions, comparing them to another type of symptomology or life experience, but at the same time the desire for 'specialness' and 'individuality' that characterises psychotic patients must be kept in mind. The patient's behaviour should be directed towards the values that are important to them, without this making them too rigid or causing them not to pay attention to present circumstances. We believe that for an intervention to be successful, it is essential that the therapist be convinced that the final goal of treatment is not about symptoms, but that the client redirects their life in a more effective and adaptable manner.

Luis's case shows how changes in the level of belief he gave to his delusions were always preceded by a change in the circumstances in his life. So as Luis began to build up a new relationship, he was gradually able to pass his courses and achieve a new circle of friends. His worries about the secret service began to dissipate, until 2 years later he was able to see them from a completely critical point of view.

Acknowledgement

This work was done in the framework of research project PSI2009-09453, funded by the Spanish Ministry of Science and Technology.

Note

1   In regard to the distinction between 'active' and 'passive' forms of experiential avoidance, following Millon's personality model (Millon, 1969), 'active' should be understood as 'self-initiating' or 'engaging', whereas 'passive' should be understood as 'appeasing' or 'reactive'.

References

American Psychiatric Association (2000). *Diagnostic and Statistical Manual of Mental Disorders* (4th edn, text revision). Washington, DC: Author.

Bach, P. (2004). ACT with the seriously mentally ill. In S. C. Hayes & K. D. Strosahl (eds). *A Practical Guide to Acceptance and Commitment Therapy*. New York: Springer, pp. 185–208.

Bach, P. & Hayes, S. C. (2002). The use of Acceptance and Commitment Therapy to prevent the rehospitalization of psychotic patients: a randomized controlled trial. *Journal of Consulting and Clinical Psychology*, 70, 1129–1139.

Bach, P. & Moran, D. (2008). *ACT in Practice: Case Conceptualization in Acceptance and Commitment Therapy*. Oakland: New Harbinger.

Bach, P., Gaudiano, B. A., Pankey, J., Herbert, J. D. & Hayes, S. C. (2006). Acceptance, mindfulness, values, and psychosis: applying Acceptance and Commitment Therapy (ACT) to the chronically mentally ill. In R. A. Baer (ed.). *Mindfulness-based Treatment Approaches: Clinician's Guide to Evidence Base and Applications*. San Diego: Academic Press, pp. 93–116.

Baruch, D. E., Kanter, J. W., Busch, A. M. & Juskiewicz, K. (2009). Enhancing the therapy relationship in Acceptance and Commitment Therapy for psychotic symptoms. *Clinical Case Studies*, 8, 241–257.

Bell, V., Halligan, P. W. & Ellis, H.D. (2007). The psychosis continuum and the Cardiff Anomalous Perceptions Scale (CAPS): are there multiple factors underlying anomalous experience? *European Psychiatry*, 22(Suppl. 1), S47.

Bentall, R. P. & Swarbrick, R. (2003). The best laid schemas of paranoid patients: autonomy, sociotropy and need for closure. *Psychology and Psychotherapy: Theory, Research and Practice*, 76, 163–172.

Bentall, R. P., Kinderman, P. & Kaney, S. (1994). The self, attributional processes and abnormal beliefs: towards a model of persecutory delusions. *Behaviour Research and Therapy*, 32, 331–341.

Bloy, S., Oliver, J. E. & Morris, E. (2011). Using Acceptance and Commitment Therapy with people with psychosis: a case study. *Clinical Case Studies*, 10, 347–359.

Bowins, B. & Shugar, G. (1998). Delusions and self-esteem. *Canadian Journal of Psychiatry*, 43, 154–158.

Bradbury, D. A., Stirling, J., Cavill, J. & Parker, A. (2009). Psychosis-like experiences in the general population: an exploratory factor analysis. *Personality and Individual Differences*, 46, 729–734.

Chadwick, P. D. J. (2006). *Person-based Cognitive Therapy for Distressing Psychosis*. Chichester: John Wiley & Sons.

Chadwick, P. D. J., Birchwood, M. J. & Trower, P. (1996). *Cognitive Therapy for Delusions, Voices and Paranoia*. Chichester: John Wiley & Sons.

Dougher, M. J. & Hayes, S. C. (1999). Clinical behavior analysis. In M. J. Dougher (ed.). *Clinical Behavior Analysis*. Reno: Context Press, pp. 11–25.

Dudley, R. E., John, C. H., Young, A. W. & Over, D. E. (1997). The effect of self-referent material on the reasoning of people with delusion. *British Journal of Clinical Psychology*, 364, 575–584.

Freud, S. (1924). Neurosis and psychosis. *The Standard Edition of the Complete Psychological Works of Sigmund Freud, Volume XIX (1923–1925): The Ego and the Id and Other Works*. London: Norton, pp. 147–154.

García-Montes, J. M. & Pérez-Álvarez, M. (2001). ACT como tratamiento de síntomas psicóticos. El caso de las alucinaciones auditivas. *Análisis y Modificación de Conducta*, 27, 455–472.

García-Montes, J. M. & Pérez-Álvarez, M. (2003). Reivindicación de la persona en la esquizofrenia. *International Journal of Clinical and Health Psychology*, 3, 107–122.

García-Montes, J. M. & Pérez-Álvarez, M. (2005). Fundamentación experimental y primeras aplicaciones clínicas de la Terapia de Aceptación y Compromiso en el campo de los síntomas psicóticos. *Revista Latinoamericana de Psicología*, 37, 379–393.

García-Montes, J. M., Luciano, M. C., Hernández-López, M. & Zaldívar, F. (2004). Aplicación de la Terapia de Aceptación y Compromiso (ACT) a sintomatología delirante. Un estudio de caso. *Psicothema*, 16(1), 117–124.

García Montes, J. M., Pérez Álvarez, M. & Cangas, A. (2006). Aproximación al abordaje clínico de los síntomas psicóticos desde la aceptación. *Apuntes de Psicología*, 24, 293–307.

Hayes, S. C., Wilson, K. W., Gifford, E. V., Follette, V. M. & Strosahl, K. (1996). Experiential avoidance and behavioral disorders: a functional dimensional approach to diagnosis and treatment. *Journal of Consulting and Clinical Psychology*, 64, 1152–1168.

Hayes, S. C., Strosahl, K. & Wilson, K. G. (1999). *Acceptance and Commitment Therapy: An Experiential Approach to Behavior Change*. New York: Guilford Press.

Hayes, S. C., Barnes-Holmes, D. & Roche, B. (2001). *Relational Frame Theory: A Post-Skinnerian Account of Human Language and Cognition*. New York: Plenum Press.

Huq, S. F., Garety, P. A. & Hemsley, D. R. (1988). Probabilistic judgements in deluded and non-deluded subjects. *Quarterly Journal of Experimental Psychology*, 40A, 801–812.

Jakes, S., Rhodes, J. & Issa, S. (2004). Are the themes of delusional beliefs related to the themes of life-problems and goals? *Journal of Mental Health*, 13, 611–619.

Jaspers, K. (1963). *General Psychopathology* (7th edn) (trans. J. Hoenig & M. W. Hamilton). Manchester: Manchester University Press.

Kinderman, P. & Bentall, R. P. (1996). Self-discrepancies and persecutory delusions: evidence for a model of paranoid ideation. *Journal of Abnormal Psychology*, 105, 106–113.

Kinderman, R. & Bentall, R. P. (2000). Self-discrepancies and causal attributions: studies of hypothesized relationships. *British Journal of Clinical Psychology*, 39, 255–273.

Kinderman, P., Prince, S., Waller, G. & Peters, E. (2003). Self-discrepancies, attentional bias and persecutory delusions. *British Journal of Clinical Psychology*, 42, 1–12.

Kohlenberg, R. J., Hayes, S. C. & Tsai, M. (1993). Radical behavioral psychotherapy: two contemporary examples. *Clinical Psychology Review*, 13, 579–592.

Maher, B. A. (1974). Delusional thinking and perceptual disorder. *Journal of Individual Psychology*, 30, 98–113.

Maher, B. A. (1988). Anomalous experience and delusional thinking: the logic of explanations. In T. F. Oltmanns & B. A. Maher (eds). *Delusional Beliefs*. New York: John Wiley & Sons, pp. 15–33.

Maher, B. (1999). Anomalous experience in everyday life: its significance for psychopathology. *Monist*, 82, 547–570.

McKay, R., Langdon, R. & Coltheart, M. (2007). The defensive function of persecutory delusions: an investigation using the Implicit Association Test. *Cognitive Neuropsychiatry*, 12, 1–24.

Millon, T. (1969). *Modern Psychopathology: A Biosocial Approach to Maladaptive Learning and Functioning*. Prospect Heights, IL: Waveland.

Motiz, S. & Woodward, T. S. (2005). Jumping to conclusions in delusional and non-delusional schizophrenic patients. *British Journal of Clinical Psychology*, 44, 193–207.

Myin-Germeys, I., Nicolson N. A. & Delespaul, P. A. E. G. (2001). The context of delusional experiences in schizophrenia. *Psychological Medicine*, 31, 489–498.

Ortega y Gasset, J. (1957). El hombre y la gente. *Obras Completas, Tomo VII (1948–1958)* (2nd edn). Madrid: Revista de Occidente, pp. 69–272.

Pankey, J. & Hayes, S. C. (2003). Acceptance and Commitment Therapy for psychosis. *International Journal of Psychology and Psychological Therapy*, 3, 311–328.

Rhodes, J. E. & Jakes, S. (2000). Correspondence between delusions and personal goals: a qualitative analysis. *British Journal of Medical Psychology*, 73, 211–225.

Rhodes, J. E. & Jakes, S. (2004). The contribution of metaphor and metonymy to delusions. *Psychology and Psychotherapy: Theory, Research and Practice*, 77, 1–17.

Shevlin, M., Murphy, J., Dorahy, M. J. & Adamson, G. (2007). The distribution of positive psychosis-like symptoms in the population: a latent class analysis of the National Comorbidity Survey. *Schizophrenia Research*, 89, 101–109.

Stanghellini, G. (2001). Psychopathology of common sense. *Philosophy, Psychiatry and Psychology*, 8, 201–218.

Veiga-Martínez, C., Pérez-Álvarez, M. & García-Montes, J. M. (2008). Acceptance and commitment therapy applied to treatment of auditory hallucinations. *Clinical Case Studies*, 7, 118–135.

Wilson, K. G. & Luciano, C. (2002). *Terapia de Aceptación y Compromiso: Un Tratamiento Conductual Orientado a los Valores*. Madrid: Pirámide.

Wolpe, J. (1970). The discontinuity of neurosis and schizophrenia. *Behaviour Research and Therapy*, 8, 179–187.

Zettle, R. D. & Hayes, S. C. (1986). Dysfunctional control by client verbal behavior: the context of reason giving. *The Analysis of Verbal Behavior*, 4, 30–38.

9

Acceptance and Commitment Therapy for Emotional Dysfunction following Psychosis

Ross White

9.1 Introduction

This chapter will focus on the emotional dysfunction that can emerge following psychosis. Even when the symptoms of psychosis have largely remitted, an individual can still experience marked difficulties with their mood. As they adjust to what has been a major life event, the individual is confronted with difficult thoughts about themselves, how others might see them, what has happened in the past and what might happen in the future. A contextual psychology perspective will be provided on how these difficulties emerge, and an acceptance and commitment therapy (ACT) approach will be presented. Key themes that can emerge in an ACT intervention for emotional dysfunction following psychosis will be discussed and suggestions will be made about how to work with these themes therapeutically. Finally, extracts from therapy sessions will be used to elaborate on how this therapeutic work is operationalised in the therapist–client interaction.

9.2 Understanding Emotional Dysfunction following Psychosis

Birchwood (2003) and Tarrier (2005) noted that three forms of emotional dysfunction can commonly occur following psychosis:

Acceptance and Commitment Therapy and Mindfulness for Psychosis, First Edition.
Edited by Eric M. J. Morris, Louise C. Johns and Joseph E. Oliver.
© 2013 John Wiley & Sons, Ltd. Published 2013 by John Wiley & Sons, Ltd.

(1) traumatic responses to the experience of psychosis and/or coercive treatment;
(2) depression;
(3) social anxiety.

The experience of psychosis can induce feelings of intense fear, helplessness or horror (Herring, 1995; Jordan, 1995), which can be sufficiently traumatic to precipitate a reaction similar to post-traumatic stress disorder (PTSD) (Williams-Keeler *et al.*, 1994). Post-psychotic PTSD (PP-PTSD), as it has been described (Shaw *et al.*, 1997, 2002), is associated with the reliving of traumatic events related to the experience of psychosis, avoidance of stimuli related to these events and overarousal. Research has consistently demonstrated an association between PP-PTSD and levels of depression (Harrison & Fowler, 2004; Kennedy *et al.*, 2002; Lu *et al.*, 2011; McGorry *et al.*, 1991; Morrison *et al.*, 1999; White *et al.*, 2009).

Research has shown that several months after an acute episode of psychosis, depression can affect 30–50% of cases (Birchwood, 2003; Whitehead, 2002). Individuals diagnosed with psychosis who develop depression appraise psychosis as an impediment to the attainment of personally valued social roles (loss), a stigmatising experience (humiliation) and a threat to their autonomy (entrapment) (Birchwood *et al.*, 2000, 2006). Depression in psychosis has been linked with an increased hopelessness and likelihood of suicide (Drake *et al.*, 1985; White *et al.*, 2007). Saarni *et al.* (2010) recently concluded that depressive symptoms are the strongest predictor of poor quality of life in psychotic disorders.

Michail & Birchwood (2009) have shown that 50% of individuals who are depressed following psychosis also meet criteria for social anxiety. The hallmark of social anxiety is extreme and persistent fear of embarrassment and humiliation (Schneier, 2003). Rates of social anxiety can be as high as 30% of individuals with first-episode psychosis (Birchwood *et al.*, 2007; Michail & Birchwood, 2009) and between17 and 36% of individuals with multiple episodes of psychosis (Cossof & Hafner, 1998; Pallanti *et al.*, 2004; Tibbo *et al.*, 2003).

9.3   Emotional Dysfunction and Experiential Avoidance

Depression has been shown to be both precipitated and perpetuated by *rumination* (Nolen-Hoeksema, 2000; Nolen- Hoeksema *et al.*, 1993): a form of self-focused attention characterised by a repetitive and passive focus on one's negative emotions (Nolen-Hoeksema, 1991, 2000; Nolen-Hoeksema *et al.*, 1999). Reflecting on the potential function of rumination, Watkins & Mould (2005) claimed that it impedes the activation of distressing emotional and somatic responses. According to Nolen-Hoeksema *et al.* (2008), evidence gathered during rumination can help bring certainty that a situation is hopeless. They propose that this is less aversive than continued uncertainty about the controllability of the situation. The manner in which rumination preoccupies attention means that the individual avoids engaging in the aversive environment that surrounds them (Ferster, 1973; Martell *et al.*, 2001). Cribb *et al.* (2006) proposed that rumination has two avoidant pathways:

(1) *A behavioural pathway.* Rumination is an alternative to engaging in activities that might entail discomfort to the individual.
(2) *A cognitive pathway.* As a mainly 'verbal' process, rumination acts to limit the distressing affect of more concrete image-based thought content.

Worry and rumination share important similarities: both are repetitive, perseverative forms of self-focused thought (Barlow, 2002; Borkovec *et al.*, 2004; Segerstrom *et al.*, 2000) and both are associated with cognitive inflexibility and difficulty in switching attention from negative stimuli (Davis & Nolen-Hoeksema, 2000; Hazlett-Stevens & Borkovec, 2001). Whereas rumination is closely associated with depression, worry is more closely associated with anxiety. Worry tends to be future-orientated and focuses on threats that might occur, whereas rumination predominantly involves past events, and wondering about their causes and implications (Nolen-Hoeksema *et al.*, 2008). Worry can provide an illusion of controllability of the situation (Alloy *et al.*, 1990; Barlow, 1988; Borkovec *et al.*, 1999). As is the case with rumination, researchers have argued that worry has an additional nonconscious function of avoiding confrontation of core negative affect and aversive images (Borkovec, 1979; Borkovec & Roemer, 1995; Borkovec *et al.*, 2004).

9.4 An ACT Conceptualisation of Emotional Dysfunction following Psychosis

Research has highlighted elevated levels of depression, PP-PTSD and social anxiety following psychosis. Furthermore, substantial overlap exists between the phenomenology of these forms of emotional dysfunction; specifically, these difficulties can be characterised by repetitive, perseverative forms of self-focused thought. The overarching theme of the particular repetitive thoughts may differ between PP-PTSD, depression and social anxiety (e.g. thoughts about personal safety, loss, negative evaluation from others), but the level of preoccupation with the thoughts is similar. Stanley Rachman (1997) claimed that the misinterpretation of thoughts as being 'very important, personally significant, revealing and threatening or even catastrophic, has the effect of transforming a commonplace nuisance into a torment' (p. 794). The ACT model adds to Rachman's work by suggesting that the reason particular thoughts are considered 'very important' and 'personally significant' is because of the individual's *values.* In ACT, values are defined as 'a special class of reinforcers that are verbally constructed, dynamic, ongoing patterns of activity for which the predominant reinforcer is intrinsic in the valued behavioral pattern itself' (Wilson & Dufrene, 2009, p. 66).

Values can help make sense of Birchwood *et al.*'s (1993, 2000) aforementioned observation that themes such as *loss, entrapment* and *humiliation* are important for emotional dysfunction following psychosis. These themes are likely to relate directly to life domains that the individual values. For example, an individual's romantic relationship can break down as a result of the occurrence of a psychotic episode. The individual may be stricken with feelings of loss precisely because they value the support and intimacy provided by the relationship. Others may worry that psychosis will limit their independence precisely because they have valued life goals they wish to achieve. Individuals who have experienced psychosis may be upset by stigmatising attitudes towards mentally unwell people precisely because they value being accepted by others.

When particular thoughts mesh with personally held values, importance is attached to the content of these thought processes and people engage in repetitive forms of self-focused thoughts (e.g. rumination or worry). The pervasiveness of these repetitive styles of thinking gives rise to cognitive fusion, whereby the individual defines themselves according to the thematic content of these thoughts (e.g. 'I am defective', 'I am doomed'). This cognitive fusion directs attentional resources away from initiating novel behaviours and promotes psychological and behavioural inflexibility, which serve to limit exposure to sources of threat and/or the possibility of being overwhelmed by levels of affect. Paradoxically, however, this also increases the asynchrony between the individual's behaviour and their values. A vicious circle then develops that serves to maintain the emotional dysfunction that the person is experiencing. Consistent with these claims, we have demonstrated that psychological flexibility (as assessed by the Acceptance and Action Questionnaire (AAQ-II); Bond *et al.*, 2011) significantly predicts large proportions of variance in the depression and anxiety scores of individuals who have experienced psychosis (White *et al.*, 2012a). An individual's experience of psychosis, the particular valued life domains that are threatened and the behavioural routines that are restricted all interact in a dynamic fashion to determine what particular form of emotional dysfunction develops: depression, PP-PTSD and/or social anxiety.

9.5   Treating Emotional Dysfunction following Psychosis

Although Wykes *et al.*'s (2008) meta-analysis found a moderately strong effect size of cognitive behavioural therapy for psychosis (CBTp) on *mood*, when studies with 'poor' methodological quality were controlled for the weighted effect size was not significant. The 'psychological flexibility' that ACT aims to facilitate makes it an obvious candidate for addressing the experiential avoidance that characterises the emotional dysfunction that can follow psychosis. Our feasibility study of ACT for emotional dysfunction following psychosis found that a significantly greater proportion of the ACT group than of a treatment-as-usual (TAU) group changed from being depressed at time of entry into the study to not being depressed at 3-month post-baseline follow-up (White *et al.*, 2011). These results are consistent with those of Gaudiano & Herbert (2006), who found a marginally significant impact of ACT – relative to enhanced TAU – on mood, as assessed by the Brief Psychiatric Rating Scale (BPRS) affect sub-score. Our case-series study of individuals with psychosis who had clinically important levels of depression found that 75% of these individuals had clinically significant changes in levels of depression following an ACT intervention (White *et al.*, 2012b).

9.5.1   Socialising the Individual to the ACT Model

In using ACT to treat emotional dysfunction following psychosis, we have found the *Matrix* approach developed by Polk & Webster (2011) to be very helpful in explaining to individuals the treatment rationale and building a formulation of their presentation. The beauty of this approach lies in its simplicity. The grid template, which is formed from two axes (one distinguishing between five-sense experience and mental experience, the other distinguishing between values and sufferings), creates a comparatively jargon-free context in which all aspects of the ACT hexagon of psychological flexibility (or *hexaflex*; Hayes *et al.*, 2004) can be explored. The Matrix method highlights the tension that exists between the struggle to move away from suffering on the one hand, and the move towards whatever it is that the individual values in life on the other. Suffering and values are presented as two sides of the same proverbial coin; what we consider important in life (e.g. feeling accepted by others, playing a particular sport or musical instrument) exposes us to the risk that we might fall short or lose out (e.g. we might be criticised by others, or have a bad performance).

9.5.2   Assessment and Formulation

The Matrix is divided into four quadrants, which can be used as points of focus during the assessment process:

(1)   Areas of difficulty experienced by the patient (suffering list).
(2)   Strategies that the patient has employed to combat these difficulties (attempts to solve suffering).
(3)   Themes and principles that guide the patient's behaviour (valued life direction).
(4)   Goals the patient can work towards that are consistent with these values (valued action).

Information relating to each of these quadrants provides a diagrammatic formulation of the individual's presentation. This formulation should be seen as an evolving, dynamic process that is reviewed and amended throughout the course of treatment. A formulation example is provided in Figure 9.1. This relates to a man

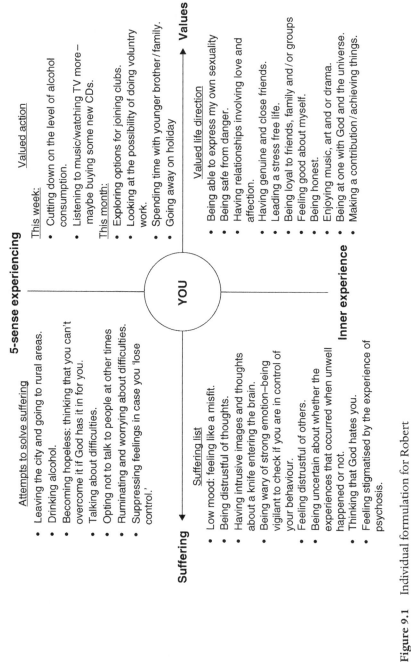

5-sense experiencing

Attempts to solve suffering

- Leaving the city and going to rural areas.
- Drinking alcohol.
- Becoming hopeless: thinking that you can't overcome it if God has it in for you.
- Talking about difficulties.
- Opting not to talk to people at other times
- Ruminating and worrying about difficulties.
- Suppressing feelings in case you 'lose control.'

Valued action

This week:
- Cutting down on the level of alcohol consumption.
- Listening to music/watching TV more – maybe buying some new CDs.

This month:
- Exploring options for joining clubs.
- Looking at the possibility of doing voluntry work.
- Spending time with younger brother/family.
- Going away on holiday

Suffering → → **Values**

YOU

Suffering list

- Low mood: feeling like a misfit.
- Being distrustful of thoughts.
- Having intrusive images and thoughts about a knife entering the brain.
- Being wary of strong emotion–being vigilant to check if you are in control of your behaviour.
- Feeling distrustful of others.
- Being uncertain about whether the experiences that occurred when unwell happened or not.
- Thinking that God hates you.
- Feeling stigmatised by the experience of psychosis.

Valued life direction

- Being able to express my own sexuality
- Being safe from danger.
- Having relationships involving love and affection.
- Having genuine and close friends.
- Leading a stress free life.
- Being loyal to friends, family and/or groups
- Feeling good about myself.
- Being honest.
- Enjoying music, art and or drama.
- Being at one with God and the universe.
- Making a contribution/achieving things.

Inner experience

Figure 9.1 Individual formulation for Robert

in his 40s named Robert (not his real name), who became unwell with psychosis in his early 20s. His last psychotic episode occurred approximately 5 years ago, coinciding with the end of a long-term relationship. Following the end of the relationship, he stopped taking medication and lost contact with his community mental-health team. He recalls experiencing paranoid symptoms at that time and believing that the radio was sending him messages. His mother had long-standing mental-health difficulties and was very disabled by her illness.

9.5.2.1 Suffering List

In assessing the sources of suffering that are of relevance to emotional dysfunction following psychosis, it is important to bear in mind the work of Birchwood and colleagues, which highlighted the important roles of loss, entrapment and humiliation in the experience of psychosis. The following questions will be helpful:

- 'What do you think caused the psychosis?' Care should be taken to explore spiritual or religious beliefs that might have important overlaps with the individual's value system.
- 'Following the psychosis, what ambitions do you worry you might not be able to achieve?'
- 'What events related to your experience of psychosis upset you the most?'
- 'Are you able to talk to other people about your experience of psychosis? How have they reacted?'
- 'What do you think other people think about you? How do you think this has changed?'
- 'Do you worry about the psychosis coming back? Can you tell me what particular worries you have?'

If the person continues to experience residual positive symptoms, it could be helpful to explore these:

- 'What upsets you most about these experiences?'
- 'What do you think those experiences prevent you from feeling or doing?'

With individuals experiencing their first episode of psychosis, it will also be important to assess any stressors that might have predated, or coincided with, the emergence of the psychosis. These factors may continue to exert an influence on the individual over and above factors related to their experience of psychosis.

The following extract from an ACT therapy session with Robert provides some insight into the nature of his struggle:

ROBERT: I mean, I was trying to think how could I describe the last 23 years of medication, and hospitalisation, and subsequent lifestyles that I've become involved in and I would have to say that basically it's been 23 years of physical, psychological and sexual abuse, and it's just going on and on and it never ends.

9.5.2.2   Attempts to Solve Suffering

Individuals may describe a variety of strategies that they have used to try and get rid of their suffering. The therapist should compassionately acknowledge the functionality of maladaptive coping strategies, while simultaneously facilitating the individual to explore the longer-term viability of these strategies. For example, drinking alcohol or using illicit drugs can provide short-term relief from low mood and/or anxiety, but can also lead to further problems if left unchecked. Care should be taken to explore whether the individual has contemplated suicide. As mentioned before, the risk of suicide in individuals who have experienced psychosis is particularly high. Compared to more conspicuous features of psychosis, such as positive symptoms, difficulties such as depression, hopelessness and suicidal ideation can develop insidiously, without drawing much clinical notice.

Attention should also be paid to attempts that the individual might have made to suppress unwanted thoughts. Research has indicated that this can have the paradoxical effect of increasing the intrusiveness and frequency of these thoughts (see Purdon, 1999; Salkovskis *et al.*, 1998). As the French Renaissance philosopher Michel de Montaigne remarked, 'nothing so fixes something in the mind as the wish to forget it'. Thus trying to control thoughts is part of the problem, not the solution. A variety of classic ACT metaphors can be used to elaborate on this, including the 'pink elephant' and the 'quicksand' (see Appendix F) metaphors (Hayes *et al.*, 1999).

9.5.2.3   Valued Life Direction

As noted earlier, the Matrix approach to ACT formulation makes much of the close association between values and suffering. By implication, the suffering list can therefore provide an insight into what values might sit below an individual's suffering. The following extract from a therapy session demonstrates the relationship between Robert's suffering and his values:

ROBERT: Six months ago I changed my medication under supervision to a new medicine. This new medication gave me severe chest pains, and after a few days of agony I phoned an ambulance and was taken to hospital, and kept in for a few days' monitoring. The medication was changed back to the original, and after a few weeks the pains were gone. At the time I was very worried about dying of a heart attack, and also, funnily enough, dying alone in my flat, where I might not have been discovered for weeks. Since then I have been worrying about my fitness and general health.

THERAPIST: As we sit here and think about that, how's it making you feel?

ROBERT: It was very hard, I find it very upsetting. I remember I phoned the ambulance, I thought I was gone. I really did. I was having breathing difficulties. And that was running through my mind all the time: I'm going to die here alone, and my body might not have been found for weeks. I thought it was kind of tragic. And yet, why worry if you die alone or in a crowded room full of people? The result is the same, isn't it?

THERAPIST: What do you think is tragic about that? What makes that scenario so tragic?

ROBERT: I keep in touch with my parents, so after a few weeks, maybe two, three, four weeks, they would obviously become concerned because I hadn't contacted them, and what happens? They phone the police, who would come and kick the door in. They would find my body in a kind of dirty, musty flat. They would do a post mortem, they would interview the neighbours: 'What was he like? Was he a loner?' 'He never had any friends or anything.' Just a tragic waste, if you like.

THERAPIST: Waste. Now, that seems to be important, because it's generating some of the heat upwards. This idea about waste: 'What a waste that would be...' We could get caught up worrying about that: 'My life, is it wasted? Is it not?' Is there maybe also a value related to that? The other side of that coin is perhaps...

ROBERT: I guess it's maybe that I want to have made a difference.

To assist with the assessment of values, Ciarrochi *et al.* (2008) produced a set of cards which individuals can sort into three piles: 'not at all important to how I live my life', 'maybe important to how I live my life' and 'definitely important to how I live my life'. We used these cards in our recent case-series study of individuals with psychosis who were experiencing clinically significant levels of depression (White *et al.*, 2012b); 50% or more identified the following values as 'definitely important' to how they wanted to live their lives:

- feeling good about myself;
- having relationships involving love and affection;
- being loyal to close friends and family;
- having genuine and close friends;
- being honest;
- being safe from danger.

In some respects, these values are almost startling in their ordinariness. It is highly likely that these values would overlap markedly with those held by the majority of people who have never experienced psychosis.

Therapists should also be vigilant to the possible development of *value-fusion*. Thinking about values should be appetitive, expansive and empowering, not aversive. Be vigilant for individuals making statements that begin with 'I must...', 'I have to...', 'I should...' Language of this type can often emerge in individuals with psychosis, who may have histories characterised by unrelenting standards and criticism from themselves and/or others. Individuals should be facilitated to think of value-consistent behaviour as something 'I can...' engage in.

It might be helpful to provide individuals with a sheet briefly summarising the values that they have identified as personally important and actions that they can perform this week, this month and this year which will be consistent with these values.

9.5.2.4   *Valued Action*

It may be that individuals who have been unwell for long periods of time have become particularly distant from their values. Consequently, discussions about engaging in value-consistent behaviour and pursuing goals might feel threatening; concerns about being able to cope may show up. Individuals may also express feelings of loss as they come to the realisation that years of struggling with their suffering have detracted from their ability to engage with what they value in life. Concerns of this type should be noted as additional sources of suffering and added to the suffering list. As with the other entries on this list, time should be spent exploring the workability of struggling with this suffering. Experiencing worry and anxiety is part of the human experience. If we are going to feel anxious and get worried, why not experience these feelings while being true to our values?

As is always the case when using ACT, care should be taken to draw a distinction between values and goals. Values should be explained as a direction of travel, rather than a destination. A value is not something that is achieved, nor completed. If someone values their physical health, for example, this does not mean that they will ever reach a point of absolute physical fitness. Goals, on the other hand, are mile markers that can be reached as one moves in a valued direction. So, someone who values their physical health might set the goal of going to the gym twice a week. They may or may not achieve this goal, but the value remains. Some individuals will be able to readily identify value-consistent goals that they can work towards, while others may require support with this. We have found that using SMART criteria (**S**pecific, **M**easurable, **A**ttainable, **R**elevant and **T**ime-limited) when identifying goals can prove helpful, as can regular reviews of progress.

9.5.3   Beyond Formulation: Progressing with the ACT Intervention

ACT therapists utilise a range of different metaphors and analogies to help explain the therapeutic processes that the therapy espouses. We have found that using an allegory or extended metaphor that incorporates different ACT metaphors into a coherent story can help individuals remember the material discussed. Using a third person in the form of the allegory's central character is a safe way to allow them to reflect on the content of their therapy. We have found that individuals are able to draw parallels between the character in a story and their own experience. The story that we have developed for this purpose is called 'See the Wood for the Trees' (see Appendix F). It charts the progress of Jeremy, who is lost in the rainforest and has to find his way back to civilization. Throughout 'See the Wood for the Trees', various scenarios are used to facilitate reflection and discussion on the six ACT processes of acceptance, defusion, contacting the present moment, self-as-context, values and committed action. The story is also compatible with the Matrix style of formulating cases.

9.5.3.1   *Showing Up to Distress*

Throughout the course of therapy, an important issue will be to address avoidant patterns of behaviour by supporting the individual to *show up* to their distress. The therapist should compassionately empathise with the individual's attempts to avoid negative affect, while simultaneously working with them to explore the life-limiting effect that avoidance can have in valued life domains. Justification for this approach is based on the understanding that vulnerability is the price of admission to a vital and meaningful life. If we are to be true to what is important to us, we will inevitably expose ourselves to some risk. Helping the individual to embody an emotion can be an effective strategy for promoting acceptance of difficult emotional experience. The individual is asked to identify where in their body they feel particular emotions.

In the following extract from a therapy session, the therapist works with Robert to help him sit with the emotion that he is experiencing:

THERAPIST:	As we sit and talk about 'miserable experiences', about 'devastating experiences'... I liked that analogy about being a boxer and going into the ring with your hands tied, while everybody else seems to have their hands free... as we sit here and talk about that, what do you feel in your body? Can you place those feelings in your body anywhere?
ROBERT:	In my stomach.
THERAPIST:	Okay. What is that like?
ROBERT:	A kind of like nauseating feeling. But before you talked to me about where you feel your mental pain... I never really thought about it before, and if I get into certain situations where I feel inadequate or nervous, I feel as if I'm going to lose control of my bowels. So it's almost in my stomach and stuff.

9.5.3.2   *Defusion*

Once the individual has started to explore in greater depth the thoughts and emotions they are experiencing, this creates a platform for them to begin to experience these thoughts and emotions in a different way. A defusion exercise that we have found to be helpful in dealing with ruminative or worrying thoughts is the 'word-processing analogy'. The individual is asked to hold a particular thought that they identify as distressing in their mind. They are asked to imagine that they have typed this thought as a sentence on a computer screen using word-processing software, and that they can manipulate the text using the software – changing the font size, colour and style, for example. This can actually be done in session on a laptop. The individual is asked to imagine that the word-processing software has a 'mind-check' facility that places a purple-dotted line under the text of their thought to emphasise that this is their mind speaking and that it is not a fact.

In the following extract from a therapy session, Robert reflects on his growing capacity to change the context in which he experiences thoughts and how this is serving to reduce the level of distress associated with these thoughts:

THERAPIST: It's good to get in touch with these feelings. Again, what we're doing is we're showing up to the feeling, we're showing up to the emotion. We're being curious about where we feel it in our body. And I know that anger has been something that has concerned you recently; some of the things that we talked about before were worrying about losing control, if you ever were to get angry... about how you would feel about that.

ROBERT: Yeah, I've been thinking about that in terms of the worst thing that I think psychiatry or my 23 years of psychiatry have given me is a fear of my own thoughts. And I think that is the thing that I'm most upset about. Because if you fear your own mind, then... I mean, you can be concerned about what you're thinking about, that's not a good way to think, but to actually be scared of it... I mean, I described to you some of these thoughts I get about maybe a knife entering my brain, that thought scares me. Whereas I was never bothered with it before... I never had thoughts like that before. And I think that's the worst aspect of my experience: to be actually scared of your own mind. Because if you're scared of your own mind and you're not sure of your mind, it makes the whole world seem like a lottery; that anything could happen, anything is possible and anything could happen. And usually when you say anything could happen, it's usually of a bad nature. But I can see, also, on the flipside of that if you like, I can see what ACT is trying to do for me. I've now got to accept that I have these thoughts, which I never had before. But I can play about with them. I can't get rid of them, but I can play about with them. So sometimes now when I get a thought like that, I try and imagine what you said about the computer screen, you can make it big, small, so I try and imagine reducing it just to a dot, so it's just a dot in my mind. And I think that helps, because it means it's not, it's not a big issue is it, it's just a dot.

9.5.3.3   *Mindful Acceptance*

We have found that practising mindfulness exercises can be helpful for individuals who are struggling with distressing thoughts about the experience of psychosis. Mindfulness exercises can be used to develop an individual's *self-as-context* capacity by helping them to notice how unruly and tangential the mind can be. The rationale for using these exercises can be explained in terms of developing the 'spectator part of the mind', which we can all use to examine what we are thinking. Allowing distressing thoughts to come and go while simultaneously bringing awareness back to the sensations of breathing through mindfulness exercises has been shown to be safe and acceptable for individuals with psychosis (Chadwick *et al.*, 2009; White *et al.*, 2011). Enhancing an individual's capacity to notice distressing recurrent thoughts while not getting caught up in reacting to them is an important step in helping them let go of the struggle with suffering. This opens the possibility of the individual orientating instead to what it is that they value in life. They should be encouraged to ask themselves, 'If I wasn't spending my time trying to get rid of these difficult experiences, what would I be doing?' They should be asked to consider the possibility that they can tolerate these experiences and still do what is important to them.

9.5.3.4 *Worries about Psychosis Recurring*

Individuals who express worries about becoming unwell in the future should be helped to identify specific concerns they might have (e.g. not being able to cope with the symptoms, having to take a long time off work). Worries of this type can lead to the development of a defensive posture, in which the agenda is set by attempts to avoid becoming unwell and being perceived as abnormal. During therapy, individuals should be supported to explore ways in which the agenda can instead be set by attempts to work towards optimising mental *wellness*. This is a much more inclusive aspiration, in that it is shared by the vast majority of people. Discussions of this type will help to operationalise what mental wellness means to the individual (e.g. helping and supporting others, feeling relaxed and refreshed, getting a good work–life balance). Talk can then centre on supporting the individual to engage in behaviours consistent with these particular values. To facilitate acceptance of particularly difficult worries about becoming unwell again in the future, and to help the individual see the values beneath these worries, the individual could be encouraged to assign specific fears to specific keys on a key ring. Each time the individual uses a particular key, they should be asked to bring the worry to mind, to notice that it is there, and to appreciate that just as a key can lock a person up, it can also set them free. It is because the future is important to them that they are worried about it. Energy should be invested in optimising mental wellness, rather than shutting themselves away from the risk of future suffering.

9.5.4 Moving Beyond the ACT Intervention

Liaising particularly closely with an individual's named nurse or support worker in the closing phases of therapy will be important. Therapists may wish to explore the possibility of seeking consent from the individual to invite their key worker to the last couple of sessions. That way, the key worker can be present during the review of the therapy and can hear about the future plans that have been identified for the pursuit of value-consistent goals. Liaising with community organisations and vocational schemes will also be invaluable in helping the individual identify goals related to their valued activities, such as music, physical exercise, gardening

an so on. In their final sessions, we have found it helpful to have individuals summarise the key points that they have taken from therapy. These can then be typed
up by the therapist to serve as a staying-well plan for the future.

9.6   Conclusion

In Section 9.2, we proposed that emotional dysfunction (e.g. depression, fear,
worry) following psychosis is the result of psychological and behavioural rigidity
that serves to minimise exposure to further sources of threat and / or the possibility
of being overwhelmed by levels of affect. Fusion with thoughts linked to themes
such as loss, entrapment and humiliation gives rise to restrictive and avoidant
patterns of behaviour that have the maladaptive consequence of producing a
discrepancy between the individual's behaviour and their values. This serves to
maintain the emotional dysfunction.

We presented growing research evidence in support of the notion that ACT
offers promise for treating emotional dysfunction following psychosis. We highlighted Kevin Polk and colleagues' Matrix approach as an effective way of formulating these difficulties. This approach draws on the distinction between the
struggle to move away from suffering on the one hand, and the move towards
what is valued in life on the other. Extracts from therapy sessions were used to
demonstrate how ACT-related processes can be operationalised to facilitate an
individual to relate differently to distressing thoughts that they have been experiencing. The importance of helping individuals to behave in ways that optimise
their mental wellness was highlighted as a way of reducing self-stigmatisation and
worries about becoming unwell in the future. Finally, it was suggested that working closely with other members of the multidisciplinary team and / or community
schemes to support the individual to engage in personally valued activity and
achieve associated goals would be important to translating the skills acquired during therapy into changes in an individual's day-to-day life.

References

Alloy, L. B., Kelly, K. A. & Mineka, S. (1990). Comorbidity of anxiety and depressive
    disorders: a helplessness-hopelessness perspective. In J. D. Maser & R. C. Cloninger
    (eds). *Comorbidity of Mood and Anxiety Disorders*. Washington, DC: American
    Psychiatric Association, pp. 499–543.
Barlow, D. H. (1988). *Anxiety and Its Disorders*. New York: Guilford Press.
Barlow, D. H. (2002) *Anxiety and Its Disorders: The Nature and Treatment of Anxiety and
    Panic*. New York: Guilford Press.
Birchwood, M. (2003). Pathways to emotional dysfunction in first-episode psychosis. *The
    British Journal of Psychiatry*, 182, 373–375.

Birchwood, M. & Trower, P. (2006) The future of cognitive-behavioural therapy for psychosis: not a quasi-neuroleptic. *The British Journal of Psychiatry*, 188, 107–108.

Birchwood, M., Mason, R., MacMillan, F. & Healy, J. (1993). Depression, demoralization and control over psychotic illness: a comparison of depressed and non-depressed patients with a chronic psychosis. *Psychological Medicine*, 23, 387–395.

Birchwood, M., Iqbal, Z., Chadwick, P. *et al.* (2000). Cognitive approach to depression and suicidal thinking in psychosis. I: ontogeny of post-psychotic depression. *British Journal of Psychiatry*, 177, 516–528.

Birchwood, M. Trower, P. Brunet, K. Gilbert, P. Iqbal, Z. & Jackson, P. (2007). Social anxiety and the shame of psychosis: a study in first episode psychosis. *Behaviour Research and Therapy*, 45, 1025–1037.

Bond, F. W., Hayes, S. C., Baer, R. A., Carpenter, K. M., Orcutt, H. K., Waltz, T. & Zettle, R. D. (2010). Preliminary psychometric properties of the Acceptance and Action Questionnaire – II: a revised measure of psychological flexibility and acceptance. *Behaviour Therapy*, 42, 676–688.

Borkovec, T. D. (1979). Pseudo(experiential)-insomnia and idiopathic(objective) insomnia: theoretical and therapeutic issues. *Advances in Behaviour Research and Therapy*, 2, 27–55.

Borkovec, T. D. & Roemer, L. (1995). Perceived functions of worry among generalized anxiety disorder subjects: distraction from more emotional topics? *Journal of Behavior Therapy and Experimental Psychiatry*, 26, 25–30

Borkovec, T. D., Hazlett-Stevens, H. & Diaz, M. L. (1999). The role of positive beliefs about worry in generalized anxiety disorder and its treatment. *Clinical Psychology and Psychotherapy*, 6, 126–138.

Borkovec, T. D., Alcaine, O. & Behar, E. (2004). Avoidance theory of worry and generalized anxiety disorder. In R. G. Heimberg, C. L. Turk & D. S. Mennin (eds). *Generalized Anxiety Disorder: Advances in Research and Practice*. New York: Guilford Press, pp. 77–108.

Chadwick, P., Hughes, S., Russell, D., Russell, I. & Dagnan, D. (2009). Mindfulness groups for distressing voices and paranoia: a replication and randomized feasibility trial. *Behavioural and Cognitive Psychotherapy*, 37, 403–412.

Ciarrochi, J. V. & Bailey, A. (2008). A CBT practitioners guide to ACT: how to bridge the gap between cognitive behavioural therapy and acceptance and commitment therapy. Oakland: New Harbinger.

Cosoff, S. J. & Hafner, R. J. (1998) The prevalence of comorbid anxiety in schizophrenia, schizoaffective disorder and bipolar disorder. *Australian and New Zealand Journal of Psychiatry*, 32, 67–72.

Cribb, G., Moulds, M. L. & Carter, S. (2006). Rumination and experiential avoidance in depression. *Behaviour Change*, 23, 165–176.

Davis, R. N. & Nolen-Hoeksema, S. (2000). Cognitive inflexibility among ruminators and nonruminators. *Cognitive Therapy and Research*, 24, 699–711.

Drake, R.E., Gates, C., Whitaker, A. & Cotton, P. G. (1985) Suicide among schizophrenics: a review. *Comprehensive Psychiatry*, 26, 90–100.

Gaudiano, B. A. & Herbert, J. D. (2006). Acute treatment of inpatients with psychotic symptoms using Acceptance and Commitment Therapy: pilot results. *Behaviour Research & Therapy*, 44, 415–437.

Harrison C. L. & Fowler D (2004). Negative symptoms, trauma and autobiographical memory: an investigation of individuals recovering from psychosis. *Journal of Nervous and Mental Disease*, 192, 745–753.

Hayes, S. C., Strosahl, K. D. & Wilson, K.G. (1999). *Acceptance and Commitment Therapy: An Experiential Approach to Behavior Change*. New York: Guilford Press.

Hayes, S. C., Strosahl, K. D., Wilson, K. G., Bissett, R. T., Pistorello, J., Toarmino, D. *et al.* (2004). Measuring experiential avoidance: a preliminary test of a working model. *The Psychological Record*, 54, 553–578.

Hazlett-Stevens, H. & Borkovec, T. D. (2001). Effects of worry and progressive relaxation on the reduction of fear in speech phobia: an investigation of situational exposure. *Behavior Therapy*, 32, 503–517.

Herrig, E. (1995). First person account: a personal experience. *Schizophrenia Bulletin*, 21, 339–342.

Jordan, J. C. (1995). First person account: schizophrenia – adrift in an anchorless reality. *Schizophrenia Bulletin*, 21, 501–503.

Kennedy, B. L., Dhaliwal, N., Pedley, L., Sahner, C., Greenberg, R. & Manshadi, M. S. (2002). Post-traumatic stress disorder in subjects with schizophrenia and bipolar disorder. *Journal of Kentucky Medical Association*, 100, 395–399.

Lu, W., Mueser, K. T., Shami, A., Siglag, M., Petrides, G., Schoepp, E., *et al.* (2011). Posttraumatic reactions to psychosis in people with multiple psychotic episodes. *Schizophrenia Research*, 127, 66–75.

McGorry, P., Chanen, A., McCarthy, E., Van Riel, R., McKenzie, D. & Singh, B. (1991). Post-traumatic stress disorder following recent onset psychosis: an unrecognised post psychotic syndrome. *Journal of Nervous and Mental Disease*, 179, 253–258.

Martell, C. R., Addis, M. E. & Jacobson, N. S. (2001). *Depression in Context: Strategies for Guided Action*. New York: W.W. Norton.

Michail, M. & Birchwood, M. (2009). Social anxiety disorder in first-episode psychosis: incidence, phenomenology and relationship with paranoia. *The British Journal of Psychiatry*, 195, 234–241.

Nolen-Hoeksema, S. (1991). Responses to depression and their effects on the duration of depressive episodes. *Journal of Abnormal Psychology*, 100, 569–582.

Nolen-Hoeksema, S. (2000). The role of rumination in depressive disorders and mixed anxiety/depressive symptoms. *Journal of Abnormal Psychology*, 109, 504–511.

Nolen-Hoeksema, S., Morrow, J. & Fredrickson, B. L. (1993). Response styles and the duration of episodes of depressed mood. *Journal of Abnormal Psychology*, 102, 20–28.

Nolen-Hoeksema, S., Larson, J. & Grayson, C. (1999). Explaining the gender difference in depressive symptoms. *Journal of Personality and Social Psychology*, 77, 101–107.

Nolen-Hoeksema, S., Wisco, B. E. & Lyubomirsky, S. (2008). Rethinking rumination. *Perspectives on Psychological Science*, 3, 400–424.

Pallanti, S., Quercioli, L. & Hollander, E. (2004). Social anxiety in outpatients with schizophrenia. A relevant cause of disability. *American Journal of Psychology*, 161, 53–8.

Polk, K. & Webster, M. (2011). A Hitchhiker's Guide to the Matrix. Workshop presented at the Association for Contextual Behavioral Science World Conference IX, Parma, Italy.

Purdon, C. (1999). Thought suppression and psychopathology. *Behaviour Research and Therapy*, 37, 1029–1054.

Rachman, S. (1997). A cognitive theory of obsessions. *Behaviour Research and Therapy*, 35, 793–802.

Saarni, S. I., Viertiö, S., Perälä, J., Koskinen, S., Lönnqvist, J. & Suvisaari, J. (2010). Quality of life of people with schizophrenia, bipolar disorder and other psychotic disorders. *British Journal of Psychiatry*, 197, 386–394.

Salkovskis, P. M., Forrester, E. & Richards, H. C. (1998). Cognitive-behavioural approach to understanding obsessional thinking. *British Journal of Psychiatry*, 173, 53–63.

Schneier, F. R. (2003). Social anxiety disorder. *British Medical Journal*, 327, 515–516.

Segerstrom, S. C., Tsao, J. C. I., Alden, L. E. & Craske, M. G. (2000). Worry and rumination: repetitive thought as a concomitant and predictor of negative mood. *Cognitive Therapy and Research*, 24, 671–688.

Shaw, K., McFarlane, A. & Bookless, C. (1997). The phenomenology of traumatic reactions to psychotic illness. *Journal of Nervous and Mental Disease*, 185, 434–441.

Shaw, K., McFarlane, A. C., Bookless, C. & Air, T. (2002). The aetiology of postpsychotic posttraumatic stress disorder following a psychotic episode. *Journal of Traumatic Stress*, 15, 39–47.

Tarrier, N. (2005) Comorbidity and associated clinical problems in schizophrenia: their nature and implications for comprehensive cognitive behavioural treatment. *Behaviour Change*, 22, 125–142.

Tibbo, P., Swainson, J., Chue, P. & LeMelledo, J.-M. (2003). Prevalence and relationship to delusions and hallucinations of anxiety disorders in schizophrenia. *Depression and Anxiety*, 17, 65–72.

Watkins, E. & Moulds, M. (2005). Distinct modes of ruminative self-focus: impact of abstract vs. concrete rumination on problem solving in depression. *Emotion*, 5, 319–328.

White, R. G. & Gumley, A. I. (2009). Postpsychotic posttraumatic stress disorder: associations with fear of recurrence and intolerance of uncertainty. *Journal of Nervous and Mental Disease*, 197, 841–849.

White, R. G., McCreery, M., Gumley A. I. & Mulholland, C. (2007) Hopelessness in schizophrenia: the impact of symptoms and beliefs about illness. *Journal of Nervous and Mental Disease*, 195, 968–975.

White, R. G., Gumley, A. I., McTaggart, J., Rattrie, L., McConville, D., Cleare, S. & Mitchell, G. (2011). A feasibility study of Acceptance and Commitment Therapy for emotional adaptation following psychosis. *Behaviour Research and Therapy*, 49, 901–907.

White, R. G., Gumley, A. I., McTaggart, J., Rattrie, L., McConville, D., Cleare, S. & Mitchell, G. (2012a). Depression and anxiety following psychosis: associations with experiential avoidance and mindfulness. *Behavioural and Cognitive Psychotherapy*, in press.

White, R. G., Gumley, A. I., McTaggart, J., Rattrie, L., McConville, D., Cleare, S. & Mitchell, G. (2012b). Acceptance and Commitment Therapy for depression following psychosis: a case series analysis. *Behavioural and Cognitive Psychotherapy*, in submission.

Whitehead, C., Moss, S., Cardno, A. & Lewis, G. (2002). Antidepressants for people with both schizophrenia and depression. *Cochrane Database Syst. Rev.*, 4, 1–40.

Williams-Keeler, L., Milliken, H. & Jones, B. (1994). Psychosis as a precipitating trauma for PTSD: a treatment strategy. *American Journal of Orthopsychiatry*, 64, 493–498.

Wilson, K. G. & Dufrene, T. (2009). *Mindfulness for Two: An Acceptance and Commitment Therapy Approach to Mindfulness in Psychotherapy*. Oakland: New Harbinger.

Wykes, T., Steel, C., Everitt, B. & Tarrier, N. (2008). Cognitive behavior therapy for schizophrenia: effect sizes, clinical models, and methodological rigor. *Schizophrenia Bulletin*, 34, 523–537.

10

Person-based Cognitive Therapy for Distressing Psychosis

Lyn Ellett

10.1 Introduction

Person-based cognitive therapy (PBCT) for distressing psychosis (Chadwick, 2006) is an integration of cognitive theory and therapy, mindfulness and Rogerian principles (particularly acceptance), in which the emphasis is on understanding and reducing clients' distress and promoting their strengths and well-being. This chapter provides an integrated summary of the PBCT approach, beginning with an overview of the zone of proximal development – the central formulation model used in PBCT. This is followed by discussion of case formulation materials (with client examples) and experiential methods of change.

10.2 Zone of Proximal Development

The central formulation model within PBCT is the zone of proximal development (ZoPD), which is used to formulate clients' distress, but also their strengths and positive characteristics. It consists of four subzones: symptomatic meaning, relationship with experience, schemata and symbolic self (see Figure 10.1), and it is defined as 'a social process, whereby with the support of a radically collaborative and skilled therapist, a client eases distress, develops metacognitive insight and achieves self-acceptance through proximal development in all four domains' (Chadwick, 2006). Proximal development occurs through a social and collaborative process; client and therapist work together in each of the four zones, placing equal

Acceptance and Commitment Therapy and Mindfulness for Psychosis, First Edition.
Edited by Eric M. J. Morris, Louise C. Johns and Joseph E. Oliver.
© 2013 John Wiley & Sons, Ltd. Published 2013 by John Wiley & Sons, Ltd.

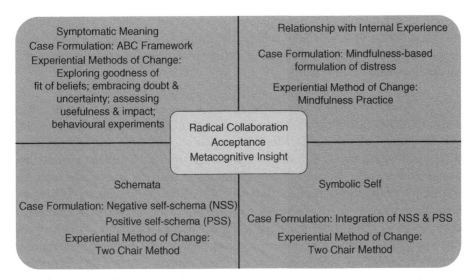

Figure 10.1 Summary of the four zones of proximal development (ZoPD). Adapted from Chadwick (2006).

emphasis on working with strengths and with distress. The zones are intentionally positioned alongside each other, promoting flexibility and movement between them during therapy, rather than 'working through' each one hierarchically. Figure 10.1 is intended mainly for therapists, to help them structure PBCT; case formulation materials that are used with clients and experiential methods of change are listed in each zone. Exploration of all four zones is infused with radical collaboration, Rogerian acceptance and development of metacognitive insights.

10.2.1 Overview of the Zones of Proximal Development

In this section, an overview of each of the four ZoPD is provided, followed by discussion of three processes that are infused across each domain: radical collaboration, acceptance and metacognitive insights.

10.2.1.1 *Symptomatic Meaning*
This domain involves working directly with symptoms, such as paranoia and beliefs about voices (Chadwick *et al.*, 1996). Working within this domain involves collaboratively exploring an individual's ability to decentre from their beliefs, which allows them not only to develop awareness of how their beliefs impact on behaviour and generate distress but also to develop new meaning that enhances well-being. The aim is to explore collaboratively the individual's capacity for proximal development in this domain, as opposed to trying to force change to occur. When working with symptomatic meaning, it can be helpful for therapists to bear

in mind that many clients may not have considered their beliefs in depth before and that working in this domain is likely to involve small change, as opposed to complete shifts in beliefs. All methods of change within this domain support proximal development.

10.2.1.2   *Relationship with Internal Experience*
In PBCT, mindfulness is used as the primary method for working within the relationship domain of the ZoPD. Mindfulness can be used both within individual therapy and within the context of mindfulness groups (see Chapter 16 for discussion of group work). By engaging in mindfulness practice, individuals learn to respond mindfully to psychotic sensations, rather than getting lost in reacting to them; being more aware of psychotic sensations and their impact allows individuals to let go of their usual reactions (e.g. experiential avoidance, rumination), which produce distress. Two main processes support the reduction of distress and enhancement of well-being through mindfulness practice: (1) decentred awareness (Segal *et al.*, 2002) and (2) acceptance of present-moment experience. This is facilitated by reflective learning (in which the role of the therapist is to draw out metacognitive insights) and guided discovery, both prior to and following meditation practice, as well as use of specific guidance during practice. Guidance during meditation and reflective learning both highlight key aspects of experience during meditation practice; for example, that sensations come and go, and that nothing stays in awareness permanently. This facilitates the acquisition of metacognitive insights, as the therapist draws out what the client notices about the nature of sensations and their reactions to them. This helps the client gain awareness of how their relationship to (psychotic) sensations impacts directly on their current emotional state. Decentred awareness and metacognitive insights form the collaborative learning process and enable clients to realise proximal development within the relationship domain of the ZoPD.

10.2.1.3   *Schemata*
In PBCT, working within the schemata domain involves reducing distress directly linked to the individual's negative schema of self and others, and enhancing overall well-being by developing positive self-schema (PSS). There are four aims when working with negative self-schema (NSS) in PBCT. First, that individuals increase their awareness of the nature and characteristics of their negative schematic experience. Second, that both client and therapist accept the NSS (although it is also important to acknowledge that there will be future times when the client's experience of self is overwhelmingly negative and all-consuming). Third, to gain metacognitive insight into the NSS (i.e. that it forms one aspect of the self, not *the entire self*). Fourth, to reduce the fear associated with negative schematic experience. Taken together, these four aims allow a new relationship with the NSS to be developed. When working with PSS, the aim is to collaboratively draw out, maintain and generalise positive schematic experience.

10.2.1.4   *Symbolic Self*

In PBCT, the symbolic self is a metacognitive model that represents an integration of both positive and negative schematic experience of self. The symbolic self brings awareness to, and facilitates acceptance of, the complex and changing nature of the experience of self. While most of us probably have moments of NSS experience, these do not tend to dominate or overwhelm the symbolic self. However, the more a person's experience of self is dominated by negative schematic experience, the more the focus of the symbolic self becomes restricted and overly negative – what Chadwick (2006) refers to as 'one-dimensional'. It is common for the symbolic self of individuals with distressing psychosis to be one-dimensional at the start of therapy; proximal development in this domain therefore involves bringing negative schematic experience into balance and elaborating and enhancing positive schematic experience, thereby 'opening out' the symbolic self and bringing awareness and acceptance of the complex and changing nature of self.

Having considered the four domains of proximal development, the three processes that are infused within each domain will now be discussed: radical collaboration, acceptance and metacognitive insights.

10.2.1.5   *Radical Collaboration (RC)*

In PBCT, the client is positioned at the heart of the therapeutic process; thus the centrality of a person-centred relationship is essential to the process of therapy. The primary task from the outset when working with clients is to develop and establish a radically collaborative relationship. A radically collaborative relationship is one that enables clients to formulate their goals within the context of an open, supportive and collaborative relationship. There are a number of characteristics that support RC, including active listening, supported discovery and open discussion of important issues such as responsibility and choice. In developing and establishing a radically collaborative relationship, it is important for the therapist to 'meet with the person', rather than their problem or symptoms. Therefore, it is essential that the therapeutic relationship is characterised by openness and collaboration. The practice of PBCT and RC is thus supported by several positive assumptions about people with psychosis and the process of therapy. Chadwick (2006) identifies five such assumptions: 'the core of people with psychosis is essentially positive'; 'psychotic experience is continuous with ordinary experience'; 'therapist responsibility is to show radical collaboration and acceptance'; 'effective therapy depends on understanding sources of distress, not sources of psychosis'; and 'therapists aim to be themselves more fully with clients'. RC thus supports a person-centred approach to examining sources of distress and potential for proximal development.

10.2.1.6   *Acceptance*

In PBCT, a central aim is to promote acceptance of unpleasant (psychotic) sensations and self-acceptance. This involves accepting that in this moment, this is my experience, without struggling against it or getting lost in reacting to it (relationship to internal experience zone) or defining the self fully in terms of it (schemata and symbolic self zones). Acceptance is a process of continually bringing mindful awareness to difficult experience, which allows an opening of awareness to all aspects of the self. This directly supports self-acceptance, because acceptance of psychosis means that it no longer defines the entirety of the individual.

It is important to note that acceptance is not just a process that we invite our clients to engage with – it is also embodied by therapists within each domain of the ZoPD. Therapists take on the unconditional acceptance of clients and the entirety of their experience, which includes psychotic experience and fixed beliefs (symptomatic meaning domain); they also accept clients' negative schematic experience (schema domain). This therapist stance facilitates clients' own acceptance of their experiences of psychosis as one facet of the self, rather than the entire self (symbolic self domain).

10.2.1.7   *Metacognitive Insights*

The process of exploring a person's ZoPD involves promoting metacognitive understanding, or insight, in all four domains. For example, when working within the zone of symptomatic meaning, individuals develop metacognitive insights about the nature of cognitive processes (e.g. 'Thoughts are not facts but hypotheses to be tested'). Within the domain of relationship to internal experience, through mindfulness practice, individuals gain metacognitive insights about the nature of experience (e.g. 'Unpleasant psychotic sensations do not stay in awareness permanently') and how their response to it maintains distress (e.g. judgement, rumination etc.). Within the domain of schemata, clients gain metacognitive insights about the nature and impact of NSS. Finally, within the domain of symbolic self, metacognitive insights are expressed through integration of negative and positive schemata, which facilitates acceptance of the complex and changing nature of the self.

10.3   Case Formulation in PBCT

The ZoPD is the central formulation model within PBCT, but there are also case formulation models within each of the four zones. These are summarised in this section, with accompanying client material.

10.3.1   Symptomatic Meaning: ABC Formulation

The main method for formulating symptomatic meaning and experience is the ABC framework. ABC formulation is a way of organising experience that clients find helpful and easy to understand. Use of the ABC formulation is flexible in PBCT – for example, it can be used as part of the assessment process, or to structure discussion of clients' experience. When using ABC formulations, it is important to isolate a specific situation

Table 10.1   Summary of the ABC formulation, with case example of paranoia and voices

	Situation (A) *Situation (e.g. low mood and isolation) and unpleasant psychotic sensation (voice, paranoia, vision)*	*Meaning (B)* *Images, thoughts, beliefs about self and others, beliefs about voices, rules*	*Distress (C)* *Emotion, behaviour, (urge and action), body state*
Example 1	Walking to get to an appointment with GP and notices a group of young people walking towards him.	Other people are unsafe When I am near others, they will try to harm me This is ruining my life I am a bad person	Fear, anxiety, powerlessness Avoids being around others, particularly groups – deliberately crosses the road to avoid the young people Feels tense in body
Example 2	Hears derogatory voice telling him to kill himself.	Voices are evil and powerful My voices control me If I do not do what the voices say, they will get worse	Tries to resist voices Partial compliance through self-harm Anger

in which clients report that distress was high. Therapists are then able to draw out symptomatic meaning (e.g. images, thoughts, beliefs about voices and self, etc.), with associated emotion, behavioural urge/action and body state. Consider the case of Jason, who experienced distressing voices and paranoid beliefs. Jason regularly heard voices telling him to kill himself. He believed the voices were evil and powerful, felt very angry when he heard them and engaged in partial compliance through self-harm. He also experienced a number of paranoid beliefs; for example, when around others, Jason believed they would try to attack him. This resulted in feelings of fear, anxiety and powerlessness and avoidance of others. He felt that he deserved to be persecuted ('bad me' paranoia) because of things that he'd done in the past, and also judged himself as bad as a result of having these experiences. Table 10.1 presents a summary of the ABC formulation, with examples that were developed with Jason during therapy.

10.3.2   Relationship with Internal Experience: Mindfulness-based Formulation of Distress

When experiencing an unpleasant psychotic sensation (voice, paranoid thought, image etc.), distress arises from a lack of clear awareness of what is being experienced due to being lost in reacting to it. Three main reactions have been identified as maintaining distress – experiential avoidance, negative judgement and rumination/confrontation

(Chadwick *et al.*, 2005). Such reactions are a result of clients feeling that they are defined by such experiences and how they react to them. In contrast, responding mindfully to unpleasant psychotic sensations involves maintaining decentred aware-ness while being open to whatever is sensed, without reacting to it or identifying with it. This conceptualises Rogerian acceptance of experience and the self. For example, consider the case of Julie, who heard distressing voices saying 'You're bad, ugly and worthless' and 'You can't do anything right, you'll never amount to anything'. At the start of therapy, Julie tried to avoid/resist her voices, and also avoided engaging in activities for fear of failure. She regularly confronted her voices by shouting and swearing back at them and got lost in depressive rumination about them. She believed what the voices told her and consequently judged herself as bad. Through mindfulness practice, Julie learned to respond differently to her distressing voices, by noting their presence (turning towards the difficult), allowing them to be there (acceptance) and not getting caught up in her usual reactions to them (letting go). Figure 10.2 shows the mindfulness-based formulation that was developed with Julie during therapy.

10.3.3   Negative and Positive Self-schema

The third formulation in PBCT is schemata, both positive and negative. Although schematic beliefs are incorporated into ABC formulations, it is also important to

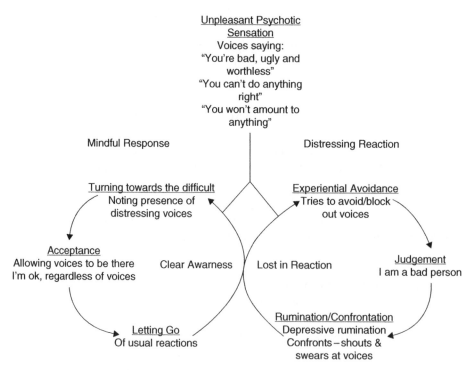

Figure 10.2   Mindfulness formulation of distressing voices. Adapted from Chadwick *et al.* (2005).

formulate them separately, as they are often extremely distressing and disabling. The emphasis when working in this domain is on acceptance of negative schematic experience as part of the self, rather than as defining the entire self. Equal importance is also placed on developing PSS. Within PBCT, formulating positive and negative schemata corresponds with the two-chair method described in Section 10.4.3.1. In addition, the fact that positive and negative experiences of self are formulated using the same basic model facilitates the development of the metacognitive insight that the symbolic self is made up of complex and conflicting experiences. Consider the case of Neil, who had a 10-year history of paranoid beliefs. Neil came to therapy believing that he was inadequate and a bad person, and that others were hostile and out to get him. He thought that others knew that he was unwell and judged him negatively as a result. The future looked bleak and Neil believed that things would never change. Neil was afraid to leave his flat, as he believed that other people might harm him, and in particular might stab him. He would often spend time ruminating when he knew he would have to leave his flat (e.g. to buy food or attend appointments) and he was hypervigilant of others when he did go out. During therapy, a number of rules for living were identified: Neil believed that if he let his guard down around others, and if they knew about his (mental-health) history, they would judge him negatively and potentially harm him. This resulted in sustained periods of isolation and fear, in which he would avoid leaving his flat. Figures 10.3 and 10.4 are examples of Neil's NSS and PSS, which were collaboratively developed during therapy.

10.4 Experiential Methods of Change

10.4.1 Symptomatic Meaning

Within the zone of symptomatic meaning, the key experiential methods of change are: exploring goodness of fit of beliefs, including exploring doubt and generating alternatives; assessing usefulness and impact; and planning and conducting behavioural tests. These are all common cognitive behaviour therapy (CBT) techniques and will be only briefly summarised here as they are discussed extensively elsewhere (see Chadwick *et al.*, 1996).

10.4.1.1 *Goodness of Fit ('Evidence') and Generating Alternative Symptomatic Meaning*
Goodness of fit concerns examining the extent to which an individual's belief, or belief system, captures the entirety of their experience. Within PBCT, the starting point for assessing goodness of fit is always an examination of the reasons behind the individual's beliefs ('evidence for the belief'). Only when a full understanding of the evidence for a belief has been gained can attention then be turned to exploring facets of experience which are less consistent with that belief ('evidence against

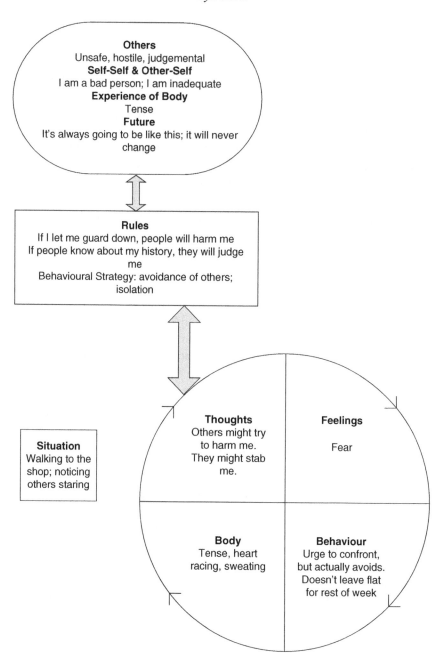

Figure 10.3   Neil's negative self-schema (NSS). Adapted from Chadwick (2006).

the belief'). Part of exploring goodness of fit, or 'evidence', involves collaboratively exploring doubt with clients. This process begins by examining the client's capacity for doubt, and includes the client and therapist offering hypothetical contradictions (offered tentatively), thereby facilitating development of alternative symptomatic

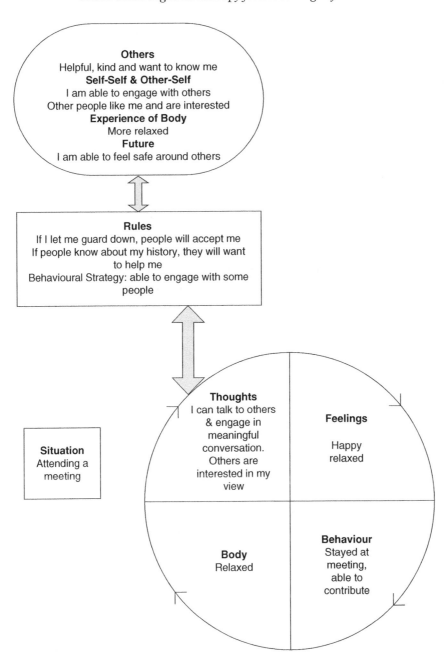

Figure 10.4   Neil's positive self-schema (PSS). Adapted from Chadwick (2006).

meaning. The symptomatic belief and alternative are assessed for consistency with the available evidence (i.e. goodness of fit) and usefulness (i.e. advantages and disadvantages of each). Within PBCT, it is important to encourage clients to fully consider both alternatives.

10.4.1.2   Behavioural Experiments

Behavioural experiments (BEs) are a method for testing hypotheses. They work best when they are formulated by clients and when there are clear predictions for both the symptomatic belief and the alternative. Their effectiveness is determined, at least in part, by the client's ability to be open to the possibility of disconfirmation, as well as confirmation. The effectiveness of any BE is enhanced when the range of outcomes has been carefully considered beforehand. Ultimately, it is the client's choice to decide whether or not to carry out the experiment.

10.4.1.3   Accepting Fixity

Therapists are often faced with the situation of a client's belief being fixed. At these times, it is helpful for the therapist to accept this – in PBCT, acceptance applies to the whole person, which includes their fixed beliefs. Although fixity can often be frustrating for therapists, it is actually informative: it reveals to the therapist that in this particular moment, proximal development in the symptomatic meaning zone is not possible. This is not to say that future proximal development in this zone will not occur, but rather, at this particular point in therapy, it may be better to turn attention to working in one of the other domains. This supports the conceptualisation of the four zones as sitting alongside each other, rather than being 'worked through' hierarchically, and allows for more flexibility and fluidity within the therapeutic process.

10.4.2   Relationship with Internal Experience

10.4.2.1   Rationale and Preparation for Mindfulness Practice

Within PBCT, mindfulness is used as the primary method for working within the relationship domain of the ZoPD. When introducing and using mindfulness with clients, it is important to initially assess and check their understanding of what mindfulness is, and to continue to do this throughout therapy. This helps uncover and correct any misunderstanding or confusion associated with practice, and supports metacognitive insights. Mindfulness is introduced as a way of enhancing well-being by learning to be aware and accepting of all experience, whether it is pleasant, unpleasant or neutral.

10.4.2.2   Overview of Mindfulness Meditation

Mindfulness practice starts by bringing awareness to sensations in the body, beginning with points of contact, such as the feeling of one's back against the chair, or the soles of one's feet on the floor. The individual is then guided to move awareness up through their body (as in a body scan), noticing whatever sensations are present (pleasant, unpleasant or neutral), as well as any tension. Having moved up through the body, awareness then turns to breathing: individuals are asked to find a place in the body where the sensations of breathing are most accessible and comfortable, such as the tips of the nostrils, or the rise and fall of chest. Breathing helps to anchor awareness, because each breath occurs in the body in the present moment, not in the past or future. Mindful awareness of breathing continues for the remainder of the practice, and individuals are gently guided to notice when their mind has wandered (e.g. to distressing voices or images) and to bring aware-ness back to the sensations of breathing. At the end of the practice, individuals are gently guided to open their eyes and settle back into the room.

10.4.2.3   *Specific Adaptations of Mindfulness Practice*
Several adaptations to mindfulness practice have been suggested when working with people with distressing psychosis (Chadwick, 2006; Chadwick *et al.*, 2005, 2009, 2011). From the outset, a strong therapeutic relationship, grounded in radical col-laboration, is essential – particularly when seen from the perspective of what the therapist is inviting the client to do: bringing awareness to difficult and distressing experiences. To date, Chadwick (2006) has identified three main adaptations to mindfulness practice for individuals with psychosis. First, practice time is limited to 10 minutes maximum, as most clients find this is the most that they can manage. Second, extended silences during meditation are avoided: therapists give brief guid-ance or comments every 1–2 minutes. This is an important grounding method, and helps clients to decentre from voices, rumination and so on and to reconnect with present experience with clearer awareness. Third, practice outside sessions is not an essential requirement, but audiotapes of 10-minute guided meditation are provided, and practice is encouraged.

10.4.3   Working with Schemata

In PBCT, a range of experiential approaches are used for working with schemata, including: (1) mindfulness, (2) shame attacking, (3) experiential roleplays and (4) two-chair methods. Mindfulness has already been described, and shame attacking and experiential roleplays are both common CBT techniques, so the focus here will be on discussion of the two-chair method (Chadwick, 2003).

10.4.3.1   *Two-chair Method*
Rationale and preparation for two-chair work   When beginning two-chair work with clients, it is important that therapists provide a clear rationale, so that the clients are fully prepared and can make an informed choice about whether to go ahead. The two-chair method usually takes around 25–30 minutes, so it can easily fit within a single therapy session. The rationale given to clients is that it provides an opportunity to explore both positive and negative experiences of self. They are also told that it involves physically moving between two chairs.

When the therapist has outlined the aims and process of two-chair work, it is important to then check in with the client to see if they have any concerns about doing it. If concerns are raised, it is important that these are discussed fully and resolved prior to commencing the exercise. In addition, when embarking on the two-chair process, particularly for the first time with a client, it is important for the therapist to identify, and reflect back to the client, a positive marker that will be used during the process. Markers are usually very brief experiences and have been defined as 'moments of emotionally positive schematic experience that indicate at least partial activation of a PSS' (Chadwick, 2006). It is important for therapists to note any markers identified from the start of therapy, as they can then be used in future two-chair work. To support generalisation and maintenance of PSS, two-chair enactments are repeated during therapy using different positive markers.

Overview of the two-chair process   When the rationale and process of the two-chair method have been outlined, and the client has decided that they want to experience it, the first step is for the client to briefly enact the NSS. Following the client's enactment, the therapist provides an empathic summary of this negative experience of self. The client is then invited to move to the second chair, while the therapist emphasises that the NSS stays in the first. The client now articulates and 'lives' a PSS in the second chair. The therapist facilitates Rogerian acceptance of both schemata, and the client and therapist together explore the complex and changing nature of the symbolic self. At the end of the two-chair process, it is important that the therapist checks in with the client, to ensure there are no continuing effects when the client returns to the chair in which the NSS was enacted. To support metacognitive insight, maintenance and generalisation, the two-chair method must be seen as a flexible process, rather than a one-off task, that will often be used many times during therapy.

10.4.4   Symbolic Self

Working with the dynamic nature of the symbolic self is achieved by: (1) bringing experientially into awareness the current focus of the symbolic self on the all-consuming nature of the NSS; (2) enhancing and elaborating on PSS experience; (3) supporting acceptance of both NSS and PSS as valid experiences of self; and (4) working directly to modify the symbolic self so that it is not solely defined by NSS experience, but also incorporates positive schemata of the self and others. The purpose of working within the domain of the symbolic self is not to get rid of or change the NSS in any way, but rather to experience the NSS as simply one aspect of the self, not the entire self. By bringing PSS more into focus, therapists can facilitate reflection on, and experience of, the changing nature of the symbolic self. They then emphasise that the client can either continue to be defined solely by their NSS or commit to further development of the positive aspects of the symbolic self. This is mainly achieved using the two-chair method.

10.5 Conclusion

PBCT is a person-centred approach, in which equal emphasis is placed on working with individuals' distress and promoting their strengths and well-being. In this chapter, an overview of PBCT for distressing psychosis has been provided. This has included consideration of the ZoPD, the central organising framework of PBCT, and of case formulation materials with linked client examples. Experiential methods of change have been reviewed, with the focus of discussion being on mindfulness practice and the two-chair method.

References

Chadwick, P. D. J. (2003). Two chairs, self-schemata and a person-based approach to psychosis. *Behavioural and Cognitive Psychotherapy*, 31(4), 439–449.

Chadwick, P. D. J. (2006). *Person-based Cognitive Therapy for Distressing Psychosis*. Chichester: John Wiley & Sons.

Chadwick, P. D. J., Birchwood, M. J. & Trower, P. (1996). *Cognitive Therapy for Delusions, Voices and Paranoia*. Chichester: John Wiley & Sons.

Chadwick, P. D. J., Newman-Taylor, K. & Abba, N. (2005). Mindfulness groups for people with distressing psychosis. *Behavioural & Cognitive Psychotherapy*, 33, 351–359.

Chadwick P. D. J., Hughes, S., Russell, I., Russell, D. & Dagnan, D. (2009). Mindfulness groups for distressing psychosis: a replication and feasibility study. *Behavioural & Cognitive Psychotherapy*, 37, 403–413.

Chadwick, P. D. J., Kaur, H., Swelam, M., Ross, S. & Ellett, L. (2011). Experience of mindfulness in people with bipolar disorder. *Psychotherapy Research*, 21(3), 277–285.

Segal, Z. V., Williams, J. M. & Teasdale, J. D. (2002). *Mindfulness-based Cognitive Therapy for Depression*. New York: Guilford Press.

11

Spirituality: A New Way into Understanding Psychosis

Isabel Clarke

11.1 Introduction

The acceptance-based therapies excel at recognising the truism that wherever you want to get to, you have to start from where you are. This assumes that we know where we are – not a safe assumption if you want to question the dominant paradigm and hence the generally received perception of where we, collectively, are. In order to grasp the relationship between psychosis and spirituality, it is necessary to question some cherished assumptions. There is little of interest to be said about that relationship when you start from the common assumption that psychosis is an illness, and a disastrous one at that, while spirituality is a good thing, possibly personally irrelevant, but which other people regard as positive. The spiritual and supernatural content of much psychotic preoccupation is just seen as pathological from this perspective. Most psychosis research is constrained by this assumption.

This constraint is achieved by ignoring a crucial element of the data: lived experience. Psychiatric diagnosis is undertaken by sampling specific data elements to fit a preordained classification system. Cognitive behaviour therapy (CBT) for psychosis privileges belief. For the person experiencing it, psychosis can plunge them into a different way of experiencing, taking them into strange, dreamlike territory and separating their reality from that of others. That separation is sometimes more insidious, more partial, but still lands them experientially in a different place. The richness of these data is lost where individual experience (as opposed to discrete answers to specific questions) is discounted.

What about spirituality? How do we know that something is 'spiritual'? The same ceremony or occasion can be labelled 'spiritual' by one person and leave

Acceptance and Commitment Therapy and Mindfulness for Psychosis, First Edition.
Edited by Eric M. J. Morris, Louise C. Johns and Joseph E. Oliver.

another cold; a location or event – say a mountain or a meal – can be deemed sacred by some, and ordinary by others. Again, it is down to a quality of experience. No objective formula can capture that distinction.

11.2   Repositioning Psychosis and Spirituality: Recognition of the Two Ways of Knowing

I appeal to cognitive science to explain this phenomenon of two ways of experiencing, and have written much about it elsewhere (e.g. Clarke, 2005, 2008a, 2010), following Teasdale & Barnard's (1993) model of human cognition, Interacting Cognitive Subsystems (ICS). ICS explains this phenomenon as follows. Detailed cognitive experimentation suggests that the human mind works through different subsystems passing information from one to another and copying it in the process. In this way, each subsystem has its own memory. Different systems operate with different coding: verbal, visual, auditory, for instance. There are higher-order systems that translate these codings and integrate the information. The crucial feature of this model is that there are not one but two meaning-making systems at the apex. The verbally coded propositional subsystem gives us the analytically sophisticated individual that our culture has perhaps mistaken for the whole. However, the wealth of sensory information from the outside world, integrated with the body and its arousal system, is gathered together by the implicational subsystem, which looks after our relatedness, both with others and with ourselves. The implicational subsystem is on the lookout for information about threat and value in relation to the self – we are, after all, social primates, and where we stand at any one time in the social hierarchy is crucial to our well-being, if not – normally – our survival

We are unaware of this gap between our two main subsystems because they work seamlessly together most of the time, passing information between them, so that we can simultaneously take the emotional temperature and make an accurate estimate in any situation. This starts to break down in states of very high and very low arousal, whether in a state of high stress or in drifting and hypnagogic states. The application of certain spiritual disciplines, or certain substances, can effect this decoupling between the two subsystems in waking life, so affording a different quality of experience, where the sense of individuality becomes distorted or merged into the whole.

This phenomenon becomes comprehensible when we consider that the propositional subsystem filters our experience to make it manageable, and in doing so, removes immediacy and supernatural glow. It enables us to grasp boundaries between people and things and logical relationships. Without this filter we lose these useful aids to navigating normal life – but can gain a dimension of experience that people seek, whether through drugs, spiritual or other practice, art and so on.

This dimension of experience embraces both valued attributes such as originality and spirituality, and the feared state of madness. Loss of boundaries, which results in the mystic's unitive experience, also underpins the persecutory experiences of thought insertion and thought broadcast of psychosis, for instance.

In summary, the two types of experience arise from the limitations of our processing apparatus. We can either achieve certainty about a limited segment or apprehend the whole but without the means to really grasp it. Science, by concentrating on the objectively verifiable, is blind to the way of knowing that captures all that is really valuable to people: relationships both inner and outer. This is the way of knowing that embraces both psychosis and spirituality.

11.3   Research Basis

Not all science has deserted this field. Over the last 10 years or so research into 'anomalous experiencing', to give it a neutral label, has started to take off. Gordon Claridge's schizotypy research (Claridge, 1997) started from an interest in vulnerability to psychopathology, but moved into establishing openness to anomalous experiencing as a universal human dimension (Claridge, 2010). High schizotypy bestowed advantages such as high creativity and spiritual sensibility, as well as the obvious vulnerability.

Students of Claridge led a strand of research that took a fresh look at psychotic experience and directly juxtaposed it with spiritual or creative experience, with startling results (Chadwick, 1992, 2010; Jackson, 1997, 2010). This married with Peters *et al.* (1999), Peters (2010) looking at the significance of context for the impact of unusual beliefs and experiences. More recently, in the work of Brett *et al.* (2007), Brett (2010) and Heriot-Maitland *et al.* (2011), comparable experiences for people in different contexts (clinical or nonclinical) have been shown to result in significantly different life adaptation. Taken together with robust epidemiological findings (Warner, 1994), these data point to the uncomfortable conclusion that much routine health-service practice is producing iatrogenic harm. At the same time, the neuroscience underpinning these phenomena has been investigated in a way that respects the spiritual dimension (Lancaster, 2010; Simmonds-Moore, 2009).

11.4   Spirituality and Mental Health

To return to spirituality and attempt to pin down this elusive concept: the description of two distinct ways of knowing available to human beings places spirituality in the holistically apprehended category. It has recently become not merely acceptable but actually required to include consideration of spirituality within health care.

The British National Health Service has started to take this dimension seriously, and much has been written on this subject both by the Department of Health (e.g. Department of Health, 2009; National Institute for Mental Health in England *et al.*, 2004) and by service user focused organisations such as the Mental Health Foundation (2006, 2007). These and other documents promote recognition of the importance of religion and spirituality within health care, and the need for staff to address this aspect of the individual with sensitivity within a holistic context, but without producing any clear definition of spirituality itself.

Acceptance and commitment therapy (ACT) has of course always recognised the importance of spirituality. In his paper 'Making Sense of Spirituality' (Hayes, 1984), Hayes locates the concept within a behavioural framework by equating it with 'you-as-perspective' (p. 104), the perspective which offers the possibility of the reflection and distance essential for the type of revision of stuck patterns sought in therapy that can be achieved through mindfulness. Hayes links this with the disruptive effects of speech and mystical spiritual traditions as follows:

> Mystical traditions are explicitly oriented toward enhancing the distinction between the verbally-held *content* in peoples' lives and the *context* of pure-perspective established in verbal organisms (p. 107).

I here propose to take this subjective knowing perspective one step further by introducing the similarly subjective experience of relationship. A sense of relationship with something (someone?) beyond, the widest and deepest, is commonly implied by spirituality and religion. This fits with a view of the human being that follows from an appreciation of the consequences of the split in human knowing. The self-contained, self-directed individual becomes only part of the story. When grounded in experiential knowing, we flow beyond individuality into relationship. Normal life is a constant intersection of the two. We make decisions and act on them. At the same time, we rely on our containing roles and relationships to define us. Sufficient rupture in these leads to breakdown (see Clarke, 2008b, pp. 118–124 for a fuller exposition of this view of the person). At times when these sustaining roles and relationships (including the internal relationship between the individual and themselves) desert or turn against us, the wider, deeper layer of relationship that many (but not all) recognise as spirituality becomes crucial, providing the meaning and coherence that enable us to carry on. This works well where we can hold on to our individuality while drawing on that wider context for sustenance. Accessing the wider dimension can aid the path of healing, constituting a transformative growth experience (Grof & Grof, 1991). Where this safe foothold is lost, however, we can become engulfed in the other way of knowing, losing our ability to function coherently with others in the world. This is a state of confusion – between inner and outer (as in voice hearing), between safety and danger (paranoia), to give but two examples. It is a state of openness and vulnerability, where the boundaries of individuality are loosened. Could it be a state in which influence from beyond the individual might actually intrude? Other cultures, subcultures and religious traditions accept notions such as possession (Tobert, 2010) and disembodied communication. Are we so sure that these must be ruled out?

11.5   Clinical Approach: The Therapeutic Alliance

This perspective offers a more sympathetic and hopeful slant on psychosis, and one which can be invaluable in forming a therapeutic alliance. Any therapy for psychosis can only proceed once there is a therapeutic alliance based on the common aim of management of symptoms to the extent that the individual can function in the world.

There are well-attested barriers to achieving such an alliance. The stigma associated with a diagnosis such as schizophrenia in our society has a lot to answer for in this respect. This stigma can produce two distinct sources of avoidance. For some, the fear of symptoms, such as aversive voices, is so great that they are too frightened to focus on them in case they return or get worse, and are therefore resistant to talking about them or working on them (see Gumley & Schwannauer, 2006 for a development of this theme). Other individuals conclude, with some justification, that society has little to offer them, and so retreat into a psychotic world, which has many disadvantages, but at least offers more status and meaning, albeit illusory. Not taking prescribed medication and using psychoactive substances such as cannabis are readily available means of perpetuating this state. Persuading these two groups to engage in a programme of coping skills, which requires them to be prepared to face their symptoms and to join the shared world, is a challenge of acceptance, and is one that our programme is designed to address.

11.5.1   The What is Real and What is Not Approach

This is delivered in our acute service as a four-session group, held in the hospital, but open to people in crisis being supported by a home treatment team and to people who have recently been discharged from hospital. The same approach is used in individual work and has been adapted for a longer group to be delivered in the community or in longer-stay settings. The programme is offered to anyone who is prepared to identify themselves as having experiences that others do not share, irrespective of diagnosis. These might be voices or visions (hallucinations, flashbacks), strongly held beliefs (delusions) or fears (paranoia). In inviting people to join the group, a new way of looking at symptoms is offered, as well as coping strategies. The fact that someone is in hospital, suggesting that others do not share their viewpoint or are concerned about them, can be helpful in persuasion. Thus the interest of people who are otherwise alienated by the mental health system can sometimes be engaged.

11.5.2   Schizotypy and 'Unshared Reality'

This approach is characterised by treating participants as the interested and intelligent adults that they are, and so presenting (briefly) research findings behind the key ideas. The programme first introduces Romme & Escher's (1989) idea of normalising voice hearing and drawing on the coping resources of experiencers for mutual support, but extended to other unusual experiences, unshared beliefs and fears. We then invite participants to give examples of how their experiences might fit into this spectrum, but with no pressure to contribute. Lack of pressure is particularly important, as it is a short group for people at the acute stage. Attending and not saying a word is perfectly acceptable, but most people feel able to share once they have got to know the other participants.

We then introduce the idea of openness to voices and strange experiences – the schizotypy spectrum, highlighting Gordon Claridge's research effort at normalising openness to this other way of experiencing given the right conditions (drugs, trauma, sleep deprivation etc.), while recognising that some are more open than others. This offers a hopeful perspective, as the research identifies positives, such as creativity and spirituality, associated with high schizotypy – along with the greater vulnerability to psychotic breakdown.

The positive and the negative aspects of high schizotypy are discussed and the group comes up with examples of famous high schizotypes: artists such as Van Gogh or celebrities such as Stephen Fry. We then introduce the specific example of a high schizotype who used this to advantage in the singer David Bowie. Bowie surmounted his vulnerability and used his high schizotypy to great effect in his act, adopting varied strange personae, with a theme of being an alien from outer space (Buckley, 2001). This example provides an accessible role model of someone who was able to inhabit both 'realities', shared and unshared; to know which he was in at any one time; and to move from one to the other and so operate creatively in a way that communicated with and was effective in the wider world.

The rest of the group programme aims to provide strategies for managing openness to unshared reality and participating in the shared world, without necessarily totally rejecting the unshared. This contrasts with other mental-health programmes, which tend to aim at elimination of 'symptoms' (i.e. unshared experiences). It respects individual values, whether they reject unshared experiencing or see it as an integral part of identity, or stages in between. Where the individual sees what others label as 'psychosis' as their access to a valued spiritual reality, this approach opens a way to dialogue. Where linked to a faith, discussion with the chaplain or other faith representative can establish whether or not someone's interpretation is normative. However, spiritual and mystical experience has always led people into unique experience, producing new insights that can be seen as challenging or heretical by orthodoxy. We are here operating beyond the realms of certainty.

In this way, the aims of the group are presented as something that will give the participants more control, but without having to reject their unique experiences or to accept a stigmatising label. Medication is recognised as one of these possible means of control, and an important one, along with psychological coping strategies. The need to commit to monitoring, to noticing whether the group members are in shared or unshared reality, is presented as essential to following the programme at this point, and monitoring sheets are handed out to be filled in between sessions. Participants are also invited to identify a personal goal for the group. This is rated at the end on a visual analogue line and represents an ideographic evaluation tool (see Durrant *et al.*, 2007, p. 123 for a description of how this is used).

11.5.3   From Conceptualisation to Coping Strategies

This conceptualisation both motivates the individual to want to cope with their symptoms and suggests priorities for doing so. The detailed programme is available in the full manual, which is downloadable from my website (www.isabelclarke.org). The first stage is to accept that some perceptions and experiences are unshared – discrepant from the norm – and therefore should not be uncritically trusted; but it often requires courage to face this. The next stage is to learn to distinguish which reality you are in at a given time. This is established by exploring the difference between the two sorts of experience through discussion in the group. People usually recognise that a sense of importance, of meaning and the supernatural, goes with the 'unshared' side. This can feel very frightening, very isolating or very grand and wonderful. Sometimes everything seems to come together – or to fall apart and be meaningless. It can be hard to know who you are: important or worthless. Every group identifies that unshared reality is buzzy and exciting, while ordinary reality is flat and boring, which explains some people's preference for the unshared.

Once someone has got their bearings, coping strategies to help them stay in the shared world and ward off unshared states of mind become relevant. Earlier in this chapter, these two ways of knowing (shared and unshared reality) were linked to the idea that the human being has distinct modes of processing. The non-ordinary way can be variously labelled as 'spiritual' or 'psychotic'. Following the ICS model (Clarke, 2010, p. 107; Teasdale & Barnard, 1993), non-ordinary experience becomes accessible at high and at low arousal. This maps nicely on to clinical experience. People's voices and delusions tend to intensify with stress, and take over in hypnogogic and drifting states. Where participants return for the second group having completed their monitoring sheets, this usually becomes apparent. The point is illustrated using an adapted version of Linehan's 'States of Mind' diagram (Linehan, 1993, p. 109), in which the wise mind represents the ability to reflect on your experience while grounded in present reality. This leads naturally into the crucial role of mindfulness, as well as discussion of arousal management – whether using breathing control, relaxation or exercise as a means of managing high arousal, or engaged activity to avoid low arousal. The latter can present a challenge in hospital!

11.5.4   Role of Mindfulness

Such strategies enable the individual to manage symptoms essentially by disengaging from them. Applied consistently, this would represent avoidance, with all its associated problems. A balancing strategy of facing the unshared experiences, however frightening or seductive, is needed. Mindfulness provides such a strategy, with a sound research base (e.g. Chadwick *et al.*, 2005, 2009). Even before mindfulness swept the board, a similar strategy had been explored by Haddock (1998) (but this was called 'focusing') in an elegant study that is now introduced to the group. Again, it is stressed that such focusing or mindfulness requires courage, whether for fear of being overwhelmed by the experience or because it means facing its unshared nature, along with the possibility that a cherished idea, even a cherished identity, is unshared. The mindfulness exercise used requires the individual to ground themselves firmly in the present and find a strong, centred place from which to embark on this challenge. Once introduced to the exercise, participants are encouraged to practise between groups.

The last session is an opportunity to review the group, to return to the goals identified in the first session and to introduce the possibility that openness to these experiences might have a role in the wider context of each individual's life. This aspect is introduced quite lightly, in what is a very brief programme, by initiating discussion of the pros and cons of using coping strategies to manage 'unshared reality', acknowledging that this is a matter of choice and that there are arguments on both sides, while emphasising that the group agenda is to try and coax people to join the shared world. This is made harder where the individuals have been offered a devalued and stigmatised position in this world by virtue of their diagnosis and unshared reality offers a more exalted position, even if it is accompanied by frightening experiences.

Another research-based idea, Mike Jackson's problem-solving hypothesis – which suggests that psychosis occurs in response to life reaching an impasse, and that if it is followed by orderly return to the shared world, it can result in new and transformative insights, illuminating a better way forward (Jackson, 2010) – is then introduced and discussed. The significance of early breakdown experiences often emerges at this point, through recognition that times of stress, specific trauma, or both, preceded the initial breakdown. This more positive, problem-solving and potentially transformative perspective is floated lightly. It resonates with some participants, but not others. We conclude with the participants marking where they have reached on their goal-setting visual analogue line and completing questionnaires.

11.6   Psychosis as a Spiritual Crisis

This positive, potentially transformative perspective draws on the spiritual emergency literature (e.g. Grof & Grof, 1991), which emphasises the transformative potential of such experience (Brett, 2010; Hartley, 2010). According to this school of thought, such crises, occurring at times when growth and development are somehow blocked, open the individual to forces either beyond or deep within themselves, or both. The foundations of the everyday sense of self can be rocked by such experiences, which are frequently deeply disturbing and frightening. The classical presentation (e.g. Grof & Grof, 1991) distinguishes such states from psychosis. Indeed, some people navigate such psychic breaks successfully in a way that enriches their lives despite accompanying disturbance, while others become lost in a psychotic state that does not confer apparent benefit and can become a recurrent affliction. However, I would argue that there is no intrinsic difference in the state itself. Such states can be understood in ICS terms as a temporary desynchrony of the two central meaning-making systems (Barnard, 2003 explores this in detail).

If we are to rethink psychosis in these terms, and Jackson, Brett and Heriot-Maitland all invite us to do so on the basis of their sound and thorough research, far-reaching and radical implications follow. 'Symptoms' are no longer an aberration to be eliminated with medication. Yes, they need managing for the sake of the individual and in order to maintain the safety and tolerance of those around them, but not necessarily to the point of obliteration, not least because the individual needs to retain some ability to navigate what is now recognised as an important process, with potential spiritual and growth implications. Services need to be prepared to support this process, even where it means greater tolerance of socially and culturally unacceptable behaviour, and this behaviour might require temporary containment, more on the Soteria model than in the current psychiatric hospital (Bola & Mosher, 2003). The role of medication is relevant here. To take a balanced approach: neuroleptic medication can release an individual from being locked in a private hell; it can make possible the management of ordinary life and inhibition of risky impulses. However, the services as they are currently set up are essentially addicted to this medication as the only solution, even where it confers little benefit. A more humane approach takes account of the individual's perspective on the process, rather than swamping it through over-sedation, reinforced by an apparatus of legal coercion. Supporting the mindful facing and accepting of inner experience, at the same time as recognising the broader perspective, offers the individual dignity and control, and ultimately choice, which is sadly often denied by current services.

At the same time as evidence builds about the limitations and harmful side effects of the medication solution (e.g. deleterious effects on motivation, see Arias-Carrion & Peoppel, 2007), the growing body of research evidence cited in this chapter recognises the spiritual/growth and transformation potential of psychosis, thus presenting a challenge to the mental-health system as currently constituted. Alternative approaches such as Soteria (www.soterianetwork.org.uk) and the Spiritual Crisis Network (www.spiritualcrisisnetwork.org.uk) provide a vital balance and an alternative perspective. Within the health service, we need to develop and make widely available a psychological therapy that offers the opportunity for the individual to take control of their own journey in this unpredictable territory. In this way, recognition that spirituality and psychosis are closely allied can lead to a transformation in the therapeutic approach to psychosis.

References

Arias-Carrion, O. & Peoppel, E. (2007) Dompamine, learning and reward seeking behaviour. *Acta Neurologicae Experimentalis*, 67, 481–488.

Barnard, P. (2003) Asynchrony, implicational meaning and the experience of self in schizophrenia. In T. Kircher & A. David (eds). *The Self in Neuroscience and Psychiatry*. Cambridge: Cambridge University Press, pp. 121–146.

Bola, J. R. & Mosher, L. R. (2003) Treatment of acute psychosis without neuroleptics:two-year outcomes from the Soteria project. *The Journal of Nervous and Mental Disease*, 191, 219–229.

Brett, C. M. C. (2010) Transformative crises. In I. Clarke (ed.). *Psychosis and Spirituality: Consolidating the New Paradigm* (2nd edn). Chichester: John Wiley & Sons.

Brett, C. M. C., Peters, E. P., Johns, L. C., Tabraham, P., Valmaggia, L. R. & Mcguire, P. K. (2007). Appraisals of Anomalous Experiences Interview (AANEX): a multidimensional measure of psychological responses to anomalies associated with psychosis. *The British Journal of Psychiatry*, 191, 23–30.

Buckley, D. (2001) *Strange Fascination: David Bowie: The Definitive Story*. London: Virgin Books.

Chadwick, P. K. (1992) *Borderline: A Psychological Study of Paranoia and Delusional Thinking*. London and New York: Routledge.

Chadwick P. K. (2010) 'On not drinking soup with a fork': from spiritual experience to madness to growith. In I. Clarke (ed.). *Psychosis and Spirituality: Consolidating the New Paradigm* (2nd edn). Chichester: John Wiley & Sons.

Chadwick, P. D. J., Newman-Taylor, K. & Abba, N. (2005). Mindfulness groups for people with distressing psychosis. *Behavioral & Cognitive Psychotherapy*, 33(3), 351–360.

Chadwick, P. D. J., Hughes, S., Russell, D. *et al.* (2009) Mindfulness groups for distressing voices and paranoia: a replication and randomized fealibility trial. *Behavioural and Cognitive Psychotherapy*, 37, 403–412.

Claridge, G. A. (1997) *Schizotypy: Implications for Illness and Health*. Oxford: Oxford University Press.

Claridge, G. A. (2010) Spiritual experience: healthy psychoticism? In I. Clarke (ed.). *Psychosis and Spirituality: Consolidating the New Paradigm* (2nd edn). Chichester: John Wiley & Sons.

Clarke, I (2005) There is a crack in everything. That's how the light gets in. In C. Clarke (ed.). *Ways of Knowing. Science and Mysticism Today*. Exeter: Imprint Academic.

Clarke I. (2008a) Pioneering a cross-diagnostic approach founded in cognitive science. In I. Clarke & H. Wilson (eds). *Cognitive Behavior Therapy for Acute Inpatient Mental Health Units: Working with Clients, Staff and the Milieu.* Hove: Routledge, pp. 65–77.

Clarke, I. (2008b) *Madness, Mystery and the Survival of God.* Winchester: O Books.

Clarke, I. (2009) Coping with crisis and overwhelming affect: employing coping mechanisms in the acute inpatient context. In A. M. Columbus (ed.). *Coping Mechanisms: Strategies and Outcomes. Advances in Psychology Research,* Vol. 63. Huntington: Nova Science.

Clarke, I. (2010) *Psychosis and Spirituality: Consolidating the New Paradigm.* Chichester: John Wiley & Sons.

Department of Health (2009). *Religion or Belief. A Practical Guide for the NHS.* London: Department of Health.

Durrant, C., Clarke, I., Tolland, A. & Wilson, H. (2007) Designing a CBT service for an acute in-patient setting: a pilot evaluation study. *Clinical Psychology and Psychotherapy,* 14, 117–125.

Grof, C. & Grof, S. (1991) *The Stormy Search for the Self. Understanding and Living with Spiritual Emergency.* London: Mandala.

Gumley, A. & Schwannauer, M. (2006) *Staying Well after Psychosis: A Cognitive Interpersonal Approach to Recovery and Relapse Prevention.* Chichester: John Wiley & Sons.

Haddock, G., Slade, P. D., Bentall, R. P., Reid, D. & Faragher, E. B. (1998) A comparison of the long-term effectiveness of distraction and focusing in the treatment of auditory hallucinations. *British Journal of Medical Psychology,* 71, 339–349.

Hartley J. (2010). Mapping our madness: the hero's journey as a therapeutic approach. In I. Clarke (ed.). *Psychosis and Spirituality: Consolidating the New Paradigm.* (2nd edn). Chichester: John Wiley & Sons.

Hayes, S. C. (1984). Making sense of spirituality. *Behaviorism,* 12, 99–110.

Heriot-Maitland, C., Knight, M. & Peters, E. (2011). A qualitative comparison of psychotic-like phenomena in clinical and non-clinical populations. *British Journal of Clinical Psychology,* doi: 10.1111/j.2044-8260.2011.02011.x

Jackson, M. C. (1997). Benign schizotypy? The case of spiritual experience. In G. S. Claridge (ed.). *Schizotypy: Relations to Illness and Health.* Oxford: Oxford University Press.

Jackson, M. C. (2010) The paradigm-shifting hypothesis: a common process in benign psychosis and psychotic disorder. In I. Clarke (ed). *Psychosis and Spirituality: Consolidating the New Paradigm* (2nd edn). Chichester: John Wiley & Sons.

Lancaster, B. L. (2010). Cognitive neuroscience: spirituality and mysticism. Recent developments. In I. Clarke (ed.). *Psychosis and Spirituality: Consolidating the New Paradigm* (2nd edn). Chichester: John Wiley & Sons.

Linehan, M. (1993). *Skills Training Manual for Treating Borderline Personality Disorder.* New York: Guildford Press.

Mental Health Foundation (2006). *The Impact of Spirituality on Mental Health.* Albany: Mental Health Foundation.

Mental Health Foundation (2007). *Keeping the Faith. Spirituality and Recovery from Mental Health Problems.* Albany: Mental Health Foundation.

National Institute for Mental Health in England, the Church of England Archbishops' Council & Mentality (2004). *Promoting Mental Health: A Resource for Spiritual and Pastoral Care.* Leeds: National Institute for Mental Health in England.

Peters, E. R. (2010). Are delusions on a continuum? The case of religious and delusional beliefs. In I. Clarke (ed.). *Psychosis and Spirituality: Consolidating the New Paradigm* (2nd edn). Chichester: John Wiley & Sons.

Peters, E. R., Day, S., McKenna, J. & Orbach, G. (1999) The incidence of delusional ideation in religious and psychotic populations. *British Journal of Clinical Psychology*, 38, 83–96.

Romme, M. & Escher, S. (1989). *Accepting Voices*. London: Mind.

Segal, Z. W., Williams J. M. G. & Teasdale J. D. (2002). *Mindfulness based Cognitive Therapy for Depression: A New Approach to Preventing Relapse*. New York: Guildford Press.

Simmonds-Moore, C. (2009) Exploring ways of manipulating/controlling pathological/ healthy anomalous experiences. Paper presented at First Conference On Health, Mental Health And Exceptional Human Experiences, Liverpool Hope University, September 2009 (to appear in an edited volume, McFarland, Jefferson, NC).

Teasdale, J. D. & Barnard, P. J. (1993) *Affect, Cognition and Change: Remodelling Depressive Thought*. Hove: Lawrence Erlbaum Associates.

Tobert, N. (2010). The Polarities of Consciousness. In I. Clarke (ed.). *Psychosis and Spirituality: Consolidating the New Paradigm* (2nd edn). Chichester: John Wiley & Sons.

Warner, R. (1994) *Recovery from Schizophrenia: Psychiatry and Political Economy* (2nd edn). London: Routledge.

12

The Service User Experience of Acceptance and Commitment Therapy and Person-based Cognitive Therapy

Joseph E. Oliver, Mark Hayward,
Helena B. McGuiness and Clara Strauss

12.1 Introduction

The chapter aims to bring current thinking and approaches about service user involvement into consideration of acceptance- and mindfulness-based therapies, specifically acceptance and commitment therapy (ACT) and person-based cognitive therapy (PBCT).

12.2 An Overview of Service User Involvement

The notion of involving the recipients of services in decisions about how the service is delivered is often both a pragmatic and a political one. Pragmatically, it has been argued that services that are tailored to the needs of recipients are likely to be more effective, more efficient and more widely used (Beresford, 2000). Indeed, there is a body of evidence to suggest that services which involve and engage with service recipients in order to help shape them produce better results (Nancarrow & Johns, 2004; Richardson, 2005; Simpson & House, 2002). In addition to the pragmatic argument, there is a political case for involving the

Acceptance and Commitment Therapy and Mindfulness for Psychosis, First Edition.
Edited by Eric M. J. Morris, Louise C. Johns and Joseph E. Oliver.
© 2013 John Wiley & Sons, Ltd. Published 2013 by John Wiley & Sons, Ltd.

users of services, which is based on the democratic right for individuals to participate in civil activities, particularly those related to public services (Taylor *et al.*, 2004). Over time, the concept of involvement has gradually been introduced to health services, and more recently into mental-health services.

Although the involvement of users in mental-health services is broadly comparable to that in other settings, there are some crucial differences that can lead to involvement becoming highly politicised and emotive. One of the central differences is that a significant number of mental-health service users have been highly traumatised by their contact with services, often because they have not had a choice about treatment, or have felt they have not needed to receive treatment. Although a large proportion of service users report positive experiences, the very negative experiences of some can lead to particularly polarised views of services. Alongside this issue, the opinions of service users about treatment provision have often been devalued or viewed as less important than professional views. People with mental-health problems have been seen as either not able to articulate their views or as holding views that are not valid or not reliable (Perkins, 1996, 2001). As a result, the views of recipients of mental-health services can often significantly diverge from those of the professionals working within the system (Dimsdale *et al.*, 1979; Perkins, 2001). This shows through even to the terminology by which recipients of mental-health services are referred to, which can include, 'patient', 'client', 'consumer', 'service user' and 'survivor'. These discrepancies are even more likely in people with serious mental-health concerns related to the experience of psychosis. Such individuals are much more likely to come into contact with mental-health services and to be detained and treated against their will.

Involving service users in the development of treatments therefore appears to make sense. However, consideration needs to be given to what constitutes successful and efficacious treatment. Traditionally, the professional viewpoint has been that an effective treatment is one that reduces symptoms experienced by the individual. However, views of wider stakeholders, including service users and carers, suggest that other outcomes are equally if not more important (Rose *et al.*, 2011): having a sense of choice and control, better social networks and fulfilling employment are often given at least as much weighting (Bond *et al.*, 1994). Carers and families place importance on treatments that involve them and provide them with the necessary support to continue to carry out their roles (Shepherd *et al.*, 1995). Evidence suggests that symptom reduction is not necessarily a precondition for these kinds of outcomes. For example, research has suggested that improvements in broader well-being indicators, such as employment and a sense of personal control, can occur independently of reductions in symptoms (Anthony *et al.*, 1995; Strauss, 1994). These findings are particularly relevant in working with people with serious mental-health problems such as psychosis, as often pharmacological and psychological interventions are not effective in ameliorating symptoms.

In addition to developing treatment protocols that target outcomes which are meaningful for service users, it is useful to consider the processes by which these outcomes can be achieved. Feedback can be used to usefully shape the development of treatments for different presenting problems. This is particularly pertinent in working with people with psychosis, who are likely to require a greater emphasis on engagement or a slower pacing in therapy (Fowler *et al.*, 1995).

12.3 The Importance of a Service User Perspective in Informing ACT and PBCT for Psychosis

Despite the apparent value of engaging with service user perspectives, there are few studies that seek to learn from service users about their experiences of psychological therapy for psychotic experiences. Berry & Hayward (2011) reviewed the literature on cognitive behaviour therapy for psychosis (CBTp) and related therapies and found only eight qualitative evaluations of service users' experiences over the past 15 years – and within these evaluations, the views of the service users were often overshadowed by the views of therapists. As a consequence, Berry & Hayward (2011) recommend that all future therapy trials should include at least an exit interview for service users, and that these exit interviews be conducted by service user researchers, so as to ensure that the experiences of service users are prioritised.

If CBTp has engaged poorly with the therapeutic experiences of service users, the challenge to ACT and PBCT is to do a lot better. This is particularly the case given the emphasis that ACT and PBCT place upon a broad repertoire of outcomes beyond symptom reduction. For ACT, there is a central focus on developing a more flexible behavioural repertoire that leads to valued actions, shifting the emphasis towards a broad range of potential treatment outcomes, which might include behaviours such as returning to work or reconnecting with family and friends. These could be broadly conceptualised as developing an increased sense of choice and control as life direction becomes more determined by steps towards desired goals and outcomes. For PBCT, the emphasis is on developing a more balanced view of the self which can facilitate engagement with the social environment and opportunities for valued roles therein.

Equally important is incorporating service user views on not only the outcomes of treatment, but on the treatment process. To date, there are no published qualitative studies relating to ACT and the actual experience of ACT therapy. Bacon *et al.* (unpublished) conducted a thematic analysis on qualitative interviews that were carried out with participants who had undergone ACT for psychosis treatment as part of the Lifengage trial at La Trobe University. Broadly, the results indicated that participants found the intervention useful and indentified the processes of mindfulness, defusion and acceptance as facilitating an ability to continue to act on values in the presence of persisting symptoms. Participants also noted that the intervention led to a change in their perspective on symptoms, which may have been related to a reduction in symptom intensity and impact.

For PBCT, there are two qualitative studies that have explored the experiences of service users, both of which have focused upon distressing voice-hearing experiences within a group-therapy format (Goodliffe *et al.*, 2010; May *et al.*, 2012). These studies were preceded by an exploration of service user experience of mindfulness groups, which was not driven by any particular therapeutic model (Abba *et al.*, 2008). Nicola Abba and colleagues used a qualitative method which allowed theory to be developed from a slowly building picture of the sense that participants were making of mindfulness. Three categories emerged from the data: (1) centring in awareness of voices, thoughts and images in the moment; (2) allowing voices, thoughts and images to come / go without reaction / struggle; and (3) reclaiming power through acceptance of voices and self. Interestingly, these issues only partially resonated with participants who reported their experience of PBCT for distressing voices (Goodliffe *et al.*, 2010). In contrast to participants in the Abba *et al.* (2008) study, who were offered regular mindfulness practice throughout therapy, those in the Goodliffe *et al.* (2010) study were offered mindfulness practice only during the second half of the programme. Logically, this led to the participants not talking about mindfulness during the qualitative interviews, as their exposure and socialisation to mindfulness had (possibly) been insufficient. Consequently, the researchers were prompted to adapt the therapy to include mindfulness practice during all sessions. This amended therapy was offered to participants within three further groups, and their experience was captured during individual post-therapy qualitative interviews (May *et al.*, 2012). These participants commented more extensively upon mindfulness as a process that enabled changed relationships towards voices, the self and others.

The benefit of having a service user perspective on when to introduce which processes into therapy is also apparent for ACT. For example, Morris and Oliver (Bloy *et al.*, 2011; Morris & Oliver, 2009), in their work on first-episode psychosis, found that service users reported that values work was often a more helpful starting point for ACT therapy than acceptance and creative hopelessness. This is because people experiencing a first episode of psychosis tend to have less experience of struggling with psychotic experiences and therefore often do not connect with the problematic aspects of an overreliance on this strategy.

12.4   A Service User Perspective on the Experience of ACT for Psychosis

David Kelly
Born: 14 May 1944
Died: 17 July 2003 (aged 59)

Cause of Death: suicide – haemorrhage from incised wounds of the left wrist, in combination with copraxamol ingestion and coronary artery atherosclerosis

It was July 2003. The newscaster was explaining in detail how David Kelly, the British scientist and UN weapons inspector, had killed himself. I didn't want to hear the details but I couldn't tear myself away. I was relieved when I heard the mention of copraxamol. That wasn't a drug which I could get my hands on.

I was watching TV in the smoking room at an acute psychiatric ward in Glasgow. I had habitually woken up to the Today programme yet the whole Weapons of Mass Destruction debate and the Iraqi war had passed me by. I had been deep in a world created by my mind which had at first offered respite from (what I then saw as) the desolation of my day-to-day life but had then overgrown my thinking abilities to a level at which I could no longer function. I was 43 and I had been admitted with psychosis.

12.4.1   Background

I had dealt with a number of intensely stressful events over 10 years, starting with having to conduct a media campaign to find my first (then ex) husband, who had been murdered while travelling alone on holiday in Turkey, and ending with my father's death from cancer. I was being bullied at work and, following separation from my 4-year-old son's father, had no partner in my life. Friends had drifted away as they found my life events difficult to handle. I felt isolated.

I was beginning to believe that my son's dad and his step-mum could offer him a 'family' life which I couldn't. I was beginning to feel that my first husband and miscarried children represented a family 'waiting' for me. I felt that I was connected more with dead people than those living.

I noticed that my vision began to be affected. I have a vivid memory of being in my living room and seeing only what was right in front of me, encircled by a grey blur. I could see my son's feet but I had to turn my head to see the rest of his body.

One day, a mature student mentioned that his wife had experienced Distance Reiki and that it had been very helpful. I browsed online and found a site which consisted entirely of one page with the word REIKI written large in the middle of the screen. When I clicked on it, nothing happened. I worried that somehow I had connected with this 'Distance Reiki' thing but didn't brood on it.

Normally I awoke in the mornings still tired and tense. Sometimes there were tears on my cheeks. On three consecutive mornings I woke up feeling refreshed; my body was tingling and I was aware of the sun on my face. This continued and I began to question how it was happening. Distance Reiki seemed like the logical answer, it seemed to be a good thing. This was confirmed when the healer, a man, communicated with me telepathically. I found that I could talk to him if I clenched the muscles around my heart and chest as I thought the words. I hadn't known that I was telepathic. I was prepared to accept the concept of Reiki – telepathy was a bit of a stretch. However, in my isolation any friendly voice was welcome. To start with, the 'friend' was welcome. I was happy and excited, as at the beginning of a romance. As my attempts to prove that this person was real didn't come to anything, I was eating irregularly and sleeping for short periods at night. I can now see that my physical health was deteriorating. I was confused and unable to focus. The 'friend', who was someone I knew in the real world and represented something which I hoped for, evolved over time through various stages. I challenged him that he wasn't real; he admitted that he was the distance healer's 'soul'. I was reasonably okay with that.

Then the 'soul' became a member of a telepathic community of souls who would surround me at night and who I found to be threatening. I began to feel scared. There were twists and turns as I followed a labyrinthine narrative created by my brain out of my hopes, fears, fantasies and experiences. My brain connected details which I had forgotten that I knew in ways which at times were hilarious. I felt that I had a talk radio station permanently switched on inside my head and that I could not think my own thoughts. I was overwhelmed.

In the latter stages, the psychosis was continuously critical and arguing with me that, for the sake of my son, I should kill myself sooner rather than later. The logic was that at the age of 5 he would be less affected than he would be if I killed myself when he was older.

At this point I phoned my GP, who decided I needed to go to hospital. As she drove me there, we went past the hospice in which my father had died. The psychosis then became his voice. I spent the first 3 weeks joyously talking with him. He told me how to behave initially. He made an acute psychiatric ward feel like a holiday. Despite this, I still wanted him to leave. I wanted my own clear thoughts. Risperidone quietened his voice.

After leaving hospital, I returned to my job determined that I was not going to lose my home and therefore potentially my 5-year-old son. I was able to perform to a degree. However, I was far from well. I managed to find counselling at a charity-run centre in Glasgow and attended for around a year in 2004. I talked about my past, trying to find a narrative with which I was comfortable. However, after finishing counselling, I continued to experience some difficulties. For some years I had been struggling with weight, alcohol and cigarettes. I started to see these as symptoms of my state of mind. I heard a programme about CBT and wondered if it could help me to approach the cause. Through my GP, I had an assessment session with my therapist, after which I was offered a course of ACT. With hindsight, having completed the course of ACT, I can describe the effect on my life as follows.

12.4.2   The Therapy

The concept of 'Acceptance and Commitment' seemed large and a little bit scary. It also seemed somehow promising. The therapy sessions took place at a meeting space in an office. I was aware that this was because my therapist was based elsewhere and had borrowed the room. However, on reflection, it's possible that the room set a helpful 'getting on with business' tone, in contrast to the 'retreat' or 'confessional' tone set by the counselling rooms which I had previously experienced. I found that there was less intensity in this set-up, which made the sessions more relaxing.

As in counselling, I was asked to define my goals. I was shown how actions which I took could be moving away from or towards my goals. Unlike in counselling, I was asked to define my values. Again, I could see how my actions worked with or against my values. Reestablishing my values was concrete. It was a yardstick of how little I had in fact changed as a person despite my perception. In short, I was not the chaos which surrounded me; I was finding my identity again. I was led towards the recognition that memory is not a video camera. I found this tremendously liberating.

I was shown simple techniques such as putting 'I think that' in front of 'they think I'm mad', which questioned my assumptions and really quite quickly led me to behave in different, more positive ways in what had been problematic family relationships.

I was shown Mindfulness, which I found to be much more achievable than meditation.

I first benefited greatly from using the technique during times when I was experiencing a sudden distressing emotion. As time has moved on, I have begun to experiment with Mindfulness when I'm commuting as an alternative to always having my mind stimulated by books.

My therapist introduced an ongoing narrative about 'Jeremy', who was apparently lost in some kind of jungle [see Appendix F for a full account of this narrative]. His journey back into civilisation somehow echoed my own journey. This was an objective but fairly lighthearted way of summarising session by session the progress being made. I'm sure that like me, he has found his way.

12.4.3   How the Therapy Helped

I believed that I couldn't change my situation. I felt that if I could operate a switch in my head which would make me look differently at my life, I would cope better. I had approached counselling with the above in mind. I ended by making changes in my activities. When the project failed, I saw that it had been just another in a line of attempts to cope.

ACT provided the switch which I had been looking for, a different, more objective vantage point. I was able to see that essentially I was still me. Although in practice nothing changed, I no longer felt that aching loneliness because I had reawoken in my own company.

To me, time had stopped. I experienced the normal awareness of how fast children grow. However, I would meet someone and talk to them with familiarity, only to find that 6 years had passed which I hadn't noticed, as if it hadn't happened. I now feel like it's only been months since my life fell apart. Everyone else has moved on.

I now have 10 years of neglect of myself and my home to catch up on. It doesn't seem to be too big a task to handle. Fortunately, my son is growing up fairly well balanced and happy, much to my relief. I have regained much of my confidence. For the first time in many years, my mind feels clear.

12.4.4   Conclusion

I am immensely grateful that I was fortunate enough to experience ACT. The day-to-day aspects of my life have changed very little, but I have a completely different point of view now. I have a clear head, I can think properly.

I am no longer in limbo, my life has started again.

12.4.4.1   *How I Felt before ACT Therapy*

- I was chronically lonely. At one point I had joined AA in order to have somewhere I could go and be around people. I felt that we would have dysfunctional lives in common.
- To me there seemed to be very little point to doing more than the minimum to get by.
- I was self-medicating, relying on cigarettes and alcohol to avoid thinking during the hours which I spent alone.
- I had no code to live by against which to make decisions.
- I believed that people did not want to relate to me.
- My family relationships were stuck in negative patterns established in childhood.
- The past was a chain of distressing narratives, which I took to be facts.
- The future was a depressing place to think of.
- The present was interminable and unfulfilling.
- I felt that I was no longer the creative, professional, capable person I had viewed myself as years earlier.

12.4.4.2   How I Feel after ACT Therapy

- I recognise that as the first person from my school and community to go to art school, I have always had different views/interests from the mainstream. People like me are hard to find.
- I initiated some community projects, a garden, a fireworks event. They haven't worked long-term, but a book group has evolved from them and neighbours speak to each other much more in the street.
- I spend many absorbing hours painting with oils. Alcohol is literally a waste of time. I drink considerably less volume and less often. I smoke half of what I did.
- I was able to reconnect with my values and see how my actions related to them. This was important in recognising who I am. I have not moved backwards.
- I realise that I was not being myself and was uncomfortable with others, always feeling that I had something to explain or justify. This is no longer an issue.
- Recognition that memory is incomplete, inaccurate and largely interpretation led me to question my beliefs. I also recognise that my sibling's beliefs are equally wrong. That fact that they don't recognise this is irrelevant. I no longer play the expected/habitual other half of the relationship, which has changed many issues much for the better.
- I am using time in ways which matter to me and stimulate me. I now have to reorder my life in order to achieve more of this creative work, which will improve the quality of my life and place me in environments where I relate to people who are similar to me. I am currently exploring the radical changes which I will have to make for this to happen.
- I am making a positive future.
- I recognised that I was and had always been that person but had believed that the context which I was living in had changed who I was.
- There are changes to my understanding of life and people, but these changes add on to what I am.
- I am now taking control of my future.

12.5   Summary of Qualitative Findings from PBCT Groups on Participant Experiences of Mindfulness Practice and What was Learned from these Studies

Service users within the Goodliffe *et al.* (2010) study were asked their views after completing an eight-session programme of PBCT groups for distressing voices (the last five sessions of which included mindfulness practices). Some of the categories that emerged from the data concerned commonly reported issues within the literature, such as sharing negative characteristics of hearing voices, developing a group identity and learning to cope with voices. Other categories and subcategories seemed to relate more specifically to the conceptual underpinnings of PBCT and offered insights into the similarities and differences between conceptually driven expectations of how therapy might be experienced and the actual experience of learning to accept voices and develop a sense of self beyond voices.

12.5.1   Acceptance of Voices

This category described the process by which service users learned to accept their voice-hearing experiences:

> I didn't really look at it as accepting, but that's probably what it was – accepting. And I suppose once you accept it it's easier for you to look at ways of coping. Because when you're fighting it, you're just scared.

Prior to joining the therapy group, participants discussed their views of the future as involving either being 'cured' or living in misery as a result of the voices, as described by Kimberly:

> I wasn't expecting to be able to cope with the voice still there. I wasn't expecting to just be in control. I was expecting to either have the voice or not have the voice.

Prior to the group, medication was seen by most people as being the only solution to alleviating voices, and voices were monitored to assess whether they were 'getting better'. The process of group members' perspectives of voices shifting from a cure to a coping model was assisted by the group facilitators' transparency regarding the aims of therapy not being to eradicate voices. Although this was described as initially causing widespread feelings of disappointment, in the longer term it increased participants' hopefulness that they would be able to manage their voices.

For some, beginning a process of accepting their voices was important in developing their ability to cope. This concept was strongly linked to self-acceptance. Participants' acceptance of their experiences began with confronting their perceived responsibility for voices, or attribution to an 'evil' personality trait. Doing so led to increased confidence and self-esteem. Of this process, James said:

> I was bitterly bitterly resentful towards myself that this illness had come into my life. And now I'm learning to accept this. I'm quite a lot happier in myself now that I've accepted it.

However, the process of acceptance was not experienced by all group members equally. Some explained that their understanding of the voices had increased but did not describe acceptance in any explicit way. For example, Rachel explained:

When I've got a lot of stress I've got voices. When less stress, less voices. And coming here my stress went down [...] It's a worry when work is too too much, too much stress I need to protect myself. Go for a walk, or take life easy – an easy life.

This reflects the way in which some participants explained the same experiences but talked about them differently – with acceptance perceived as both a way of coping *per se* and (through increased understanding) a catalyst for the deployment of coping strategies.

12.5.2   Development of Sense of Self beyond Voices

This category describes the development of group members' understanding of the experience of hearing voices as affecting their selves. A pivotal aspect of this process was reevaluating their sense of personal identity with voices as part of their sense of self. Martin said:

I am not the illness. I am a person with a certain illness.

Meeting others who heard voices had an impact on group members' beliefs about mental illness, about other people who experience voices and consequentially about themselves. Prior to the group, several participants expressed their wish to distance themselves from the concept of madness, and others they perceived to be mad. This changed over the course of the group, as they began to see similarities between their own situations and those of other group members.

Group members also began to alter the perceived relationship between voices and their mental health. For example, for some, feeling overwhelmed by voices came to be viewed as part of the process of recovery, rather than a sign of impending relapse. Doing so allowed members of the group to acknowledge hearing voices as being part of an illness, rather than an aspect of their personality, as Gina explained:

It's just one of those things that we've got with our illness, you know. And it can be overcome. It's just learning different strategies to change things around.

One of the main benefits that participants described gaining from the group was the recognition that their voices were separate to their personality. This was linked to the normalising effect of being given information regarding common symptoms that people with their respective diagnoses might experience. Danielle explained the ways in which such information helped address her understanding of her difficulties:

I found it very hard to understand why I couldn't stop [the voices] if it was me doing them. And the group's helped me understand that yes, it is me, but also it's not really me, it's my mind.

Spotting links between stress and voices was noted to be a powerful tool in viewing voices as a symptom rather than a personality trait. Through this process, group members were able to develop the concept of their voices as interacting with the self, rather than being an integral part of it.

Group members experienced their sense of self being challenged with respect to their negative and positive perceptions. Negative beliefs about self were challenged through a comparative process within the group:

> It wasn't until we were in the group that we started to realise that you haven't done anything bad. You know? But all of them were saying, 'Yeah, well, I must have done something to make me have these voices' [...] We can't all be evil. We can't all be wrong.

Receiving feedback on their positive qualities provided most group members with an alternative perspective on themselves, leading to increased self-esteem. Some group members also described having altered their self-perspective through reevaluating their ability to cope with voices. James explained:

> You learn new things about yourself. That you've got resources and assets to call on to help you deal with your illness. I never thought I was going to be working on something that I've already got.

The findings of Goodliffe *et al.* (2010) resonated strongly with the research team in both expected and unexpected ways. As anticipated, there was a sense of some of the elements of the PBCT model being corroborated by participants' experiences: voices and self were being accepted and related to differently and in more balanced ways. However, unexpectedly, mindfulness was mentioned by few participants and there was only a limited sense of the mindfulness practices and linked reflection playing a role in the participants' experience of the therapy and associated changes to perceptions of voices and self. This may reflect the limited time made available to mindfulness practices during the therapy, resulting in limited impact.

The research team reflected upon the rationale for the introduction of mindfulness practice at the midpoint of therapy and wondered if this somewhat conservative decision had been made due to concerns that participants might feel uncomfortable and alienated by mindfulness. Anecdotally, there was no evidence within the accounts of the therapists to corroborate this view. Yes, participants may have found the mindfulness practices a little unusual and uncomfortable in the early sessions, but this generated the need to begin practices earlier in therapy to allow these feelings to be overcome. Consequently, the therapy protocol was extended from 8 to 12 sessions, and mindfulness practice was offered during every one. Participants' experiences of this revised protocol were captured by May *et al.* (2012), who individually interviewed 10 participants across three groups.

May *et al.* (2012) identified three therapy-specific themes within partici-pants' accounts that referred to changed relationships: with voices, the self and other people.

12.5.2.1   *Relating to Voices*

Many group members highlighted the mindfulness practice as being useful. For most, mindfulness was a new technique that they learnt within the group. A few participants described having previously known about mindfulness, or having had brief past experience of it, but the way in which it was outlined in therapy groups was described as being more helpful than previous experiences.

Richard described acquiring a different attitude to voices through mindfulness:

> ... we learnt to, um, not put our voices out of our head, but work with them rather than try and get rid of them... cos I had always been taught to try and get rid of them, but they-they said, 'don't try and get rid of them, work with them'... [that was] unusual to start with, very unusual. But it does work.

Another participant, Anna, reflected on this changed attitude to voices, despite the voices still being present:

> Um, the voices are still quite bad now, so, but I have ways of dealing with them now, which I didn't have before like, like the mindfulness practice, so if things get too much, which they often do, then I'll do a mindfulness and sort of like give myself a break for, for 15 minutes. [...] Which doesn't sound a lot, but it's sort of like, when you're used to, you know, listening to them all the time [...] 15 minutes is like a lifetime.

Despite voices remaining, most participants talked about mindfulness practice enabling decreased fighting against voices, increased confidence in coping with voices and increased perceived ability to cope with voices, as well as making them feel less negative towards voices. This different attitude reflects some acceptance of voice-hearing experiences.

While some participants described little change in voice characteristics, others spoke of changes to voices through mindfulness practice, such as the voices becoming quieter and more distant. Adam described how voice-hearing experi-ences changed during mindfulness practice:

> Mindfulness – that for me was a, was a main event, and, if you do mindfulness then... if you can reach a mindful state – if you know what that is – then everything slowly begins to relax and... and when your voice talks to you, I find that, um, I'm able to absorb it rather than, rather than have it hit me.

Some participants described difficulties in using mindfulness, particularly at first. For example, Susan said that after the first group 'mindfulness ... made me feel very upset', but that week by week mindfulness got 'better and better'. With practice, most participants described becoming accustomed to the technique and finding it easier to engage in. Many participants talked about continued use of mindfulness between sessions and after the group had ended.

Only one participant, Phil, talked about not finding mindfulness helpful, preferring instead to use distraction techniques to cope with his voices:

> It didn't suit me, you know what I mean, um… I suppose it could have helped other people but it just didn't, didn't help me.

He did not describe finding mindfulness increasing distress, but rather that mindfulness was not 'my cup of tea'. Phil described discussing this within the group and receiving positive feedback from facilitators that mindfulness practice was different for different people and that he should use the coping strategies that were helpful for him.

12.5.2.2   *Relating to Self*

Prior to the group, several participants described feeling a sense of lost identity through the experience of hearing voices, often feeling defined by their diagnosis or the content of their voices. Some participants described being entirely defined by voices. The process of being in the group and having their experiences normalised helped group members to develop a new understanding of themselves as a person who experienced voices, rather than being defined by their voices, and therefore helped them reconnect with a self as separate from their symptoms. Rachael described the change in how she thought about herself:

> I feel that, that, you know, that I am a person at the end of it, even despite these voices, I'm still, you know, Rachael, and I'm still a person, still have my own, my identity. But, um, I was beginning to lose that a bit, you know, before I did the group. You know, I was beginning to lose my identity just seeing myself as a, constantly as an ill person – mentally ill person, and I was becoming very depressed by that.

Participation in therapy groups also allowed some group members to reevaluate beliefs about hearing voices and the concept of 'madness'. Through repositioning their experiences outside an illness, participants started to feel less stigmatised and began to view themselves as 'normal' and less defined by their voice-hearing experiences:

TOM:	I'm normal and stable now.
INTERVIEWER:	You're normal and stable?
TOM:	Um hmm.
INTERVIEWER:	That's how you, how you think of yourself now?
TOM:	Uh huh.
INTERVIEWER:	And what makes you normal and stable?
TOM:	Um, knowing who I am, basically.

The process of being involved in the group and hearing feedback from other group members aided a different or more positive sense of self, as it allowed participants to reevaluate views of themselves as 'bad' or as being in some way to blame for their voices. Through having negative beliefs about themselves challenged and having their feelings validated by other participants with similar experiences, group members were provided with an alternative perspective to the views they had developed through being isolated in their experiences. This was particularly important for group members who experienced their voices telling them to harm themselves or others. Anna described the impact that receiving feedback from other group members had on her beliefs about herself:

> I think it did affect the way I was feeling about myself because, um, mainly because of the group sort of like feeling the same as I did, cos one thing is if you hear voices that tell you to kill people you feel quite evil and quite horrible as a person and to just have somebody saying, 'well, no you, it's not you that's evil, it's the voices' [...] so I didn't feel quite as bad about myself.

Participants described the experience of sharing positive qualities with others in the group, and their surprise at the positive feedback they received. Receiving feedback provided participants with an alternative view of self to the one often presented by their voices. As a result, group members were again encouraged to reconstruct views of themselves and develop a more balanced self-identity. Jason described developing a more balanced view of himself:

> People have good points and bad points. [...] And even though the voices don't really – they tell me about my bad points, I've still got good points as well. [...] And it's... trying to remember those good points.

12.5.2.3   *Relating to Others*

Participants described reevaluating their social identity and capacity for social functioning. Prior to therapy, many participants described feeling isolated in their experience and avoided socialising. Engaging socially in the therapy group and receiving positive feedback from group members had a positive impact on participants' social confidence.

For many, the process of universality and the feeling of being able to talk safely within the group facilitated this, as it gave them a positive experience of talking to others, which they were able to model outside the group. Indeed, some participants said that their ability to talk to others about their experiences outside the group had developed. Some group members also described feeling more able to accept, or feel worthy of, support from others, through removal of the blame associated with hearing voices. Thus the establishment of a positive sense of self enabled some participants to be ready to accept relationships with other people. By continuing to talk to others about their (often distressing) experiences outside the group, group members described positive changes to their personal relationships and feeling less isolated in their experience of hearing voices. Rachael described this:

I found my relationship with my boyfriend a little better. [...] I had it out with him one day, I said that, you know, he didn't listen to me and, you know, he wasn't listening to me, you know, you know, my experiences enough, you know, he's supposed to be my carer but he wasn't listening to me enough. So we had a really good discussion one night and, er, I told him all about, er, um, we discussed, um, I was abused as a little girl, sexually abused and I talked this out with Danny and, um, we really had a good conversation about it. And I told him all about the hallucinations and how they affected me, what I'm seeing and, er, I found that I've got a little closer to him, I'm a little closer with him now and I feel that, not so frightened to talk to him about things, you know, if I have a bad day, what I'm experiencing and, you know.

The development of increased strength and power over voices also appeared to be generalised to social situations, where some participants talked about becoming more assertive about expressing their needs. For others, the use of mindfulness, and the positive impact this had on reducing voices and anxiety, made them feel better able to concentrate on conversations with others and engaging socially with them. As a result, participants described a shift from seeing themselves as an isolated individual, whose social identity was defined by their voices, to seeing themselves as a person who was 'open' to socialising with others. Patricia described this:

I think when I go to the group, it changed dramatically, I wanted to go out, I wanted to meet people and be, you know, interested in people.

Through developing a social identity, group members described changing their socialising behaviour outside the group context. For example, a number of participants talked about remaining in contact with other group members, and arranging to meet up socially or speak to each other on the phone. Others talked about improved socialisation with family members or friends, as Anna described:

Um, I think I'm more – more open at the moment. [...] I tend to talk to people a lot more. [...] Whereas before I, I was quite reclusive before. Now I'm sort of like, I go to my parents quite often, which is something I didn't do before. [...] And I tend to phone my mum quite a lot now, so. I, I go out with friends a lot more. [...] Which is again something I didn't do before.

However, all participants did not share this motivation for continued socialising. Some group members described a sense of fragility around their social identity, which they felt was dependent on the group. As a result, once therapy groups had finished, these participants felt that their social support network had been taken away, reducing their motivation for continued socialising. This left them feeling low in mood and fearful that they would return to being isolated and unable to cope with their voices. For these participants, it is possible that developments in their social identity were dependent on the group and had not sufficiently general-ised to other social relationships at the end of the therapy.

12.5.3 The Value and Challenges of Seeking Service User Views

By seeking and capturing participants' experience of PBCT groups, the researchers were both corroborated in their approach and challenged. Elements of the PBCT model were clearly influencing the experience of the service users and their sense of what was changing for them. This was particularly evident within the changing perceptions of self in relation to voices. However, challenges were also evident. Mindfulness practices were evidently not frequent enough in the early groups, and this was changed – to good effect. There also remains the question of what happens at the end of the therapy, as participants suggested that even the 12-session approach did not enable changes in relating to others to be developed to a point of being sustainable for all. Does this suggest that therapy should be further extended (pos-sibly to the 16 sessions that NICE recommend for individual CBTp), that later ses-sions should be staggered to reduce the end of therapy being experienced as abrupt or that booster sessions should be provided? These are issues the research team must consider as a result of having invited the service users to express their views.

12.6 Conclusion

Together, these perspectives provide valuable information about the content and process of psychological interventions for psychosis, which can supplement research data to improve the overall experience for service users. This chapter exemplifies the significant shift in the field of psychology over the past 20 years, as service users have become recognised as much more than the passive recipients of a service, and instead as active collaborators who have a key role in developing interventions, in terms of both content and process of delivery. We anticipate that this kind of collaborative role will become more mainstream as service user com-munities become more vocal and services increasingly recognise the benefits and utility of developing interventions in partnership with their users.

References

Abba, N., Chadwick, P. & Stevenson, C. (2008). Responding mindfully to distressing psychosis: a grounded theory analysis. *Psychotherapy Research*, 18, 77–87.

Anthony, W. A., Rogers, E. S., Cohen, M. *et al.* (1995). Relationships between psychiatric symptomatology, work skills and future vocational performance. *Psychiatric Services*, 46, 353–357.

Bacon, T., Farhall, J. & Fossey, E. (submitted). The active therapeutic processes of acceptance and commitment therapy for persistent symptoms of psychosis: clients' perspectives.

Beresford, P. (2000). Service users' knowledges and social work theory: conflict or collaboration. *British Journal of Social Work*, 30, 489–503.

Berry, C. & Hayward, M. (2011). What can qualitative research tell us about service user perspectives of CBT for psychosis? A synthesis of current evidence. *Behavioural and Cognitive Psychotherapy*, 39, 487–494.

Bloy, S., Oliver, J. E. & Morris, E. (2011). Using acceptance and commitment therapy with people with psychosis. *Clinical Case Studies*, 10, 347–359.

Bond, G. (1994). Psychiatric rehabilitation outcome. In Publication Committee of IAPSRS (ed.). *An Introduction to Psychiatric Rehabilitation*. Columbia, MD: International Association of Psychosocial Rehabilitation Services, pp. 490–494.

Dimsdale, J., Klerman, G. & Shershow, J. (1979). Conflict in treatment goals between patients and staff. *Social Psychiatry*, 14, 1–4.

Fowler, D., Garety, P. A. & Kuipers, L. (1995). *Cognitive Behaviour Therapy for Psychosis: Theory and Practice*. Chichester: John Wiley & Sons.

Goodliffe, L., Hayward, M., Brown, D., Turton, W. & Dannahy, L. (2010). Group Person-Based Cognitive Therapy for distressing voices: views from the hearers. *Psychotherapy Research*, 20, 447–461

May, K., Strauss, C., Coyle, A. & Hayward, M. (2012). Person-based cognitive therapy groups for distressing voices: a thematic analysis of participant experiences of the therapy. Psychosis, doi: 10.1080/17522439.2012.708775.

Morris, E. & Oliver, J. (2009). ACT early: acceptance and commitment therapy in early intervention in psychosis. *Clinical Psychology Forum*, 196, 27–31.

Nancarrow, S. & Johns, A (2004) 'The squeaky wheel get the grease': a case study of service user engagement in service development. *Journal of Integrated Care*, 12, 14–21.

Perkins, R. E. (1996) Seen but not heard: can 'user involvement' become more than empty rhetoric? *The Mental Health Review*, 1, 16–19.

Perkins, R. (2001) What constitutes success?: the relative priority of service users' and clinicians' views of mental health services. *British Journal of Psychiatry*, 179, 9–10.

Richardson, L. (2005) User engagement in public services: policy and Implementation. *Benefits*, 13, 189–197.

Rose, D., Evans, J., Sweeney, A. & Wykes, T. (2011). A model for developing outcome measures from the perspectives of mental health service users. *International Review of Psychiatry*, 23, 41–46.

Shepherd, G., Murray, A. & Muijen, M. (1995). Perspectives on schizophrenia: a survey of user, family care and professional views regarding effective care. *Journal of Mental Health*, 4, 403–422.

Simpson, E. L. & House, A. O. (2002) Involving users in the delivery and evaluation of mental health services: systematic review. *British Medical Journal*, 325, 1265–1267.

Strauss, J. S. (1994). The person with schizophrenia as a person. II. Approaches to the subjective and complex. *British Journal of Psychiatry*, 164, 103–107.

Taylor, G., Brown, K., Caldwell, K., Ghazi, F., Henshaw, L. & Vernon, L. (2004). User involvement in primary care: a case study examining the work of one patient participation group attached to a primary care practice in north London. *Research Policy and Planning*, 22, 21–30.

13

Acceptance and Commitment Therapy for First-episode Psychosis

Joseph E. Oliver and Eric M. J. Morris

13.1   Introduction

As described in previous chapters of this book, acceptance and commitment therapy (ACT) is a transdiagnostic model of behaviour change, with a broad applicability across multiple problems and disorders (Morris & Oliver, 2012). ACT, combining the development of mindfulness skills with values-based behavioural activation, presents a recovery-orientated approach that fits with the broader aims of early intervention (Morris & Oliver, 2009): to enhance functioning, help young people achieve meaningful social roles and improve quality of life. Our work in developing ACT as this type of flexible, mindfulness-based intervention has been influenced by the broader literatures on early intervention in general, as well as the developments emerging from cognitive behavioural therapies for psychosis within the United Kingdom. It is our view that ACT is broadly consistent with established cognitive behavioural therapies for psychosis (CBTp), while also bringing unique aspects that are advantageous when working with younger people recovering from psychosis.

In the last 15 years there has been increasing international interest in the possibilities of intervening early with psychotic disorders to prevent long-term disability (Birchwood, 1999), and potentially to prevent the onset of psychosis itself (e.g. Broome *et al.*, 2005). A first episode of psychosis typically occurs in late adolescence/early adulthood, usually following a period of mood and cognitive changes, and the presence of anomalous experiences (unusual perceptions, preoccupations, increased salience) (Parnas, 1999). Prior to the early-detection and -intervention paradigm (Birchwood & MacMillan, 1993; McGorry & Killackey, 2002), young people could experience significant delays in receiving effective treatment for a psychotic episode,

Acceptance and Commitment Therapy and Mindfulness for Psychosis, First Edition.
Edited by Eric M. J. Morris, Louise C. Johns and Joseph E. Oliver.
© 2013 John Wiley & Sons, Ltd. Published 2013 by John Wiley & Sons, Ltd.

with the associated risk that this treatment might occur through a crisis, resulting in a hospital admission, against the background of social and functional decline and family and relationship discord. Following discharge from hospital, many people recovering from a first episode of psychosis were lost to follow-up by community mental-health teams, and this group has a high risk of relapse, functional decline and suicidality without assertive community treatment (Birchwood, 2003; Malla & Payne, 2005). Additionally, it has broadly been found that providing pharmacological treatments and contact with standard community treatment alone does not optimise recovery and long-term functioning (Peterson *et al.*, 2005). Rather, there is a need for a flexible 'wraparound' of psychosocial interventions with this population, which can take into account the different needs of young people and the various phases of recovery, and provide a consistent thread throughout a young person's care with the mental-health team (McGorry *et al.*, 2008).

13.2   Recovery from a First Episode of Psychosis

Based on studies from traditional treatment settings for psychosis, young people can face a challenging period following their first episode, with up to 80% experiencing a relapse within 5 years (Linszen *et al.*, 2001), and there is a growing risk of treatment-resistant symptoms with each subsequent relapse. In addition, 20% will show persisting positive symptoms from the first episode (Mason *et al.*, 1995). Progressing in social roles can be challenging: 50–70% of those recovering from a first episode will continue to be unemployed/out of education 12 months after starting treatment, and there is a strong risk of long-term poor social recovery (Harrison *et al.*, 1996; Malla & Payne, 2005; Whitehorn *et al.*, 2002). Unsurprisingly, mood and anxiety problems are common, with over 50% of young people reporting significant depressive and anxiety symptoms, secondary to the psychosis (Birchwood, 2003). More worryingly, young people recovering from psychosis present with one of the highest risks for attempted and completed suicide of any group with mental-health problems (Power *et al.*, 2003).

It is important to consider the developmental tasks and social environments that are the contexts for young people recovering from a first episode of psychosis. Late adolescence and early adulthood is often a period of significant change in terms of role and identity. Typically young people are negotiating achievement of greater personal autonomy through education, training and work. Peer and intimate relationships have great importance, as do having children and parenting effectively for some individuals. Harrop & Trower (2001) describe the effect of a psychotic illness as 'stalling' development of the important social roles that signify adulthood in developed nations; an awareness of the developmental tasks of young people can inform an understanding of the social contexts in which these tasks are situated. Any psychological intervention needs to be sensitive to these contexts.

13.2.1   At-risk Mental States

People with at-risk mental states (ARMS) are deemed to be at ultra high risk of developing psychosis by virtue of experiencing one or more of the following: attenuated psychotic symptoms; brief, limited intermittent psychotic symptoms (BLIPS); and a decline in functioning, in addition to either meeting the criteria for schizotypal personality disorder or having an immediate relative with a psychotic disorder (Phillips *et al.*, 2000). This is a fast-moving area of research and clinical interest, and not without controversies with regard to the identification and treatment of young people who do not meet criteria for a diagnosis of a psychotic disorder.

In recent years there has been research interest in the potential role that emotional dysfunction, avoidance and metacognitive beliefs play in making the *transition* to psychosis (Morrison *et al.*, 2006). Certainly young people who are experiencing ARMS can appear very worried about the implications of changes in perceptions and thinking, and try to cope by avoiding situations that appear to make these experiences more intense and prolonged. Experiential avoidance can be supported by engaging in worry and rumination, and acting on the belief that certain internal experiences need to be controlled and eliminated; similarly, the stigma associated with having unusual experiences can result in the young person keeping their concerns to themselves, supporting social avoidance.

13.3   Using ACT to Enhance Recovery from a First Episode of Psychosis

In this section we will outline the major areas in which ACT is used when working with young people recovering from a first episode of psychosis, and the typical approach we can take with individuals, families and carers.

13.3.1   Assessment and Formulation

In many respects, the way in which we start with first-episode clients (FE clients) in using ACT is similar to most therapeutic approaches to working with young people and those with psychosis. Key to the assessment process is engagement. As a group, younger people experiencing or recovering from their first episode of psychosis tend to be wary of mental-health professionals and particularly psychological therapists, and as such engagement and relationship building are vital in the early stages. To this end, as is recommended within CBTp, we proceed very slowly and approach potentially sensitive subjects, such as psychotic experiences, only once we are confident that a good therapeutic rapport has been established.

In initial sessions we build in a structure that sets expectations and guidelines for how therapy works, as most of the clients we see have no previous experience of therapy. To set the scene for ACT, we suggest to clients that therapy is often about helping people to 'manage difficult thoughts, feelings or experiences more effectively in order to help you to get more out of your life, in a way that suits you'.

In terms of assessment, the central areas described in Chapter 4 would be covered, with some differences. While discussion of values is an integral part of the assessment, more room is made for this to evolve over the course of therapy. As described earlier, because a first episode can disrupt important developmental tasks (such as establishing an identity as separate from family or parental figures), interruptions in this process often mean that FE clients come to therapy with less well-formed notions of what is important to them and their personal values. As such, assessment and construction of values often takes place over the course of therapy, and may form a core part of the intervention.

As with any ACT assessment, it is important to consider the function, rather than form, of the client's behaviours. We find that this is particularly important because many actions that younger people engage in may overtly look dysfunctional but have additional functional properties. For example, drug use may serve as a method of avoiding difficult experiences, but also function to facilitate engagement with a peer group. Similarly, 'sealing over' (McGlashan *et al.*, 1975), or the apparent reluctance to talk about issues related to psychotic experience, may be an unhelpful method of avoiding unpleasant emotional or cognitive experiences. However, this could also function as a useful method of titrating such experiences, so as not to be overwhelmed by them. Therefore, key to an initial ACT assessment is to not take particular behaviours at face value, but to consider the functions they have for each individual in context.

As outlined in Chapter 4, a broad aim of the assessment is to understand what it means for the client to live a full, rich and meaningful life in light of their goals and valued directions. Alongside this, we also consider what thoughts, emotions or experiences that the young person struggles with might function as barriers to taking steps in these directions and the workability of efforts to control these experiences (e.g. Bloy *et al.*, 2011; Valmaggia & Morris, 2010). In addition, it is appreciated that clients are recovering from a psychotic illness, which can be understood from a stress-vulnerability framework (Zubin & Spring, 1977). This may help to normalise and destigmatise the experience of psychosis and, for some clients, provide a more helpful way of understanding what they have been through.

Once this formulation has been developed, work then begins in helping the client experiment with relating to the barriers differently (mindfulness and willingness), to see if this fosters more effective action consistent with their values. Therapy broadly focuses on three key areas: assisting the client to become more aware of and present with their internal experiences, helping them to open up to these experiences and assisting them to take active steps towards what matters. In the next section, we will discuss the different ways in which we work in each of these areas with FE clients specifically.

13.3.2   Being Aware and Present

Mindfulness-based interventions have so far demonstrated mixed outcomes in early intervention (Ashcroft *et al.*, 2011; van der Valk *et al.*, 2012). We think that what can be taken from these studies is the importance of therapists being clear about the purpose of introducing present-moment awareness exercises to young people: we would suggest that the purpose is to build psychological flexibility, rather than to eliminate symptoms. For many young people, exercises such as contemplative meditation are less engaging than finding alternative ways of noticing in the present moment and practising nonjudgemental awareness. As such, we find it is important to use creative, flexible approaches that take into account the kinds of difficulty likely to be experienced by FE clients, while adhering to the principles of mindfulness. In our experience, introducing these skills involves:

(1)   Discussing what it is like to be on 'automatic pilot' and contrasting this with moments of being connected, engaged in sensory experience and doing things that are meaningful.
(2)   Introducing the idea of 'noticing': deliberate ways of becoming more present, more involved in your activities and slowing down.
(3)   Practising the skill of noticing in regular activities, such as walking, doing chores, eating things and listening to music.
(4)   Suggesting noticing as an option in any situation, by linking it with an anchoring experience such as breathing or feeling the ground beneath your feet.
(5)   Reinforcing any efforts by the young person towards noticing.

As suggested by Chadwick (2006), we have altered our exercises to provide more instruction and reduce the amount of silent time, in order to compensate for limited attention spans and distractibility. We tend to favour brief exercises over longer ones. We find that for some individuals, cultivating a more open, present-moment focus can be a key component in active relapse prevention. By developing this stance, we encourage clients to be more aware of symptoms, emotions or sensations that may be indicative of increased stress as a potential precursor to relapse. This can allow for more proactive and responsive planning and action. We find that some attention must almost always be given to helping clients practising greater openness to difficult experiences, particularly as the typical response is to be both cognitively and emotionally avoidant. The combination of these approaches allows for the development of more meaningful relapse-prevention plans.

We find that mindfulness work is particularly important in assisting FE clients in developing a more self-accepting and compassionate stance towards themselves. Mindfulness exercises that encourage clients to notice, make room for and open up to difficult thoughts, feelings, sensations and experiences, without deliberate attempts to change them, naturally foster self-compassion, as individuals become more willing to accept all parts of their self-stories, without necessarily getting entangled in them. Further support for this process can be given by the use of exercises or metaphors that help the client distinguish aspects of their experience that are transitory (self as content: thoughts, sensations, beliefs, emotions) from the observing self. The stage-show metaphor (Harris, 2009a), for example, introduces these aspects of the self as either the whole theatre, the part that watches the show or the contents of the show itself. Such metaphors can be highly useful for clients who do not have a resilient sense of self or who have been highly attached to self-beliefs that are unhelpful ('I'm a psycho who can't ever be trusted').

13.3.3 Opening Up

Here we seek to develop two core skills to help promote acceptance and defusion, in order to broadly assist clients in becoming more open and flexible to the full range of their internal experiences.

It is our clinical observation that young people (including those with persisting symptoms) have not yet had the sense of 'stuckness' towards these experiences that can motivate those in long-term services to seek psychological therapy. For instance, the young people we see have not tried all of the medications available, and have options in this area. Similarly, they may have expectations that these symptoms might still resolve 'with the just the right dose' – these are not unrealistic hopes. As a result, FE clients often remain invested in experiential avoidance strategies, as they have less direct longer-term experience of these approaches preventing them from doing what matters. Therefore, we generally (although not always) find it more fruitful to work on acceptance and defusion skills once the client has completed some work in clarifying values and developing mindfulness skills.

In addition to the types of acceptance and defusion work outlined in other chapters within this volume, we find self-stigmatisation particularly important to target, as young people appear especially susceptible to self-stigmatising beliefs about mental illness (such as, 'I'm mad/crazy/mental/a nutcase'). Self-stigmatisation is the internalisation of negative societal stereotypes (Link, 1987); this process has been shown to be particularly relevant to people with psychosis (Corrigan, 2004). Given exposure to dominant societal attitudes about mental illness and psychosis, it is likely that FE clients will apply these judgements to themselves. This can manifest in self-critical views of self and a lack of trust in one's own judgements and identity, and can ultimately lead to self-limiting choices, based upon fear of recurrence (Gumley & Schwannauer, 2006). It can be useful early in a person's experience of mental-health services to introduce the idea of responding flexibly to both the dominant messages about what psychosis 'means' and fears and concerns about what the future holds. Therefore, defusion exercises can help clients notice the processes of thinking, so as to get better at responding in ways that are more likely to facilitate movement in valued directions (for example, 'I am crazy and will never amount to anything' versus 'There goes my mind again, telling me I'm crazy and will amount to nothing'). It is important to recognise the power and pervasiveness of these social messages about mental illness, and not to invalidate the client's experience. Rather, the purpose of defusion is to help the client have more 'wiggle room' between themselves and such thoughts, so that they are still able to do what matters.

Metaphors are a key vehicle in the delivery of ACT and are particularly important in assisting FE clients grapple with concepts, such as defusion, that they might not have encountered before. We tend to use a range of metaphors, and work to ensure that they map on to the client's experience, with elements that are familiar and recognisable. As most of our work is with young people who live in a densely populated urban area, we adapt metaphors to reflect this. For example, as our client group can relate less to experiences of nature, we have modified the 'leaves-on-the-stream' exercise (see Appendix B) to 'buses on Brixton Road' or 'trains at Waterloo Station'. We find that roleplaying or acting out metaphors (such as 'passengers on the bus', see Appendix C) can be particularly useful in ensuring that they are fun, accessible and memorable.

Alongside such defusion work, we aim to promote acceptance (although typically we would not use the word 'acceptance') with regard to the often problematic emotions associated with self-stigma. Particularly important are feelings of shame or humiliation (Birchwood *et al.*, 2005) linked to being viewed by others as having mental-health problems. We would work to assist the client to notice and bring such feelings into awareness, make room for them and drop the struggle with them, all with the overall purpose of helping the client engage in a different, more values-based, set of behaviours in response to such emotions. This could lead to conversations like:

THERAPIST: So, tell me what it was like thinking about going to meet your friends.
CLIENT: It was awful, I couldn't do it.
THERAPIST: Tell me a little about what came up when you thought about meeting your friends.
CLIENT: I couldn't, I knew that if they saw me, they would know something was wrong, that I was mental. Which is true, I am mental.
THERAPIST: Okay, sounds tough. Tell me a little about the feelings that came up.
CLIENT: I just ended up feeling rubbish, like really depressed.

THERAPIST: I can see these are difficult feelings that come up here. And some sticky thoughts, too! First, it's great that you're able to notice these and bring attention to them right now. I think these feelings are really important and, if it's okay, I'd like us to spend some more time with them, perhaps gently observing them, to see if we can make a little room around them. To see if we can find a different way of holding them so they don't completely take over when you take steps towards doing stuff that's important to you, like being with your friends.

13.3.4   Being Active

Vital to any ACT intervention is assisting clients in clarifying what matters to them and taking active steps to reflect these key values. As described earlier, with FE clients we have found that adaptations are necessary, given the developmental stages that young people are often tackling. As such, values work often needs to be highly flexible, and clarifying values is frequently a task that continues over the course of therapy. The focus therefore may be on helping clients to approach engaging in values-based actions in the spirit of discovery, so they can experientially contact what works for them personally, rather than on what family, peers or society says should be important. This can be analogous to trying on a new wardrobe until the person gets a feel for what particular style suits them best.

A particular challenge that often arises is the tendency for FE clients to want to feel or think a certain way before taking steps towards values. Commonly, clients will say, 'I must feel less stressed/anxious/depressed' or 'I have to feel more motivated/normal/energetic' before taking steps forward. Adherence to such rules can significantly interfere with a client's ability to actively engage in valued action, particularly as steps in these directions initially often increase the likelihood that problematic experiences will occur. After some defusion and acceptance work, we might invite a client with the suggestion, 'I wonder if we could play with this a little and maybe see if we can bring these experiences "along for the ride" as you take some steps towards doing the things that you really care about.'

We find that roleplay is a particularly useful approach in helping clients discriminate between what they would habitually do (give in, block out, argue with) and what it might be like to take actual steps towards their goals and values, while choosing to carry difficult experiences with them.

In taking steps forward, we normally focus on helping clients to develop small, achievable goals that are closely linked to important values. In this way, we help clients to have early successes and use these to build on increasing larger patterns of committed action. Because of the problems with memory, concentration and organisation often experienced by FE clients, we invariably follow up any committed action plan with a phone call, text message or reminder. In order to avoid these reminders being seen as 'checking up' or punitive, particularly if the activity is not completed, we often frame them as opportunities to notice thoughts, experiences and emotions associated with coming into contact with values. We would add that if the activity is completed, that is the 'icing on the cake'. In this way we are able to frame any activity, including even thinking about undertaking the task, as a step in a valued direction.

Finally, a key part of the work is developing a values-based relapse-prevention plan. Typical methods for relapse prevention in early intervention involve some variant of the back-in-the-saddle approach, developed by Birchwood *et al.* (2000). ACT can be used to enhance the typical approach, by introducing a values-based focus to relapse prevention, emphasising engagement in activities that are likely to support and supplement well-being and recovery, thereby minimising the likelihood of relapse. An ACT-based relapse-prevention plan includes skills in active acceptance and defusion as a means of facilitating early detection (rather than avoidance and sealing over) and thus effective and appropriate management of potential early-warning signs.

13.4   ACT in Different Modalities

13.4.1   Group Work

Our group therapy approach emphasises normalisation of unusual experiences and focuses on the effects of efforts to control these experiences through avoidance and worry. The nature of a group therapy fosters a context in which young people can discover that others share similar struggles with their minds, and validation of the resulting cost of trying to 'deal with' unusual experiences. The ACT model, which points to a set of constructive actions through which to pursue life meaning, easily allows for group universality to be reinforced, an important component in reducing stigma. In the group, we discuss in ACT-consistent ways how we rarely know how other people feel or think inside, and how we can feel odd or fraudulent when observing how we struggle with private (unusual) experiences. This struggling can be reinforced by our lack of knowledge and limited sharing about what it is like to be a human being who achieves while having unwanted or distracting experiences. In Chapter 15, our colleague Louise Johns briefly describes the content of the ACT groups we run with FE clients, which are based upon the central metaphor of the 'passengers on the bus' (see Appendix C for a description of this metaphor). Group work with young people requires creativity and skills in developing a therapeutic environment that is engaging, collaborative and flexible, allowing for considerable variation in the capacity to participate in the group session (depending on mental state).

13.4.2   Working with Families and Carers

Cognitive behavioural approaches to family interventions for people with psychosis have a good evidence base, having been shown to reduce relapse rates and hospital admissions, and to improve social impairment and family communication (Pharoah *et al.*, 2006). Although the evidence base is much smaller, reports have suggested similar benefits for FE clients and their families (Bird *et al.*, 2010). Such interventions typically involve a combination of psycho-education, problem solving, enhancement of communication and adjustment of carer appraisals of the illness.

There is evidence of a relationship between avoidance-based coping and carer distress (Onwumere *et al.*, 2011), and carer burden and distress are elevated in early psychosis (Onwumere *et al.*, 2008). As such, we speculate that family intervention may be enhanced by the introduction of acceptance-based and values-enhancing relationship techniques, similar in manner to integrative behavioural couples therapy (IBCT) (Jacobson *et al.*, 2000) and the ACT clinical literature for relationship work (Harris, 2009b). Acceptance-based family intervention may provide more options therapeutically: as well as the usual interventions to help carers develop more helpful appraisals of their relative and their situation, values work could provide greater clarity about the goals of therapy and acceptance/defusion may foster less judgemental communication styles and avoidant coping.

Our experience has been that discussions about the values that families hold are enormously helpful from the outset of family work. This can involve asking families questions such as, 'What things are important to each of you as a family?', 'In 5 years' time, where would you like to see your family?' and 'What are the things you personally do that help your family do the things that are important?' Often we find that the values that families bring up fall into two broad (but not exclusive) categories: 'improving relationships' and 'assisting in recovery'.

Once a set of shared family values has been clarified, they can be used as a framework for understanding problems or obstacles for the family. For example, intrafamily communication is often a key issue for family members and a reduction in hostile or critical communication (with a corresponding increase in warm, supportive communication) is a key treatment target. While it may make sense for a family member to point out problems and concerns, the usefulness of this communication style can be evaluated in terms of the degree to which it helps the family to work towards family values. For example, a family member, out of best intentions or concerns, may berate an individual about their lack of activity, inadvertently reducing the warmth and closeness in the relationship. Such behaviour can therefore be assessed in terms of its function in assisting the individual in moving towards important goals. By introducing this notion of workability, families can begin to develop a more flexible and mindful stance towards communication that more usefully aligns members with central values.

Absolutely essential in this work is to validate the family's attempts to manage what is often an extremely difficult situation and explicitly link these attempts with underlying values, by using statements such as 'I can see that you have your son's best interests at heart here, and you're really concerned that if you don't keep highlighting these problems, he may get worse and I know you want the best for him'. Normalising such behaviour as reasonable attempts to problem solve, which would work under normal circumstances, can help to minimise and reduce fusion with unhelpful, stigmatising or blaming thoughts. Such explicit discussion of the values 'alive' in these relationships may help to clarify actions that are more consistent with how each person wants to act within the family. This can be particularly helpful in negotiating some of the common problems that arise for FE clients and families, including establishing a commonly understood language with which to talk about mental-health experiences or disagreements about appropriate levels of activity related to household chores, study or work.

Problem solving and communication may be enhanced by introducing active acceptance and compassion towards self and relatives as alternatives to judgemental and critical attempts to solve problems. Validation and active acceptance of the feelings that arise from stressful family conversations may open the possibility of defusion from thoughts and memories that act as barriers. This is particularly important in relation to appraisals of guilt or shame, which are common in both carers and clients. An emphasis on acceptance can assist families in not getting so entangled in these emotions, thereby allowing more focus on valued action. For example, parents who feel deeply guilty that they somehow caused their daughter's illness may push her excessively to return to pre-illness levels of functioning in order to avoid those feelings of guilt. Making room for such painful feelings and reducing attempts to avoid them may allow the parents to be more appropriately supportive of their daughter and responsive to her current abilities and needs.

13.5   Case Study

In this section we will describe a case study in which we used ACT to enhance the general early-intervention approach. This vignette is an amalgam of various people seen in our setting, in order to protect confidentiality.

Sarah was a 23-year-old woman who was referred to our early-intervention-for-psychosis community team, following the onset of a number of distressing symptoms of psychosis, which had resulted in an admission to an acute psychiatric unit. During her admission, she described experiencing a number of problems, largely associated with her belief that other people could hear her thoughts and that she could hear the thoughts of others. She was not sure how this happened but wondered if a microchip had been inserted into her brain, through which thoughts were broadcast and received.

She described the onset of these problems as occurring shortly after a breakup with a boyfriend. She said that after the breakup her ex-boyfriend and his circle of friends, whom she had become close to, had been verbally abusive and bullying towards her. Sarah found this particularly distressing, in part because she had not experienced it before and had been profoundly shocked that people could be so cruel. Soon after this, Sarah started to experience a stream of negative, critical thoughts, which she strongly believed were not from her own mind. She eventually concluded that these thoughts were coming from her ex-boyfriend and his friends.

Over a period of a few months, Sarah became increasing distressed and preoc- cupied by these experiences, particularly as the thoughts she heard from others were typically about her and tended to be very negative and critical. She said she often became highly anxious when in social situations and felt very strongly that this anxiety was a sign there was something very wrong with her. Although Sarah was a very social person, she gradually withdrew, and became increasingly lonely and depressed. During this time she also increased her use of cannabis, which she found helped her to relax. When she came into the service, Sarah lived at home with her mother and father. She described her relationship with each of them as good, and felt they were supportive of her, although they did not always under- stand how difficult her life had become. Before her admission, Sarah had been studying fashion design but had dropped out.

Sarah was unsure as to the origin of the external thoughts. When she was in a social situation, she found the visceral nature of the thoughts highly convincing and was sure they came from an external source. However, once out of the situation, she typically found she was much less convinced by the experience. She also noted that, if the experiences were real (due to others), this would be validating, but her options for managing the situation would be limited. Alternatively, she felt that if the experiences were the result of mental illness, she would have some options for coping, but at the cost of dealing with the stigma of being mentally ill. Sarah would spend long periods of time ruminating about whether her experiences were 'real' or not, particularly after smoking cannabis. This also led to ambivalence with regard to taking medication, as she felt it confirmed to her that she had a mental illness. As a result, she tended to take her medication only infrequently.

When Sarah was first referred for psychology, she stated that her main aims were to find a way to stop feeling so anxious and to block out the thoughts from other people. In terms of an initial formulation, it was evident that Sarah was highly experientially avoidant, particularly of anxiety. She tended to overutilise control strategies (thought blocking, avoidance of anxiety-provoking situations, rumina- tion, smoking cannabis) in response to unwanted experiences, which, although often highly successful in the short term, had increased the overall incidence of these experiences. In terms of cognitive fusion, there were a number of thoughts that Sarah was unhelpfully fused with, including 'There is something wrong with me' and 'I have to figure my situation out before I can move forward with my life'. As a result of these experiences, Sarah's behavioural repertoire had been consider- ably narrowed and, importantly, she now had limited opportunities to engage in values-based activities.

As we have often found with young people with psychosis, Sarah was initially reluctant to consider the effects of avoidance behaviours in maintaining her difficulties. She felt very strongly that her anxiety needed to be controlled and that she simply needed to refine her current methods. As such, we spent time in the initial sessions discussing what she found important in her life, in terms of personal values. While her studies and family were important, being able to spend time with and be there for friends was vital for Sarah. We discussed obstacles to being with her friends and Sarah identified several key areas, including the presence of external thoughts and anxiety. Sarah was very focused on eliminating these experiences before she felt she could reengage with friends, which was understandable given the associated distress. However, this approach meant that she lost the opportunity to be with her friends, and this loss negatively impacted on her.

In our work we introduced the metaphor of a ship sailing through a storm (an adaptation of the swamp metaphor from Hayes *et al.*, 1999), as Sarah knew about sailing due to her father doing it. The metaphor suggested that sometimes, in order to head in a direction that is important, it can be necessary to sail through stormy territory. Going through storms just for the sake of it doesn't make sense, but if the direction leads to something worthwhile, storms can be weathered. Using this metaphor, we discussed the possibility of Sarah 'weathering' some difficult experiences for the purpose of being able to spend more time with her friends. We began practising mindfulness exercises, increasing her ability to make space and reduce her struggle with difficult experiences. Sarah expanded on the sailing metaphor, considering how it is important to roll with the natural movement of the boat, rather than constantly fight it. She used this to develop her ability to let go of the struggle with difficult experiences and to practise willingness. We also discussed the important of 'setting a course' and noticing when we get pulled off it by struggling with experiences.

Sarah began to recognise that her rumination and worry about the origin of the external thoughts, although very reasonable, often took her off course, preventing her from being with her friends. She eventually decided to leave the question as unresolved, which she found difficult initially. She began to spend a greater amount of time with her friends, which led to an initial increase in anxiety and the frequency of external thoughts. However, at the same time, she also felt both proud of herself and pleased to be acting more like the friend she wanted to be, and this made 'being in the storm' more manageable. She eventually spoke to two of her friends about what she had been through and found they were supportive, particularly after one friend disclosed that her brother had been through a similar experience. At this point she described a significant lift in her mood.

Sarah also reconsidered her stance towards medication after she decided to put the question regarding the origin of the external thoughts aside. She decided to take her medication more regularly in order to see if it would help her manage her 'storms' more effectively. Interestingly, she noticed that, over the next few months, the external thoughts reduced in terms of frequency. Although Sarah remained unsure about their origin, and was at times convinced they resulted from a microchip, she was much less distressed and preoccupied. Shortly after this point, she decided to finish therapy. She said she had had 'enough of talking' and wanted to get on with her life. She soon returned to college full time.

13.6   Conclusion

In summary, we think that the use of values-based acceptance and mindfulness approaches has much to offer in working with young people to assist them in recovering from their first episode of psychosis, and can be of value to their families. The experience of psychosis can be highly distressing and disruptive, for both individuals and their families, particularly at a stage of life characterised by significantly change and development. Developing broad skills in openness, awareness and engagement with values can help to maintain flexibility in the face of such an experience, giving hope that life can still be filled with richness and vitality.

References

Ashcroft, K., Barrow, F., Lee, R. & MacKinnon, K. (2011). Mindfulness groups for early psychosis: a qualitative study. *Psychology and Psychotherapy: Theory, Research and Practice*, 85(3), 327–334.

Birchwood, M. (1999). Early intervention in psychosis: the critical period. In P. D. McGorry & H. J. Jackson (eds). *The Recognition and Management of Early Psychosis: A Preventive Approach*. Cambridge: Cambridge University Press.

Birchwood, M. (2003). Pathways to emotional dysfunction in first-episode psychosis. *The British Journal of Psychiatry*, 182(5), 373–375.

Birchwood, M. & MacMillan, F. (1993). Early intervention in schizophrenia. *Australian and New Zealand Journal of Psychiatry*, 27(3), 374–378.

Birchwood, M., Spencer, E. & McGovern, D. (2000). Schizophrenia: early warning signs. *Advances in Psychiatric Treatment*, 6, 93–101.

Birchwood, M., Iqbal, Z. & Upthegrove, R. (2005). Psychological pathways to depression in schizophrenia. *European Archives of Psychiatry and Clinical Neuroscience*, 255(3), 202–212.

Bird, V., Premkumar, P., Kendall, T., Whittington, C., Mitchell, J. & Kuipers, E. (2010). Early intervention services, cognitive-behavioural therapy and family intervention in early psychosis: systematic review. *British Journal of Psychiatry*, 197, 350–356.

Bloy, S., Oliver, J. E. & Morris, E. (2011). Using acceptance and commitment therapy with people with psychosis. *Clinical Case Studies*, 10, 347–359.

Broome, M. R., Woolley, J. B., Johns, L. C., Valmaggia, L. R., Tabraham, P., Gafoor, R., Bramon, E. *et al.* (2005). Outreach and support in south London (OASIS): implementation of a clinical service for prodromal psychosis and the at risk mental state. *European Psychiatry*, 20, 372–378.

Chadwick, P. D. J. (2006). *Person-based Cognitive Therapy for Distressing Psychosis.* Chichester: John Wiley & Sons.

Corrigan, P. W. (2004). How stigma interferes with mental health care. *American Psychologist, 59,* 614–625.

Francey, S. M., Nelson, B., Thompson, A., Parker, A. G., Kerr, M., Macneil, C., Fraser, R. et al. (2010). Who needs antipsychotic medication in the earliest stages of psychosis? A reconsideration of benefits, risks, neurobiology and ethics in the era of early intervention. *Schizophrenia Rresearch, 119,* 1–10.

Gumley, A. & Schwannauer, M. (2006). *Staying Well After Psychosis: A Cognitive Interpersonal Approach to Recovery and Relapse Prevention.* Chichester: John Wiley & Sons.

Harris, R. (2009a). *ACT Made Simple: An Easy-To-Read Primer on Acceptance and Commitment Therapy.* Oakland: New Harbinger.

Harris, R. (2009b). *ACT with Love: Stop Struggling, Reconcile Differences, and Strengthen your Relationship with Acceptance and Commitment Therapy.* Oakland: New Harbinger.

Harrison, G., Croudace, T., Mason, P., Glazebrook, C. & Medley, I. (1996). Predicting the long-term outcome of schizophrenia. *Psychological Medicine, 26*(4), 697–705.

Harrop, C. & Trower, P. (2001). Why does schizophrenia develop at late adolescence? *Clinical PsychologyRreview, 21,* 241–265.

Jacobson, N. S., Christensen, A., Prince, S. E., Cordova, J. & Eldridge, K. (2000). Integrative Behavioral Couple Therapy: an acceptance-based, promising new treatment for couple discord. *Journal of Consulting and Clinical Psychology, 68,* 351–355.

Link, B. G. (1987). Understanding the labelling effects in the area of mental disorders: an assessment of the effects of expectations of rejection. *American Sociological Review, 52,* 95–112.

Linszen, D., Dingemans, P. & Lenior, M. (2001). Early intervention and a five year follow up in young adults with a short duration of untreated psychosis: ethical implications. *Schizophrenia Research, 51*(1), 55–61.

Malla, A. & Payne, J. (2005). First-episode psychosis: psychopathology, quality of life, and functional outcome. *Schizophrenia Bulletin, 31*(3), 650–671.

Mason, P., Harrison, G., Glazebrook, C., Medley, I., Dalkin, T. & Croudace, T. (1995). Characteristics of outcome in schizophrenia at 13 years. *The British Journal of Psychiatry, 167,* 596–603.

McGlashan, T. H., Levy, S. T. & Carpenter, W. T. Jr (1975). Integration and sealing over: clinically distinct recovery styles from schizophrenia. *Archives of General Psychiatry, 32,* 1269.

McGorry, P. D. & Killackey, E. J. (2002). Early intervention in psychosis: a new evidence based paradigm. *Epidemiology and Psychiatric Sciences, 11*(4), 237–247.

McGorry, P. D., Hickie, I. B., Yung, A. R., Pantelis, C. & Jackson, H. J. (2006). Clinical staging of psychiatric disorders: a heuristic framework for choosing earlier, safer and more effective interventions. *Australian and New Zealand Journal of Psychiatry, 40*(8), 616–622.

McGorry, P. D., Killackey, E. & Yung, A. (2008). Early intervention in psychosis: concepts, evidence and future directions. *World Psychiatry, 7*(3), 148–156.

Morris, E. & Oliver, J. (2009). ACT Early: Acceptance and Commitment Therapy in early intervention in psychosis. *Clinical Psychology Forum, 196,* 27–31.

Morris, E. & Oliver, J. E. (2012). Acceptance & Commitment Therapy. In W. Dryden (ed.). *Cognitive Behaviour Therapies.* London: SAGE.

Morrison, A. P., French, P., Lewis, S. W., Roberts, M., Raja, S., Neil, S. T., Parker, S. *et al.* (2006). Psychological factors in people at ultra-high risk of psychosis: comparisons with non-patients and associations with symptoms. *Psychological Medicine*, 36(10), 1395–1404.

Onwumere, J., Kuipers, E., Bebbington, P., Dunn, G., Freeman, D., Fowler, D. & Garety, P. (2011). Coping styles in carers of people with recent and long-term psychosis. *Journal of Nervous and Mental Disease*, 199, 423–424.

Onwumere, J., Kuipers, E, Bebbington, P., Dunn, G., Fowler, D., Freeman, D., Watson, P. & Garety, P. (2008). Care-giving and illness beliefs in the course of psychotic illness. *Canadian Journal of Psychiatry*, 53, 460–468.

Parnas, J. (1999). From predisposition to psychosis: progression of symptoms in schizophrenia. *Acta Psychiatrica Scandinavica*, 99, 20–29.

Petersen, L., Nordentoft, M., Jeppesen, P., Øhlenschlæger, J., Thorup, A., Christensen, T. Ø., Krarup, G. *et al.* (2005). Improving 1-year outcome in first-episode psychosis OPUS trial. *The British Journal of Psychiatry*, 187(48), s98–s103.

Pharoah, F. M., Mari, J. J. & Steiner, D. (2000). Family intervention for schizophrenia. *Cochrane Database System Review*, 2, CD000088.

Phillips, L. J., Yung, A. R. & McGorry, P. D. (2000). Identification of young people at risk of psychosis: validation of Personal Assessment and Crisis Evaluation Clinic intake criteria. *Australian and New Zealand Journal of Psychiatry*, 34, 164–S169.

Power, P., Bell, R., Mills, R., Herrman-Doig, T., Davern, M., Henry, L., Yuen, H. *et al.* (2003). Suicide prevention in first episode psychosis: the development of a randomised controlled trial of cognitive therapy for acutely suicidal patients with early psychosis. *Australian and New Zealand Journal of Psychiatry*, 37(4), 414–420.

Valmaggia, L. R. & Morris, E. (2010). Attention training technique and acceptance and commitment therapy for distressing auditory hallucinations. In F. Larøi & A. Aleman (eds). *Hallucinations: A Guide to Treatment and Management*. Oxford: Oxford University Press, pp. 123–141.

Van der Valk, R., van de Waerdt, S., Meijer, C. J., van den Hout, I. & de Haan, L. (2012). Feasibility of mindfulness-based therapy in patients recovering from a first psychotic episode: a pilot study. *Early Intervention in Psychiatry*, doi: 10.1111/j.1751-7893.2012.00356.x.

Whitehorn, D., Brown, J., Richard, J., Rui, Q. & Kopala, L. (2002). Multiple dimensions of recovery in early psychosis. *International Review of Psychiatry*, 14(4), 273–283.

Zubin, J. & Spring, B. (1977). Vulnerability: a new view on schizophrenia. *Journal of Abnormal Psychology*, 86, 103–126.

14

Acceptance and Commitment Therapy for Psychosis in Acute Psychiatric Admission Settings

Gordon Mitchell and Amy McArthur

14.1 Introduction

The goal of this chapter is to explore how an acceptance and commitment therapy (ACT) approach can enhance the treatment of people with psychosis who are resident in hospital settings, specifically focusing on acute psychiatric admission wards. We will begin with a discussion of the challenges encountered in terms of the common profiles of individuals who experience acute psychosis and the obstacles inherent in this particular treatment setting. This is especially important in implementing ACT-consistent interventions within a complex clinical service system. We will then present a detailed clinical case vignette to illustrate our attempts to integrate an ACT approach into an acute admission environment. Finally, we will review examples of convergence between ACT and other psychological approaches that are pertinent to the client group in this clinical setting and summarise areas for future research.

14.2 Acute Psychosis and ACT Interventions

It is a well-established clinical observation that when individuals experience acute episodes of psychosis, they actively search for explanations for them (Drury *et al.*, 1996). Their search for causation may be disordered, highly biased

Acceptance and Commitment Therapy and Mindfulness for Psychosis, First Edition.
Edited by Eric M. J. Morris, Louise C. Johns and Joseph E. Oliver.
© 2013 John Wiley & Sons, Ltd. Published 2013 by John Wiley & Sons, Ltd.

and chaotic, but nevertheless they actively try to make sense of what is happening to them. Many first-person accounts of acute psychotic experiences reflect this drive for explanation (Maher, 1988), and how this can lead to progressively more suspicion if the individual does not receive opportunity for reflection.

> … the more I thought my ideas were extraordinary, the more I began to think that others were going to try to steal my ideas from me. Then I felt afraid my adversaries might disagree with my thoughts and understandings of life, or be jealous of my creative ideas – wanting to suppress them or introduce them as their own. Then I wondered too if I was being controlled by my persecutors in their efforts to tap into my creative thinking process (Chapman, 2002).

This is in stark contrast with the phenomenon of 'sealing over' that is generally associated with the post-acute phase (McGlashan *et al.*, 1975). In this state, people avoid reference to their psychosis and show little curiosity or motivation to reflect and integrate their experiences into a wider context. There are several significant psychological factors influencing this. For example, individuals learn not to refer to psychotic experiences so that they can be discharged from acute facilities. This reflects the emphasis given to equating recovery primarily with evidence of a reduction in positive symptoms (McGorry *et al.*, 2010). In addition, there is the paradoxical effect of acute services concentrating on containment of distress rather than engagement in dialogue about the personal experience of psychosis. In such a context, patients will most likely become less inclined to share their search for an explanation and become even more fused into their own inner world, through increased avoidance and suppression. Individuals will thus become increasingly dominated by their illness, often retreating from previously valued activities and aspirations. In this sense, the acute phase offers an important opportunity for psychological intervention.

ACT aims to enable individuals to accept difficult internal experiences such as psychosis and to move to behave in ways that are consistent with personally held values (Hayes *et al.*, 1999). However, the extremes of psychopathology frequently witnessed when individuals experience an acute exacerbation of psychosis make it difficult to conceptualise how an ACT perspective can aid and guide psychological interventions. Individuals requiring acute admission to hospital regularly display poor insight and have high levels of disorganisation, severely reducing their ability to receive and reflect rationally on feedback from their environment (Byrne, 2007). Is it possible for the ACT therapist to work around the bizarre content often expressed during the acute phase in order to promote the type of psychological flexibility required to increase an individual's sensitivity to their inner and external environments? The profound influence of psychotic processes regularly dominates over direct experience. If the individual experiencing acute psychosis is aware of environmental contingences, their interpretation of causation is hugely biased towards supporting psychotic beliefs (e.g. Garety *et al.*, 2011).

If the goal of ACT in psychosis is to encourage individuals to live more adaptively with their condition (Mcleod, 2009), is it contraindicated to attempt interventions while they are in an acute state? It may be more prudent to refrain from such psychological intervention until the individual is stabilised on medication and less consumed by their psychosis. Indeed, it is argued by some that the function of an acute inpatient service should be to act as a last resort and 'contain' associated levels of distress and dysfunction that cannot be managed in community settings (as summarised by Clarke, 2009). Linked to this primary aim is the associated goal of returning individuals to their community as quickly as possible. It seems reasonable to assume that psychological interventions will have more impact when an individual has recovered from the acute exacerbation and is back within their own community, rather than in the rather artificial context of a busy admission unit.

While an acute phase may offer a context for greater integration and reflection, if this is not actively fostered, the trauma associated with an acute exacerbation of psychosis may become more prominent. Feelings of stigma, depression, fear and shame intrude and develop a momentum of their own (Gumley & Schwannauer, 2006). Psychological pain associated with these emotions is difficult to cope with, making it even harder for individuals to process their original psychotic preoccupations in an adaptive manner. This is an extremely important issue, as such factors clearly influence the maintenance of social anhedonia amongst the client group, with a major impact on recovery (White *et al.*, 2007).

All these factors contribute to work against the core ACT requirement of encouraging individuals to be more 'open' to distressing internal events (Luoma *et al.*, 2007). In fact, the prevailing ethos and culture in many acute inpatient settings rewards the very human tendency to avoid such a psychological stance. Unfortunately, within an acute setting, individuals with psychosis often develop comorbid problems, which tend to become the prime focus of clinical discussion and intervention, in place of the core issues associated with their psychosis. For example, patients will manifest associated substance abuse, self-harm or so-called 'borderline' personality issues as a maladaptive attempt to cope with their experiences. Services themselves become 'fused' and increasingly preoccupied by behaviours that are relatively distant from the original presentation. It is obviously essential that comorbidity issues be addressed, but services need to ensure that their overall perspective integrates the various strands of psychopathology. This is where an ACT formulation can link fundamental factors associated with the psychosis and any additional comorbid conditions that may have developed from further experiential avoidance. Clinical interventions are often hampered by a lack of integrated formulation in individuals with so-called multiproblem presentations (e.g. Strosahl, 2004).

14.3   ACT in the Acute Psychiatric Admission Ward

For staff working on the front lines of busy and demanding inpatient acute wards, it is draining enough just providing individuals with safe containment, without the additional expectation of encouraging them to learn from and reflect upon their psychotic episodes. However, Pinto (2009) describes the problems which arise from an excessively protective attitude on the part of mental-health services. He cites the prominence of the stress–vulnerability model as promoting the necessity to create a 'protective belt' around the idea of vulnerability, rather than encouraging psychological interventions based on a climate of acceptance and abstention of judgement. Pinto describes this openness as a necessary prerequisite to enabling patients to experience new ways of relating to their own experiences and the outside world.

It is a considerable challenge to promote a psychologically informed and planned therapeutic environment which consistently fosters openness to others' distressing experiences, the basic requirement underpinning ACT interventions in an acute setting. Acute psychiatric wards are complex locations, in which increasingly medical models of mental illness dominate (Pilgram, 2009) and various professionals coexist, each with their own unique theoretical and training histories. Patients may have relatively short admissions, mitigating against the adoption of psychological interventions. To expect diverse professionals to embrace ACT as the main anchor to psychological formulation and intervention seems unrealistic. However, if ACT can contribute to counter the unworkable consequences of acute exacerbations of psychosis, by promoting improved perspective taking, empathy and compassion while individuals are actively searching for personal meaning, then it is critical for ACT therapists to work alongside other professionals.

There are three key strands to our attempts to implement this approach in the acute settings in which we have worked:

- Providing brief experiential ACT training to direct-care staff, in order to influence the environment systemically.
- Providing opportunities for staff to work alongside ACT therapists in group settings, in order to develop relevant knowledge and skills (see Chapter 15).
- Providing ACT-based interventions in individual and group settings, in order to foster reduced experiential avoidance and increased contact with valued living as a means of moving beyond unworkable behavioural patterns.

14.4   Case Study

The following case vignette illustrates an attempt to explore whether the aforementioned challenges can be addressed and ACT for psychosis can be relevant in an acute setting. This vignette is an amalgam of various people seen in our setting, in order to protect confidentiality.

David is a male in his late 40s with a long history of psychosis and multiple previous acute admissions. His main presenting symptoms are extremely distressing command hallucinations which consistently tell him to harm his elderly mother, Rose, with whom he lives. The onset of David's psychotic symptoms occurred when he left home to study at university. The only recorded evidence of David partially responding to these commands was some years ago, when, for a period of a few weeks, he prevented health professionals from visiting his mother at home and withheld some of her medication. This series of events culminated with a brief admission to hospital. During his admission, David often requested ever-increasing dosages of psychotropic medications and additional 'as-required' medication in an attempt to 'numb out' the experiences of the voices. David has never acted on the voices' instructions to directly cause physical harm to Rose.

Following this episode, David felt great concern that he couldn't trust himself to resist the voices, which remained despite high maintenance dosages of various medications. As a consequence, David sought considerable reassurance from his siblings and community mental-health team, and tried to minimise the amount of time he and his mother spent alone together by arranging for family and friends to visit frequently and for her to have regular visits from health-care and voluntary agencies. On a number of occasions over the last few years, David has harmed himself as a result of his difficulty in coping with the presence of the voices, which has led to further unplanned admissions to hospital for assessment and stabilisation. David was previously referred for cognitive behavioural therapy for psychosis (CBTp) while in the community, but failed to engage, citing his inability to talk about his psychotic experiences, as this would, in his view, activate them further.

It was decided to offer David an ACT-based psychological intervention during another acute admission. The rationale presented to David was that this would allow him to explore his feelings associated with the voices rather than directly discussing their content. There was also an emphasis on providing supports for him to 'move on' in his life in ways he could identify as being relevant and important.

The nursing staff from the care team was provided with introductory ACT workshops and follow-up clinical supervision in an attempt to ensure consistency in encouraging David to explore and learn from his experiences, rather than focusing on containing and reducing his distress. The workshops and supervision were extremely well-received by the direct-care staff. Although no one had had previous exposure to ACT models of psychopathology and clinical intervention, the approach appeared to make intuitive sense to the staff group, as they recognised the clinical presentations that resulted from or were maintained by experiential avoidance. Most interestingly, the workshops introduced these issues from a normative, continuum perspective, acknowledging the human tendency to avoid difficult experiences. Members of the direct-care staff recognised they were working with individuals at the extremes of this continuum, with additional complicating factors thrown in, and that the model highlighted human commonalities which would help them see these individuals in the whole.

The values emphasis also appeared to strike a chord. Values were introduced by exploring staff members' own personally held values (in particular those linked to mutual professional and organisational issues) and then reflecting on how easy it was to lose sight of them as a constant source of guidance and motivation. The care team members seemed to naturally see a valued role for themselves as professionals acting as mentors or coaches, encouraging David to expand his behavioural repertoires towards more values-based ones.

One member of the care team was available to act as a co-therapist during all the ACT sessions. It was envisaged that having a member of the direct-care staff as a co-therapist would help further generalise ACT-consistent approaches outside the actual sessions. This was particularly important as David tended to cope with distress by requesting additional as-required medication, or by resorting to self-harm in more extreme situations. David's consultant psychiatrist was also kept informed, and progress was discussed in detail during clinical ward rounds.

David was informed that the ACT sessions would take place twice a week, with additional opportunities to speak with key workers when they were on duty. During the initial sessions, he was encouraged to remain present with his emotions associated with the occurrence of auditory hallucinations. We expected some degree of resistance towards this, considering the chronic nature of his presentation. However, David appeared to be reassured simply by knowing the structure of the sessions, which we reinforced by providing him with written summaries. It seemed as if a safe and trusting environment had been created in which he could ventilate his feelings, even though he was in the midst of an acute relapse. The emphasis here was on promoting contact with the present moment and taking a more accepting stance towards his experiences.

David reported various delusional ideas regarding his attempts to make sense of why he was being persecuted by the voices, but we continued to focus on his associated emotional responses, using phrases such as, 'How does that make *you* feel?', 'How would *you* describe the feeling *you* experience when that occurs?' It soon become apparent that David had been harbouring significant negative affect associated with his sense of self, which he had never been able to adequately process. Indeed, it came pouring out, and both therapists acknowledged their personal discomfort at witnessing the levels of distress and the tendency to intervene or 'rescue' David from that pain.

The co-therapist arranged with colleagues from David's care team to provide additional half-hour daily sessions in which he could further ventilate his experiences during this stage of accepting and being more present. What was soon noticeable during the sessions was a dilution of the psychotic preoccupations and an accompanying increase in David's willingness to show up with core emotional issues. This apparent shift seems to echo Bentall's (2001) assertion that psychosis can manifest as a result of experiential avoidance, rather than as an experience to avoid in itself. These additional sessions were used appropriately, and staff members reported a decline in requests for as-required medication and a cessation of previous self-harm behaviours. ACT metaphors such as the 'tug-of-war with the monster' (see Appendix H) and the 'computer screen' (see Chapter 9) (Harris, 2009) were used to reinforce defusion from these core experiences. David was provided with illustrated examples of both metaphors, with empty monsters and computer screens which he could complete with his own descriptions of unpleasant internal experiences. David appeared to be more willing to show up with his pain, but also found appropriate ways to 'let it go', such as by practising stepping back and 'noticing' his internal experiences in the moment, rather than responding to them automatically.

As the therapy progressed, it was clear that David was moving from relating mainly to self-as-content to relating to self-as-process, and from there was shifting further to self-as-context (Foody *et al.*, 2012). In the course of this work, values were identified as David's contact with painful affect brought to the surface evidence of what was personally important to him. This was particularly connected to his underlying desire to be a good son and brother, despite his reservations over his ability to fulfil such roles. Without prompting, David provided information from his developmental history to suggest the historical context behind his underlying poor sense of self and subsequent vulnerability to psychotic experience. David was able to describe this history in a very reflective and compassionate manner. He provided a powerful story of his past learning context that allowed him a sense of being able to add new chapters. He could adjust the story to have more to do with his own agenda, rather than functioning to keep him stuck in reason-giving. All this seemed to promote a greater sense of purpose and choice, reflecting his exploration of self-as-context and perspective taking, and undermining attachment to his self-concept as being dangerous, insofar as he was dominated by the voices.

It was not lost on either therapist that it was probably a unique situation for David to be in an environment he found safe and trusting, allowing him to connect with these issues. We speculated over whether he could ever have achieved this as an outpatient, as the necessary 'rawness' of presentation would have been replaced by entrenched, defensive experiential avoidance. It was worthy of notice that the admission unit created a safe and trusting environment with sufficient access to contact and supports: something that wouldn't have been possible in an outpatient setting. On this occasion, we did not have input from other potentially appropriate clinicians; it would have been useful to have an art therapist use their specific skills to aid David in further engaging with present-moment experience.

David began to identify specific valued goals associated with his desire to be a good son, which were consistently supported by the care team, even with the continued presence of his psychotic experiences. He planned more activities with his mother and other family members during periods of leave from the ward. David quickly progressed through these planned activities in a hierarchical fashion, eventually being able to take his mother out for the day without a chaperone being present. This in particular was a momentous achievement, as David acknowledged his voices were present during the walk, and that they informed him of opportunities to harm Rose. This occasioned a considerable shift for the whole clinical team as David described this event at his review meeting. The team members recognised their uneasiness at the risk involved, but also acknowledged that David was able to discriminate between his psychotic experience and his ability to pursue his own valued behaviours.

When he was discharged, David's community psychiatric nurse was briefed regarding the progress he had made, and they ensured further opportunities were available to maintain similar supports. David was also able to see the same clinical psychologist and consultant psychiatrist who had supported him during therapy, providing further continuity from the hospital to the community setting. His psychiatrist was able to negotiate reductions in dosages and multiple medication prescriptions, a situation that had previously been unthinkable.

However, during a routine appointment for blood tests, David, now used to speaking openly with staff about his voices, described a recent occasion on which the voices had encouraged him to harm his mother. The phlebotomist unfortunately was not one of the staff in the communication loop acquainted with the ACT approach. They did have some information about David's original symptoms, and understandably felt it prudent to ask the duty doctor to see him. The duty doctor had no available case notes but was informed by the phlebotomist about past concerns regarding the possibility of David harming his mother. The duty doctor thus asked if David would arrange for another family member to look after his mother and wait to see a social worker who could assess the situation further.

These were understandable reactions by the staff involved, given the circumstances. Unfortunately, they created an equally comprehensible response from David: he retreated back into a failsafe 'don't say anything' mode. This was interpreted as resistance due to psychotic preoccupation, and David was observed to be agitated and distressed. The social worker thus suggested contacting his consultant psychiatrist, who was available, and who suggested a member of the ward staff accompany David to the hospital for interview. David's initial reaction was one of failure: he had always been a bad son and he shouldn't have kid himself to the contrary. The voices amplified this belief, and by the time David arrived at the hospital, he was in a state of acute distress, with emphasis once more on the power and dominance manifested by the voices.

The consultant and ward staff reminded David of the substantial progress he had made and suggested he stay in hospital for a few days, just to help him regain confidence. This was very different from his emergency admissions under the mental health section in the past: David was able to use the short stay productively to once more process his distress, reflect on it rather than get hooked in and reconnect with allowing his personal values to guide him rather than being dominated by illness. David himself was able to comment that the recent event was something to learn from, rather than a return to experiential avoidance.

14.5   Convergence of Mindfulness/Metacognitive-based Cognitive Therapy Approaches

This vignette illustrates both the potential for ACT approaches to benefit an individual with psychosis in acute settings and how challenging it is to create a consistent approach which constantly encourages a willingness stance instead of avoidance. Nevertheless, the type of clinical environment that creates a safe and enhancing context within which individuals can explore their psychotic experiences echoes a recent review of advances in cognitive treatments for psychosis. Freeman (2011) stresses how simply allowing individuals to talk about their psychotic experiences, in a systematic manner, can in itself be incredibly therapeutic. Psychotic symptoms are viewed as being perpetuated by associated worry and ruminations, which impact on emotional processing of the psychotic experience. Freeman (2011) notes that there is often a lack of opportunity for patients being 'carefully listened to, for their distress being taken seriously, and for the clinician not being shocked, blaming or rejecting' (p. 137).

This description is very similar to ACT formulations of psychosis. Pankey & Hayes (2003) speculate that the main source of negative impact associated with psychosis comes from patients becoming 'entangled in the literal content of their own unusual and at times frightening thoughts and emotions, because contexts that encourage said entanglement are common, while those that weaken it are rare. As entanglement increases, the transfer of negative emotional functions increases' (p. 316).

Interestingly, both approaches stress the need for psychological interventions to avoid directly disputing the validity of psychotic beliefs. ACT views attempts to control or change verbal relations as potentially counterproductive, as they might increase entanglement within existing networks. From a different theoretical perspective, Freeman and his colleagues developed a similar intervention, emotional processing and metacognitive awareness (EPMA). Hepworth *et al.* (2011) report on key elements of this approach. Patients are helped to distance themselves from their experience by describing it in a narrative form, with a first-person present emphasis (e.g. 'I am thinking he is looking at me' rather than 'Why is he looking at me?') The whole narrative process is slowed down to promote the identification and labelling of associated thoughts, sensations, memories and images. Decentring, acceptance and letting go of experiences are promoted by using the 'leaves-on-the-stream' metaphor (see Appendix B). Other elements of the intervention also echo attempts to promote acceptability/willingness to directly connect with difficult but core internal experiences. Finally, perspective-taking techniques are used to encourage defusion and self as context.

The focus on encouraging clients to develop a richer narrative about their lives and to be mindful of the process of thinking in order to promote psychological flexibility resembles recent arguments by Lysaker *et al.* (2010), who advocate the development of therapeutic interventions that go beyond symptom- or problem-focused approaches and address larger issues around self-experience, helping individuals to construct a personal narrative in which the self is viewed as more multifaceted and more integrated. They argue that this emphasis can create the basis for people to develop new behaviours that evolve positive self-experience and gain greater capacity to reflect about thinking rather than being trapped by inner experiences.

These themes echo our own experience of introducing ACT into a busy acute inpatient unit. Given adequate training, support and continuing clinical supervision, the direct-care staff readily adapted to a role akin to providing a cognitive prosthesis, encouraging David to process and label his self-experience and to become aware of the process of thinking beyond unhelpful attempts at correcting maladaptive beliefs. The staff aided David in thinking about his particular experience of life and its challenges, but in a supportive compassionate way, which further enabled him to reconnect with personal values.

14.6   Reflections on Developing Systemic Applications of ACT

In our case vignette, the direct-care staff responded to an ACT approach and was keen to incorporate it. It seemed important that individual staff members made a 'personal' connection to ACT, were able to share clinical experiences of its application and felt sufficiently 'safe' within themselves and their clinical environments to move from a pro-containment, risk-aversive stance towards encouraging patients to actually 'learn from' their difficult experiences.

Based on the experiences gained from this case study, we have proceeded with a proposal to develop a 'whole-system' ACT training study. This includes all members of the nursing staff employed in the same acute psychiatric admission unit. The practicalities of providing a sufficient level of training and supervision to all staff members operating on a shift system in a busy admission ward are considerable. It has been acknowledged that the process will take almost a year to complete. Cohorts of four staff members each (eventually covering a total of nearly 30) will attend 10 hours of training over five weekly 2-hour sessions. Each cohort will receive 4 hours of ACT workshops aimed at promoting personal flexibility/resilience (Flaxman & Bond, 2010). These sessions will also look at enhancing the values base of the team working within the acute psychiatric unit and how its members can work more effectively together (Bethay *et al.*, 2009). Each cohort will then receive 4 hours of training on how to use ACT as a clinical formulation tool. Part of this segment of the package has been influenced by Strosahl & Robinson's (2009) recent work describing practical examples of teaching ACT to diverse health-professional groups. Finally, 2 hours of clinical supervision will be provided, encouraging staff members to reflect on their work with current patients under their care. The emphasis is on how they perceive their level of 'openness' towards coping with the distress expressed by their patients and how they can use ACT in formulating clinical presentations.

Evaluating psychosocial interventions within inpatient settings is notoriously difficult (Durrant & Tolland, 2009). At this stage, there is no expectation of staff members becoming ACT therapists; rather, the aim is to explore how an ACT model can enhance levels of confidence and competence regarding working with individuals who experience acute exacerbations of severe mental illness. Therefore, repeated outcome measures over the period of training will reflect assessments of clinical confidence, work engagement and psychological resilience/flexibility. In addition, all individuals receiving inpatient care on the unit over the period of the study will be invited at their discharge to complete measures of satisfaction with and perceptions of the appropriateness of their treatment. Finally, patients will be asked to complete a short measure on how they perceive services as meeting their attachment needs (that is, providing them with a secure and positive relationship while in hospital). All measures will be initially collected for a baseline period prior to training interventions, then completed monthly and at all discharges during the intervention, and finally for a sufficient post-intervention period.

The aim is to explore the extent of changes in both staff and patient experience on the unit over the period of training, in order to ascertain the impact of introducing ACT as a significant model of an integrated clinical approach in an acute psychiatric inpatient setting.

14.7 Conclusion

This chapter provides arguments to support the use of ACT interventions for acute psychosis within psychiatric admission facilities. However, it is important to recognise the particular challenges that exist for individuals with acute psychosis and within the environment of the ward setting. It is especially critical to ensure interventions are supported by the broader context of the ward system. This is not unlike the tradition of therapeutic communities (www.therapeuticcommunities. org), which place importance on the creation of 'psychologically informed planned environments'. In this case, the particular psychological theory is based on ACT. Each service system will have its own particular history and context. Creating ACT-consistent therapeutic environments requires not only sound knowledge and relevant clinical experience of delivering ACT to this client group but also innovative approaches to training and development. It is crucial to evaluate such initiatives but at the same time to remain sensitive to the unit's own history and context. Any approach requires networking in a nonhierarchical manner, adopting as open an approach to service development and evaluation as possible.

References

Bentall, R. P. (2001). Social cognition and delusional beliefs. In P. W. Corrigan & D. L. Penn (eds). *Social Cognition and Schizophrenia*. Washington, DC: American Psychological Association.

Bethay, S. J., Wilson, K. G. & Moyer, K. H. (2009). Acceptance and commitment therapy training for work stress and burnout in mental health direct care providers. In J. T. Blackledge, J. Ciarrochi & F. P. Deane (eds). *Acceptance and Commitment Therapy: Contemporary Theory, Research and Practice*. Bowen Hills: Australian Academic Press.

Byrne, P. (2007). Managing the acute psychiatric episode. *British Medical Journal*, 334, 686–692.

Chapman, R. K. (2002). First person account: eliminating delusions. *Schizophrenia Bulletin*, 28(3), 545–553.

Clarke, I. (2009). Introduction. In I. Clarke & H. Wilson (eds). *Cognitive Behaviour Therapy for Acute Inpatient Mental Health Units: Working with Clients, Staff and Milieu*. Hove: Routledge.

Drury, V., Birchwood, M. & Cochrane, R. (1996). Cognitive therapy and recovery from acute psychosis: a controlled trial. 1. Impact on psychotic symptoms. *British Journal of Psychiatry*, 169, 593–601.

Durrant, C. & Tolland, A. (2009). Evaluating short term CBT in an acute adult inpatient unit. In I. Clarke & H. Wilson (eds). *Cognitive Behaviour Therapy for Acute Inpatient Mental Health Units: Working with Clients, Staff and Milieu*. Hove: Routledge.

Flaxman, P. E. & Bond, F. W. (2010). A randomised worksite Comparison of acceptance and commitment therapy and stress inoculation training. *Behaviour Research and Therapy*, 48, 816–820.

Foody, M., Barnes-Holmes, Y. & Barnes-Holmes, D. (2012). The role of self in acceptance & commitment therapy. In L. McHugh & I. Stewart (eds). *The Self and Perspective Taking: Contributions and Applications from Modern Behavioral Science*. Oakland: Context Press.

Freeman, D. (2011). Improving cognitive treatment for delusions. *Schizophrenia Research*, 13, 135–139.

Garety, P., Freeman, D., Jolley, S., Ross, K., Waller, H. & Dunn, G. (2011). Jumping to conclusions: the psychology of delusional reasoning. *Advances in Psychiatric Treatment*, 17, 332–339.

Gumley, A. & Schwannauer, M. (2006). *Staying Well after Psychosis: A Cognitive Interpersonal Approach to Recovery and Relapse Prevention*. London: John Wiley & Sons.

Harris, R. (2009). *ACT Made Simple: An Easy-to-Read Primer on Acceptance and Commitment Therapy*. Oakland: New Harbinger.

Hayes, S. C., Strosahl, K. D. & Wilson K. G. (1999). *Acceptance and Commitment Therapy: An ExperientialAapproach to Behaviour Change*. New York: Guilford Press.

Hepworth, C., Startup, H. & Freeman, D. (2011). Developing treatments for persistent persecutory delusions. The impact of an emotional processing and metacognitive awareness intervention. *Journal of Nervous and Mental Disease*, 199(9), 653–658.

Luoma, J. B., Hayes, S. C. & Walser, R. D. (2007). *Learning ACT: An ACT Skills Training Manual for Therapists*. Oakland: New Harbinger.

Lysaker, P. H., Wilkness, S. M., Glynn, S. M. & Silverstein, S. M. (2010). Psychotherapy and recovery from schizophrenia: a review of potential applications and need for future study. *Psychological Services*, 7(2), 75–91.

Maher, B. A. (1988). Anomalous experience and delusional thinking: the logic of explanations. In T. F. Offman & B. A. Maher (eds). *Delusional Beliefs*. New York: John Wiley & Sons.

McGlashan, T H., Levy S. T. & Carpenter W. T. (1975). Integration and sealing over. Clinically distinct recovery styles from schizophrenia. *Archives of General Psychiatry*, 32(10), 1269–1272.

McGorry, P., Johanessen, J., Lewis, S., Birchwood, M., Malla, A., Nordentoft, M., Addington, J. & Yung, A. (2010). Early intervention in psychosis: keeping faith with evidence based health care. *Psychological Medicine*, 40(3), 399–404.

McLeod, H. J. (2009). ACT and CBT for psychosis: comparisons and contrasts. In J. T. Blackledge, J. Ciarrochi & F. P. Deane (eds). *Acceptance and Commitment Therapy: Contemporary Theory, Research and Practice*. Bowen Hills: Australian Academic Press.

Pankey, J. & Hayes, S. (2003). Acceptance and commitment therapy for psychosis. *International Journal of Psychology and Psychological Therapy*, 3(2), 311–328.

Pilgram, D. (2009). *Key Concepts in Mental Health* (2nd edn). London: Sage.

Pinto, A. (2009). Mindfulness and psychosis. In J. Kabat-Zinn & F. Didonna (eds). *Clinical Handbook of Mindfulness*. New York: Springer.

Strosahl, K. D. (2004). ACT with the multi-problem patient. In S. C. Hayes & K. D. Strosahl (eds). *A Practical Guide to Acceptance and Commitment Therapy*. New York: Springer.

Strosahl, K. D. & Robinson, P. J. (2009). Teaching ACT: to whom, why and how. In J. T. Blackledge, J. Ciarrochi & F. P. Deane (eds). *Acceptance and Commitment Therapy: Contemporary Theory, Research and Practice*. Bowen Hills: Australian Academic Press.

White, R., McGlerry, M. & Gumley, A. (2007). Hopelessness in schizophrenia. The impact of symptoms and beliefs about illness. *Journal of Nervous and Mental Disease*, 195(12), 968–975.

15

Developing Acceptance and Commitment Therapy for Psychosis as a Group-based Intervention

Amy McArthur, Gordon Mitchell
and Louise C. Johns

15.1 Introduction

The rationale for developing acceptance and commitment therapy (ACT) as a group-based intervention for individuals who experience psychosis has three main strands. First, the relevance of the ACT model to the needs of individuals who experience psychosis is a strong imperative, as has been described elsewhere in this volume (e.g. Chapters 1 and 5). Second, there is evidence that group-based psychological therapies improve outcomes for this population. Research has shown the effectiveness of group cognitive behaviour therapy (CBT) for a number of difficulties associated with psychosis, including psychotic symptoms, mood and functioning (Wykes *et al.*, 2008). Wykes *et al.*'s (2008) meta-analysis also indicates that group treatment may be as effective as individual CBT in terms of outcomes. Saksa *et al.* (2009) concluded that, specifically in relation to the early stages of psychosis, CBT delivered in a group may even be more effective than CBT in individual format. They suggest that factors contributing to this finding include the benefits of peer-to-peer relating, plus the possibility that a group format might be less interpersonally intense or anxiety-provoking for the early psychosis client group, enabling them to engage more effectively with the therapeutic work. The equivalent, or in some circumstances superior, outcomes for psychological therapies delivered in group format to a psychosis client group supports the pragmatic position that group interventions may offer an effective way of delivering psychological interventions

Acceptance and Commitment Therapy and Mindfulness for Psychosis, First Edition.
Edited by Eric M. J. Morris, Louise C. Johns and Joseph E. Oliver.
© 2013 John Wiley & Sons, Ltd. Published 2013 by John Wiley & Sons, Ltd.

to this population using limited resources. Working in groups with a co-facilitator also provides a useful training model, in which a more experienced lead therapist can provide a model to, and observe the practice of, a more junior colleague, thus meeting the common service development need to disseminate expertise and skill in the practise of psychological therapies.

The third specific strand of the rationale for developing these interventions is based on the proposed therapeutic value of the group process. We would contend, as indeed have many group-process theorists (e.g. Yalom, 1995), that when skilfully managed, the group process can offer benefits that can be difficult, if not impossible, to foster in individual psychological therapy. Prior (2007), for example, writes about the importance of processes such as universality of experience (after Yalom, 1995) for individuals who have experienced psychosis in identifying and connecting with others, which may eventually form the basis for a more compassionate stance towards the self. Prior (2007) also identifies the importance of working within a group format to enable individuals who have experienced psychosis to remain in contact with their reality-based pain and build a broader awareness of self – processes that are also prioritised from an ACT perspective.

In addition, there is a developing body of research which supports the acceptability and feasibility of delivering other mindfulness- and acceptance-based psychological interventions in a group format to individuals who experience psychosis (Jacobsen *et al.*, 2010; Chadwick *et al.*, 2009; Chapter 16 of this volume), together with positive and clinically relevant outcomes following group-based mindfulness training (Chadwick *et al.*, 2005) and group-based compassionate mind therapy for individuals with psychosis (Laithwaite *et al.*, 2009). The growing evidence for the successful delivery of these interventions in a group setting for participants who experience psychosis, as well as the favourable outcomes, offers some support to efforts to develop ACT for this client base in a group format.

ACT has been adapted to be delivered in a group format for a wide range of clinical presentations, including depression, anxiety and trauma, as well as a range of nonclinical issues (Walser & Pistorello, 2004), and it continues to demonstrate benefits for participants in a growing number of outcome studies (e.g. Ossman *et al.*, 2006). A very useful recent addition to the literature is the brief group ACT-for-anxiety protocol presented by Glaser *et al.* (2009), which outlines a six-session group intervention and discusses a number of key considerations for the delivery ACT in a short-term structured group format.

Walser & Pistorello (2004) summarised several aspects of ACT that lend themselves to delivery in group format, including the following:

- Many of the metaphors and experiential exercises are very interactive in nature and can benefit from the involvement of more than two individuals, when well managed, such as the passengers-on-the-bus exercise (see Appendix C).
- Listening to others' reactions and responses to the exercises and materials can contribute to participants' understanding of these materials.

- It is often easier to notice when other people are becoming 'hooked' by their content than it is with oneself. This may contribute to an overall awareness and understanding of this process that can gradually be applied to oneself.
- Observing others being present and practising willingness can serve as a form of exposure to these processes, and can be a powerful thing to witness.
- Making commitments towards valued actions within a social context is likely to strengthen the power of those commitments.

When considering group work with clients who experience psychosis, one reservation that often crops up for clinicians is how to manage psychotic content expressed within a group format. However, given that ACT seeks to foster defusion from such content while developing a focus on valued directions, this issue may not present as many challenges to the group process as anticipated when managed in an ACT-consistent way. This is perhaps another reason why an ACT approach to group work is a good fit for this client group.

We are currently aware of a small but growing number of clinicians using ACT in group format for individuals with psychosis, and evaluating this work. In terms of developing the protocols presented here, we have found Walser & Pistorello's (2004) chapter on general considerations and issues in developing ACT group work very useful, together with the literature and protocols on applying individual ACT to the needs of individuals who experience psychosis (e.g. Bach, 2004; Bach & Hayes, 2002; Bach *et al.*, 2006; Pankey & Hayes, 2003). We have also drawn on the work of Kevin Polk and colleagues (e.g. Polk *et al.*, 2008, 2009) and their group work with patients with complex and long-term mental-health problems across a range of diagnoses.

15.2   A Six-session ACT-for-Psychosis Group Protocol

Before outlining the protocol, it is important to note that it has now evolved through several iterations and will doubtless continue to do so. We have incorporated new approaches and exercises over time as we have learned about these from others in the ACT community. To date we have run our groups as closed programmes, as this has been the best fit with our context and allows us to progressively develop the model and approach with participants across several sessions.

Wherever practicable, when individuals are either put forward by a member of staff or self-refer to a group, we arrange at least one preparatory meeting. This meeting serves as an opportunity to gain informed consent, after first providing the individual with some initial information about the group and the ACT approach. We have used brief information sheets or leaflets to support this process. The initial meeting also allows the clinician to begin to assess the individual's presentation and consider the appropriateness of the proposed intervention, while at the same time beginning to build rapport and completing any planned pregroup measures.

The protocol has been used flexibly and in a number of different formats according to what the specific context affords and the needs of those involved. The protocol was initially designed to be delivered in six (1.5–2.0 hour) sessions but could be delivered across more sessions of shorter duration. We have delivered the approach over a short time span, such as in six sessions over a 2-week period for inpatients during a short acute admission (see Chapter 14 on inpatient work) or in weekly sessions with outpatients, often with a follow-up or 'booster' session a few months after the regular sessions have concluded, in order to promote ongoing functional progress. Our experience suggests that both approaches have benefits and can work well, but the key issue is to consider your context and the functioning and needs of the participants in determining how to deliver the content. It is important to consider balancing the intensity of the intervention with any potential barriers to maintaining engagement or perhaps with retention of key aspects of the therapy when sessions are spread over a longer period. We would always encourage a flexible approach to the material and would stress the need to be present with and responsive to what participants 'show up' with in sessions.

We work in a group with at least two facilitators. As noted by Walser & Pistorello (2004), one of the benefits of doing so is that the facilitators can support each other to remain defused from the content of what is developing within the session. Polk *et al.* (2008) have also suggested that when undertaking intense experiential exercises that actively involve several group members (e.g. passengers on the bus), having two facilitators enables a division between them of the key tasks involved in managing the exercise and the experience of the participants.

The following provides a brief summary of the themes, approach and exercises used in the group sessions.

15.2.1   Session 1: Introducing the ACT Approach and Exploring the Workability of Current Strategies for Managing Distress

As with any kind of group work, we begin the first session with introductions, the setting of some standard group rules and a brief discussion of the participants' aims and expectations for the group. We then move on to introducing the ACT model through the 'Matrix' from Polk *et al.* (2009, 2011) (outlined in Chapter 9).

15.2.1.1   The Matrix
The first step in developing the Matrix involves supporting participants in an exercise of 'tuning in' to the part of themselves that is always present and which can notice the distinction between direct sensory experiences and mental experiences. This is done using a brief exercise involving noticing the various sensory properties of a particular object, often a pen, and then moving on to relating to the object in terms of mental experience, following which participants are asked to reflect on the difference and who it was that noticed this. Participants thereby begin to develop processes of defusion, contact with the present moment and self as context.

We then move on to ask participants to reflect on the experience of behaviour being driven by a desire to avoid pain versus the experience of behaviour driven by values. Participants are encouraged to contribute to the discussion based on their own experience and we tend to find that this distinction is very intuitive for most people and can lead to an initial discussion around the processes of acceptance or avoidance of pain, together with values and committed action. In addition, the Matrix is drawn out using a board or flip chart, and this process in itself seems to contribute to the overall efforts to develop a defused stance: looking 'at' one's mental experiences rather than looking 'from' them (Bloy *et al.*, 2011). We provide worksheets and encourage and support individuals where appropriate to person-alise the Matrix to represent their experiences, although this can require some additional input outwith the group session.

In our experience, the Matrix provides a nontechnical way of initiating a group discussion of the key ACT processes that also allows one to draw out examples of participants' own experiences. Here we find that the group process can be very positive in recognising individuals' efforts to cope and offering them compassion for the struggle they are engaged in. Woven through this work will be the begin-nings of an exploration of workability and an introduction to the validating idea that while this 'problem-solving' approach is an understandable human response, it isn't suited to human pain and suffering. This work provides the beginnings of an ACT-based individual formulation, which we find generally to be very accessible to clients who experience psychosis, and starts to point towards values that can be worked on during the group. In our experience, when beginning to explore what group participants struggle with, although some will identify positive psychotic phenomena, many will identify other issues such as an absence of satisfying inter-personal relationships or highly critical attitudes to the self, perhaps in relation to specific past behaviours. We ask participants to build on the work done in the group sessions by undertaking an experiential task between each session. This gives an opportunity to develop the processes initiated within the session and provides material for experiential learning to be shared in the next session.

15.2.1.2   Between-session Task
Between today and the next meeting, periodically 'step back' and notice whether your behaviour is being driven by values or the desire to avoid experiencing pain.

15.2.2   Session 2: Exploring the Impact of the Struggle for Control and Introducing Willingness as an Alternative

From Session 2 onwards, we usually begin the sessions with a brief mindfulness exercise (3–5 minutes), wherein participants are guided to pay attention (with eyes closed or open as preferred) to various aspects of their present-moment sensory and mental experiences from a nonjudgemental stance. We approach these exercises with the principles developed by Paul Chadwick (2006) for using mindfulness approaches with individuals who experience psychosis very much in mind (see Chapter 16).

We then move on to a more detailed exploration of the impact of struggling with content, using metaphors and exercises picked according to the particular context in the group. There are several metaphors used in ACT to illustrate the impact of struggle and the often paradoxical effect it can have on a problem, as well as the way it can increase disconnection from positive activity in one's life. We tend to use metaphors that lend themselves best to acting out within the group, as our experience has been that these tend to harness the group process most effectively.

Most often we use the 'tug-of-war-with-the-monster' metaphor (see Appendix H) (Hayes *et al.*, 1999), which is acted out with a willing group member playing themselves and the lead facilitator representing their personal monster. Struggling with difficult psychological experiences is framed as being like engaging in a tug of war with a monster: we put all our energy into pulling away from the monster, as we are scared to come into contact with it. However, the monster is strong and we are not free to give our energy and attention to other things. Also, paradoxically, while our main objective is to get away from the monster, the nature of the struggle is such that it actually keeps us engaged with and attached to the monster. For this client group psychotic experience may well be woven through the particular nature of an individual's 'monster', but in a lot of cases we find the monster more often represents a negative view of the self.

The facilitators set up the exercise, bring in a group member and ask them to act out the struggle, after spending a short period supporting them to explore exactly what their own monster consists of. After the participant has experienced the struggle for a short time, a facilitator asks them and the other group members to reflect on and discuss the impact and workability of the struggle. Following this, we discuss alternative ways of relating to the monster and act out suggestions from the participants, which might include continuing to pull on the 'rope' with one's back turned/eyes closed and so on. Often the suggestion will be made spontaneously to 'drop the rope' and allow the monster to move freely in one's space. If not suggested by the group members, a facilitator will make this suggestion. This is then acted out by one of the facilitators and the group member, and the workability of this option is reflected on by the group. Following the active portion of this exercise, we spend some time discussing it and making links with other group members' experiences, and then go on to have a more explicit discussion around the theme of willingness and what willingness might mean for individuals in practice.

Other metaphors which can be used as alternatives to the 'tug-of-war' (or in addition to it) include the quicksand (see Appendix F) and the Chinese fingercuffs metaphors (Hayes *et al.*, 1999). We have found the Chinese fingercuffs metaphor works particularly well when participants are given a set of fingercuffs so that they can directly experience the sense of 'stuckness' that occurs when pulling away versus the easier movement that comes from 'leaning in' to the experience. In the past we have more often used the 'pain circle' exercise (Walser & Pistorello, 2004) to explore the cost of the struggle and the impact of control efforts.

In addition to acting out metaphors in the sessions, we have also found it helpful to use cartoons of various ACT metaphors (http://www.acceptandchange.com/visual-metaphors/), which serve as very useful visual summaries, particularly with client groups who experience difficulties of concentration and memory.

15.2.2.1 Between-session Task
Notice when you engage in a tug-of-war with your own monster. What are you struggling with and what does this struggle look like?

15.2.3 Session 3: Identifying Personal Valued Directions

We start the session with a brief noticing exercise to develop present-moment awareness and practise willingness to remain in contact with this.

We begin to encourage the participants to tune in to and discuss more of their own values. In the ripple exercise (see Section 15.2.3.1), which forms the main focus of Session 3, we discuss in more depth the concept of values as life directions that are 'freely chosen' and never fully attained, and which guide our actions. The distinction between values and committed action is clarified, perhaps using an established metaphor that distinguishes between travelling west and reaching a specific location. We also discuss how outcomes from committed action cannot be guaranteed but how there is perhaps some satisfaction to be gained from the sense of living life consistently with ones values, regardless of the outcome.

It is important to be aware that it can be distressing for participants to explore and reconnect with their personal values, as this may involve a process of recognising how their life has become increasingly disconnected from them. Therefore, this process requires careful management and pacing by the therapists and may require some additional support in between sessions. Nonetheless, this is an essential component of ACT and can harness a powerful source of motivation, as well as allowing individuals to connect emotionally with the costs of their avoidance and thereby possibly shift their sense of workability.

15.2.3.1 The Ripple Exercise
The ripple (Figure 15.1) is a modified version of the 'bull's eye' exercise (http://contextualpsychology.org/values_bulls_eye) (Harris, 2009), which we adapted following feedback from one of our participants in an earlier group. The participant had suggested that the idea of a 'ripple', with the circles spreading outwards and with the committed actions fanning out from the centre to the outer circles, seemed more consistent with the idea of values having no end point or final goal and a broadening of action and experience. We were very struck by this insight and modified the exercise accordingly.

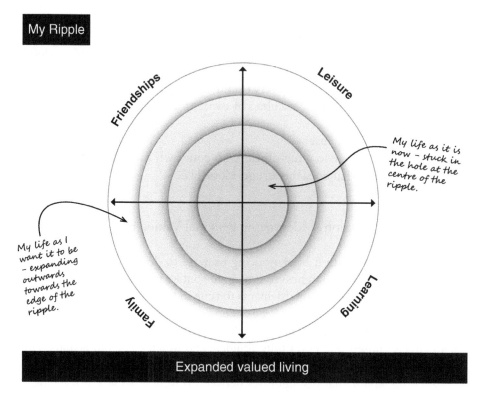

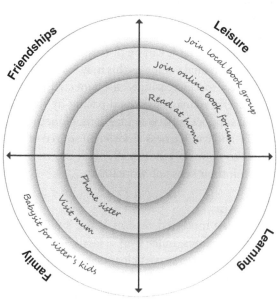

Figure 15.1   The ripple exercise. Adapted from the 'bull's eye' exercise (http://contextual psychology.org/values_bulls_eye) (Harris, 2009)

The ripple exercise is first introduced and discussed as a group, then individuals are given some time in session to begin to fill in the worksheets. The group members are then brought together again to reflect on what they have written. The exercise focuses on four of the life domains, in order to make the work more focused and manageable within the group setting. These are usually relationships, work/education, leisure and personal growth, but this can be modified to fit with individual priorities. The worksheet begins by asking the individual to explore and identify personally relevant values and progressive committed actions associated with them. They then use the visual representation of the 'ripple' to place these actions in a hierarchy of difficulty, working from the centre outwards. In part two of the worksheet, participants are asked to consider and record potential barriers and difficulties, and to begin to develop an action plan for how they might approach these, even when the usually avoided content is present. Group facilitators are able to provide some one-to-one support during this exercise, according to individual need. Participants are also encouraged to take the worksheets away and work on them further, with assistance from a key worker, friend or family member where appropriate. The group facilitators liaise with other staff involved to support this work and seek to ensure that the values and committed actions identified can be fed in to other ongoing care and support.

15.2.3.2   *Between-session Task*
Ensure that you have fleshed out values for at least one life domain on the ripple and identified some relevant committed actions (assistance from community staff with this process can be agreed to where needed).

15.2.4   Session 4: Moving in Valued Directions

The session begins with a brief guided exercise based on noticing present-moment experience.

We then spend some time reviewing group members' progress with the ripple exercise and any additional work done on this between sessions, and discussing participants' experiences of attempting to put any of the identified steps towards their values into practice. There is an open discussion of the challenges involved and any barriers encountered, such as content or symptoms with which individuals find it difficult to remain in contact.

We then initiate a brief group discussion, seeking to bring together the themes that have been developed over the previous three sessions around the workability of different ways of relating to painful content, the impact of the struggle and reconnection with values. This prepares the ground to move on to the next exercise.

15.2.4.1   The Passengers-on-the-Bus Exercise

This ACT metaphor (originally described in Hayes *et al.*, 1999 and reproduced in Appendix C, and presented in sources such as Glaser *et al.*, 2009; Polk *et al.*, 2008; and Walser & Pistorello, 2004) can serve as a powerful method for individuals to use to gain some experience in session of relating differently to distressing content while sustaining efforts to move in a valued direction when acted out '*in vivo*'. This experimental use of the metaphor is something we have developed since we attended workshops run by Kevin Polk and colleagues (e.g. Polk *et al.*, 2008) and experienced the approach in action. This exercise forms a central part of the remaining group sessions.

One of the group facilitators sets up the exercise with an initial outline of the metaphor, describing the client as the driver of a bus called 'My Life'. Along the route, the driver has picked up a collection of unruly, bullying passengers (representing distressing thoughts, memories, sensations etc.), which harass them and tell them to change the direction of the bus away from where they wish to head (their personal values). The central thrust of the exercise is of course to support clients to continue to 'drive' in the valued direction, regardless of what is thrown at them by the problematic passengers. It essentially encourages, and crucially provides some '*in vivo*' experience of, choosing action based on values rather than the content of private experiences. Beneficial use of the passengers-on-the-bus exercise is contingent on group participants having meaningfully connected with the ACT processes as developed thus far in the group sessions.

The task for the therapist at this stage is to gain an impression of which participants might tolerate a little more intensity in terms of playing the bus driver. It is of course essential to gain individual consent to participate in the roleplay and to support all the individuals involved appropriately. The volunteer is asked to stand with the main facilitator and identify a personally valued direction. The group members are then asked whether they also connect with this value, and another group member is selected to represent the value in some way – for example, by standing across the room from the driver and periodically calling, 'I care about being a good son / daughter' or holding up a sign that simply says 'Family'. The facilitator then begins to explore with the 'driver' what a specific committed action towards this value might be, which can be written on a piece of paper and placed part way across the room towards the person representing the value.

Next the facilitator begins to explore what unwanted experiences might show up as the individual carries out the committed action. The various aspects of this content are assigned to other group participants to act out in the exercise; for example, one person might be chosen to represent the main physical sensation that shows up, another to represent the key thought and another to represent a memory of a previous failed attempt to carry out the committed action. This should be done using the 'driver's' own language and phrases.

We then work through a process of 'acting out' the scenario, with the client playing the driver trying to relate to those playing the content in different ways while also physically moving towards the identified committed action and value. First, we might ask them to act out their usual way of relating to the content, usually some form of struggle such as arguing back or deliberate suppression. The 'driver' and/or the group members are then asked to come up with alternative modes of responding to this content. After reflecting on how these approaches are experienced and what their impact and cost is, we then move on to trying an alternative way of relating, based on the principle of noticing without struggling – hopefully this option will be elicited from the group following discussion, but if not it is suggested by the facilitators. Once again, the experience and impact of this is reflected on in further group discussion.

The two facilitators need to continually assess and manage the level of intensity involved in the exercise, in order to ensure that it remains safe and facilitates learning, rather than leading to aversive reactions. One approach suggested (Polk *et al.*, 2008) is that the first facilitator focuses on the driver while the second facilitator takes responsibility for observing the participants who play the passengers (as well as the observing participants) and managing the exercise as required based on these observations.

In our experience, working through this exercise can be a very powerful process for individuals when well set up and managed by the facilitators. Given the common underlying process of experiential avoidance, we generally find that most group members, including those not directly involved in the exercise, take some useful reflections and learning from it. For the exercise to work well, around six participants and two facilitators are needed, and there are benefits to those not directly involved acting as observers and feeding back to the rest of the group.

15.2.4.2   *Between-session Task*

Notice examples of these processes of avoidance and willingness to approach at work in your own experiences. What are the passengers on your own bus like?

15.2.5   Session 5: Continuing to Develop Self-as-Context and Willingness to Move towards Values

The session begins with a brief sitting mindfulness exercise, followed by an opportunity to share reflections on the previous session, the passengers-on-the-bus exercise and the between-session task. The facilitators seek to draw out the key ACT processes and themes in this discussion. We then spend some time discussing the concept of self-as-context in an accessible and meaningful way, using metaphors such as the sky versus the clouds/weather (Harris, 2009) to illustrate what is meant by self-as-context as contrasted with self-as-content. We encourage participants to share their views and experiences and again seek to link these to the model where appropriate.

We then spend some additional time working on the passengers-on-the-bus exercise, as outlined in Session 4. This provides the opportunity for other group members to gain experience of playing the driver, value and passengers, and hopefully will prompt further useful group reflection on the processes involved. This experience, albeit a roleplay within a therapy context, can serve as an initial step in reducing avoidance of difficult private experience and thereby be the first step towards real behavioural movement.

15.2.5.1 *Between-session Task*
Notice how you relate to difficult experiences and any opportunities you have to move towards your values.

15.2.6 Session 6: Summarising the Themes of the Course and Reviewing Experiences of the Work

We once again begin with a brief adapted mindfulness exercise. In this session the facilitators endeavour to summarise and draw together the main themes of the group and provide an opportunity for the group members to reflect on their experience of it: the ending and the ACT model in particular. We also revisit progress with the committed actions identified on the individuals' ripple worksheets and ask them to ensure they have identified specific actions to be taken going forward after the group is concluded. We discuss ongoing support that group members might harness to assist them with this process. We also discuss and agree upon any follow-up sessions, where relevant.

15.2.7 Optional Follow-up Session

This session usually takes place between 2 and 3 months following the conclusion of the regular meetings. Its main purpose is to refresh the participants' awareness of the key ACT concepts and processes and to review their progress with identified valued directions. Where individuals have begun to return to unhelpful patterns of experiential avoidance, this session can provide an opportunity to share experiences of the challenges of moving in valued directions, and to reflect and renew commitment.

In general, the follow-up session has proved to be surprisingly well attended and well received. Individuals seem to value the opportunity to come back together to share their experiences of trying to move in valued directions. Inevitably there is considerable variation in the extent to which participants have been able to progress with reducing avoidance and engaging with valued living, but with careful management by the therapist(s) this can be a beneficial and noncritical encounter, perhaps of most use to those who have struggled to make progress following the conclusion of regular group meetings.

As is the case with any psychological intervention, it is crucial that there is liaison and integration of this work with the other professionals involved in each individual's care and support. This is important to ensuring that the model of care is as consistent with the approach taken in the group as possible (a considerable challenge in some areas of a predominantly medical and disease/symptom-elimination-based health-care system), but also allows the individual's valued directions and associated committed actions to be shared and understood by all professionals involved in supporting them. We have found that this approach can fit in well with the care programme approach (CPA) (an approach to identifying, managing and meeting the care needs of individuals with severe mental-health problems used in the UK), and CPA meetings can provide a useful opportunity for liaison and for dissemination of the work an individual has undertaken in the groups.

15.3   Case Study

Mary was a woman in her 40s who had experienced psychotic episodes characterised by derogatory auditory hallucinations and passivity experiences. Her voices persisted between acute episodes. There was a considerable history of mental illness in Mary's family; she experienced poor developmental attachment to her mother and recalled an entrenched sense of personal vulnerability from an early age. Over the years, Mary had experienced numerous admissions. She had aspirations to work in retail as a shop assistant but was unable to sustain efforts in this direction. Although she didn't do well academically at school, she reported enjoying the process of learning, but again she had been unable to engage with adult-education options.

Mary agreed to participate in an ACT-based group programme, which began using the Matrix (Polk *et al.*, 2009). Mary appeared to connect at a very early stage to the difference between mental and direct sensory experience and how she herself could take that perspective. When the group moved on to explore the experience of moving towards values, Mary was able to give a personal example of how at times her behaviour could remain essentially the same but be driven by different motivations. For example, she would make a more active, strategic choice to maintain certain valued behaviours such as listening to music that was initiated by herself, regardless of her voices. She was able to notice how this contrasted with using music as part of distraction attempts that were more motivated by efforts to avoid voices.

When undertaking the 'pain circle' exercise, Mary displayed her openness by not only contributing core pain experiences such as her fear of rejection but also acknowledging the very human tendency to attempt to push this pain away. Mary also actively contributed during the tug-of-war-with-the-monster exercise to the

232   *Amy McArthur, Gordon Mitchell and Louise C. Johns*

collective group realisation that the real problem wasn't with the monster itself but what resulted from the struggles associated with picking up the rope. The reality of choosing the option of dropping the rope was felt at an intense emotional level for the group, and the compassion required to make this a positive and productive stance was helped by Mary's contribution. She was able to acknowledge that she and indeed most of the other participants could readily support and accept other participants' pain but that significant challenges exist in extending this compassionate stance to themselves.

However, probably the strongest clinical advance for Mary was in her participation with the passengers-on-the-bus exercise. Mary volunteered to be the bus driver. She was very clear about her chosen value regarding pursuing educational opportunities. Mary's stated committed action for the exercise appeared relatively modest: being able to attend a meeting to explore supportive educational opportunities at a local college. However, 'opening any new door' was fraught with anxiety and inevitably prompted malevolent auditory hallucinations. Mary actively directed other group members to be her various passengers, who created obstacles in the way of this valued move. The passengers did not make it easy for her, particularly as they readily identified with the various voices described by Mary.

As the exercise progressed, Mary adopted familiar attempts at distraction, fighting back and obeying the voices, and experienced how these inevitably led to her losing sight of her values and specific goal. There was then a truly awe-inspiring 'drop the rope' move when Mary experimented with looking directly into the eyes of her various passengers, acknowledging their presence and then spontaneously moving with purpose towards the previously nominated college office door with them in tow, but clearly following her own personal agenda. The door actually entered the kitchen next to the group room but the symbolism was not lost on Mary or the other group members. Mary herself suggested the move did not depend on getting rid of the passengers but rather that by making such moves she now had the opportunity to take aboard some new passengers. Exposing herself directly to new contingencies did not guarantee the new passengers would all be positive, but she described a feeling of being more alive, more of her own agent. This was the opposite from her vulnerability to passivity feelings, which she associated with the consequences of chronically 'not driving her bus'.

In subsequent individual clinical follow-ups, Mary often used the bus metaphor to describe her progress. She joked of sometimes forgetting to put her bus driver's hat on when she had episodes of losing herself to the voices, which remained part of her experience, but gave increasing accounts of activities that were based on her own personal choices. Some ended in disappointments, but regardless Mary was definitely more involved with the overall process. She maintained a heightened sense of personal agency and although she continued contact with services, the relationship was more as an active service user steadily moving on in her own recovery.

15.4 Reflections on the Experience of Developing and Delivering the Groups

There are a number of practical and systems challenges in developing group work, some of which are generic issues and some more specific to using an ACT model. Among the generic issues to consider is the challenge of carving out sufficient reflective space within which to undertake reflective therapeutic work, both for staff involved in specific psychotherapeutic roles and particularly for staff such as mental health nurses who have more general roles and responsibilities and for whom workloads can be particularly challenging. This has implications for the availability of facilitators to prepare for and run the groups and to supervise and reflect around the experience of running the group. Clearly it is crucial to seek to have an intervention such as this supported by and embedded in the broader service systems, which in itself can require considerable work around training and communicating the model.

A more specific issue in relation to developing therapeutic approaches based on an ACT model is the tensions that exist between some of the principles and philosophies underpinning ACT and those that underpin a medical model. For example, there is a clear tension between the approach of remaining in contact with difficult experiences in ACT and the conceptualisation of distress as a symptom of an illness, which should be reduced if not eliminated, from a medical standpoint. Introducing an ACT approach into a broader health-care system will highlight some of these tensions; the extent and degree to which these might interfere with the work will of course vary considerably depending on the approach and philosophy of individual workers and particular services.

We have found that offering the possibility to individuals of repeating the group at different stages in their recovery is beneficial in several ways. In our experience of clients doing so, an initial experience of the group can serve to pave the way for a deeper engagement with the processes at a later stage in individuals who were perhaps not fully open to the approach at first. In addition, having a group member who has more familiarity with the model in the group, participating in the exercises and sharing in reflections may well have more resonance with other participants than when concepts are conveyed by a facilitator. Therefore, we believe there can be benefit to both the individual themselves and other group members in their repeating the group.

There are a range of challenges involved in developing the therapeutic processes in the group in a way that is faithful to the ACT model. For example, it can be a considerable challenge to balance working in a group format with a protocol while being open to and sufficiently present to learn from the participants in the moment. Working in a group setting means there can be a great deal going on for different participants and therefore just the level of contextual information they must be open to can be quite overwhelming for facilitators, especially combined with the need to balance the needs of and processes going on for different members. These are, of course, issues for group work in every therapeutic model, but in ACT, where one is working specifically on fostering contact with present-moment experience, on the part of both the client and the therapist, this is perhaps a particular consideration. In our experience, this is where co-facilitators are so crucial to the group process. The lead facilitator and co-facilitator(s) can agree on a 'division of labour' for each exercise, whereby the lead facilitator is supported by the others perhaps observing those group members less directly involved in the exercise and cueing the lead facilitator to moderate the exercise or involve others as appropriate. This also points to the importance of having co-facilitators available who are suitably trained in the model and building training into any process of service development along these lines.

We have also observed that the group process naturally offers a valuable opportunity to develop compassion for the self, through the experience of being offered compassion by others. There have been some powerful examples in our group of clients validating and normalising the suffering and struggles of others, often with little or no guidance from the facilitators. We have found the work of Paul Gilbert (2005) of particular relevance to understanding how experiencing the receipt of compassion from another person can be facilitative for beginning to internalise such a compassionate stance and later offering it to oneself, and we have sought to foster and reinforce such processes within the group wherever possible.

In terms of supervision for the delivery of the groups, we have used a number of different approaches, including scheduling 30-minute reflective sessions for the staff involved directly after each session and longer reflective supervision sessions for all staff following each iteration of the group. We have found the former to be extremely difficult for nursing staff due to various other time pressures, but we continue to believe that reflection while the experience of the session is still quite 'live' is likely to be most helpful. In order to try and facilitate this kind of reflection, we have used audio recordings of the sessions (with appropriate consent from participants) to cue reflections at other times. We have also used the model developed by Polk *et al.* (2008, 2011) in supervision and training, whereby therapists are encouraged to conceptualise the therapy process according to a reciprocal interaction between their own process and what is being offered by the client in terms of the broader categories of 'showing up', 'letting go' and 'moving on', representing the more specific ACT processes.

15.5   Other Protocols

There are a few other ACT-for-psychosis and related group protocols described in the literature. For example, Adria Pearson and colleagues (Pearson & Tingey, 2011) have developed an 18-session protocol for working with psychosis clients within a psychosocial rehabilitation and recovery centre. Pinto (2009) has described his mindfulness-based group work with clients who experience psychosis, which incorporates an awareness of ACT processes.

15.5.1 ACT for Life Group

The ACT for Life group has been developed in South London as part of a study evaluating the transferability of ACT from the USA to routine mental health services in the UK, in terms of feasibility, acceptability and clinical outcomes. Part of the rationale is to increase the availability of evidenced-based psychological therapies for psychosis. Despite NICE recommendations (National Institute for Health and Clinical Excellence, 2009), CBT is not accessible to all individuals with schizophrenia, due to lack of capacity. Group interventions can reach more clients and be cheaper to provide, and ACT is a brief cognitive behavioural intervention that readily lends itself to group format. The current project (Johns *et al.*, unpublished) is evaluating group-based ACT for psychosis, with the hypotheses that service users who attend an ACT group will show improvements in daily functioning, mood and relationship with symptoms (willingness to experience symptoms, distancing from symptoms and choices and actions less influenced by symptoms).

The study includes participants from across the spectrum of psychosis: chronic psychosis, first-episode psychosis and those at high risk of developing psychosis. All these clients experience prominent cognitive intrusions, in the form of negative thoughts, worries, delusional ideas, voices or other hallucinations. The tendency to struggle with these internal experiences is common to all clients, irrespective of the stage of psychosis. The effectiveness of the intervention is being evaluated using measures of values, behaviour, mood and service use, and possible mediators of change are examined by measures of fusion, acceptance and mindfulness. These assessments are administered by a research assistant at various points before and after group attendance, and satisfaction with the group is also assessed post-intervention.

The ACT for Life group comprises four 2-hour sessions held on a weekly basis. This number of sessions was decided upon following earlier pilot work with six- or eight-session groups, where it was found that attendance frequently dipped after the fourth session. We aim to have six to eight participants in each group, and the groups are run within services rather than across them; that is, there are separate groups for the different client groups (at-risk mental state, first-episode psychosis, long-standing psychosis). There are typically two to three facilitators for each group (a mixture of clinical psychologists, occupational therapists and CBT therapists), all of whom have some knowledge and experience of ACT and have attended at least one experiential training day on delivering the group intervention.

The group manual has been developed over several years, based on earlier work in both inpatient and community settings. It is available from http://is.gd/actgroup.

The group aims to encourage a more flexible (accepting, mindful, defused) response to symptoms of psychosis and associated thoughts and emotions in order to increase values-based behaviour. The main components of the group include values clarification, mindfulness/noticing exercises, willingness, defusion and committed action. In helping clients to get in touch with their values and identify barriers, we start by discussing 'what's important in our life' and 'what gets in the way of us doing what's important'. The sessions tend to focus on key areas, such as relationships with other people, work/study, health, meaningful activity, leisure and spirituality. The group uses lots of 'scaffolding' to support people in talking about difficult content, including the experiences of 'friends', as well as therapist self-disclosure and watching and commenting on a video (an actor roleplaying a service user, Tom). We also make use of small-group work within the sessions, breaking into groups of two or three plus a facilitator. This enables more detailed discussion of valued actions and barriers, particularly for those clients who feel anxious about talking in the bigger group. All the mindfulness exercises included in the group are brief, typically 5–10 minutes, and participants are given a CD of these exercises so they can practise at home. Based on prior experience of running ACT groups for psychosis clients, the session content is mainly based around one metaphor (passengers on the bus) for simplicity. The metaphor is introduced in first session, and then acted out in Sessions 2 and 3, and summarised again in the last session. In acting out the metaphor, facilitators focus on noticing passengers, the workability of struggling with passengers, 'adding in' alternative ways of being with passengers (e.g. inviting them along for the ride, observing without necessarily engaging with them) and noticing opportunities to base actions on values, rather than what passengers say.

From Session 1, we ask clients at the end of each session to identify a valued action for the week and discuss the associated goal and underlying value, together with possible barriers or 'passengers'. This is done in small groups with the aid of an 'out-of-session planning worksheet' and is framed as a noticing exercise; that is, 'Notice what happens when you try to do this values-based action'. With permission, facilitators telephone the participants during the week to see how they have been getting on with their stated action and what they have noticed. We tend to find that group members make good progress with their actions and like to receive the call between sessions. Again with permission, immediately after the group a facilitator liaises with a key health professional working with each client (e.g. care coordinator, psychologist, occupational therapist) for continued support, feeding back the client's values, goals and barriers to moving forward.

Clients have reported high levels of satisfaction with the group, and the positive feedback has clustered into three areas:

(1) The process of being in a group: 'Knowing there are other people with the same problems'.

(2)   Which ACT processes/interventions seem to help: 'Being the driver of the bus and focusing on a direction I wanted to go in'.

(3)   The active, behavioural-change aspect of the group: 'It helped me to leave the house and go out with my sister'.

15.6   Conclusion

There are a number of exciting clinical developments in ACT-based group work which offer the potential to be effective psychological interventions for individuals who experience psychosis, although research into the clinical impact of these interventions is at a relatively early stage. We have presented details of the development of our groups, together with reflections on the clinical experience of undertaking this work. There are a number of contextual factors that can present challenges to taking these developments forward. In our local services, we are continuing to explore the relative benefits of psychosis/diagnosis-specific groups versus transdiagnostic groups, but we recognise that group membership will depend on how services are structured and planned in different areas. In addition, our initial involvement in developing this work has served to reinforce the importance of training and working with the system to ensure the interventions are supported by the broader context. This is where our current energies are being focused, in order to ensure that future efforts to embed and evaluate this work are meaningful and sustainable.

Acknowledgement

The ACT for Life study was funded by a grant from Guy's & St Thomas' Charitable Foundation, New Services and Innovations in Health Care.

References

Bach, P. (2004). ACT with the Seriously Mentally Ill. In S. C. Hayes & K. D. Strosahls (eds). *A Practical Guide to Acceptance & Commitment Therapy*. New York: Springer.

Bach, P. & Hayes, S. C. (2002). The use of acceptance and commitment therapy to prevent the rehospitalisation of psychotic patients: a randomized controlled trial. *Journal of Consulting and Clinical Psychology*, 70(5), 1129–1139.

Bach, P. A., Gaudiano, B., Pankey, J., Herbert, J. D. & Hayes, S. C. (2006). Acceptance, mindfulness and psychosis: applying acceptance and commitment therapy (ACT) to the chronically mentally ill. In R. A. Baer (ed.). *Mindfulness-Based Treatment Approaches: Clinician's Guide to Evidence Base and Applications*. Academic Press.

Bloy, S., Oliver, J. E. & Morris, E. (2011). Using acceptance and commitment therapy with people with psychosis: a case study. *Clinical Case Studies*, 10, 347–359.

Chadwick, P. (2006). *Person Based Cognitive Therapy for Distressing Psychosis*. Wiley, New York.

Chadwick, P., Taylor, K. N. & Abba, N. (2005). Mindfulness groups for people with psychosis. *Behavioural and Cognitive Psychotherapy*, 33(3), 351–359.

Chadwick, P., Hughes, S., Russell, D., Russell, I. & Dagnan, D. (2009). Mindfulness groups for distressing voices and paranoia: a replication and randomized feasibility trial. *Behavioural and Cognitive Psychotherapy*, 37, 403–412.

Eifert, G. H. & Forsyth, J. P. (2005). *Acceptance and Commitment Therapy for Anxiety Disorders*. Oakland: New Harbinger.

Gilbert, P. (2005). *Compassion: Conceptualisations, Research and Use of Psychotherapy*. London: Routledge.

Glaser, N. M., Blackledge, J. T., Shepherd, L. M. & Deane, F. P. (2009). Brief group ACT for anxiety. In J. T. Ciarrochi & F. P. Deane (eds). *Acceptance & Commitment Therapy: Contemporary Theory, Research & Practice*. Blackledge: Australian Academic Press.

Harris, R. (2009). *ACT Made Simple: A Quick Start Guide to ACT Basics and Beyond*. Oakland: New Harbinger.

Hayes, S. C., Strosahl, K. D. & Wilson, K. G. (1999). *Acceptance and Commitment Therpay: An Experiential Approach to Behavior Change*. New York: Guilford Press.

Jacobsen, P., Morris, E., Johns, L. & Hodkinson, K. (2010). Mindfulness groups for psychosis; key issues for implementation on an inpatient unit. *Behavioural and Cognitive Psychotherapy*, 39(3), 349–353.

Johns, L. J., Morris, E. M. & Oliver, J. E. (unpublished). ACT for Life: evaluation of a group intervention for people with psychosis.

Laithwaite, H., O'Hanlon, M., Collins, P., Doyle, P., Abraham, L., Porter, S. & Gumley, A. (2009). Recovery After Psychosis (RAP): a compassion focused programme for individuals residing in high security settings. *Behavioural and Cognitive Psychotherapy*, 37(5), 511–526.

National Institute for Health and Clinical Excellence (2009). *Schizophrenia: Core Interventions in the Treatment and Management of Schizophrenia in Adults in Primary and Secondary Care. Quick Reference Guide*. London: NICE.

Ossman, W. A., Wilson, K. G., Storaasli, R. D. & McNeill, J. W. (2006). A preliminary investigation of the use of Acceptance and Commitment Therapy in group treatment for social phobia. *International Journal of Psychology and Psychological Therapy*, 6(3), 397–416.

Pankey, J. & Hayes, S. C. (2003). Acceptance and Commitment Therapy for psychosis. *International Journal of Psychology and Psychological Therapy*, 3(2), 311–328.

Pearson, A. N. & Tingey, R. (2011). ACT for psychosis: a treatment protocol for group therapy. Paper presented at the Association for Contextual Behavioral Science World Conference IX, Parma, Italy.

Pinto, A. (2009). Mindfulness and psychosis. In J. Kabat-Zinn & F. Didonnna (eds). *Clinical Handbook of Mindfulness*. New York: Springer.

Polk, K., Hambright, J., Drake, C. E., Mocciola, K. & Agee, J. (2008). ACT gone wild: the adventure continues. Workshop presented at the ACT Summer Institute IV, Chicago, IL, USA.

Polk, K., Webster, M., Schoendorff, B & Hambright, J. (2009). Creative confusion: an idiot's guide to ACT in groups. Workshop at Association for Contextual Behavioural Science World Conference III, Eschede, Netherlands.

Polk, K. & Webster, M. (2011). A Hitchhiker's Guide to the Matrix. Workshop presented at the Association for Contextual Behavioral Science World Conference IX, Parma, Italy.

Prior, J. (2007). Psychosis in the group. *Therapy Today*, 18(10), 40–42.

Saksa, J. R., Cohen, S. J., Srihari, V. H. & Woods, S. W. (2009). Cognitive behavior therapy for early psychosis: a comprehensive review of individual vs. group treatment studies. *International Journal of Group Psychotherapy*, 59(3), 357–383.

Walser, R. D. & Pisotorello, J. (2004). ACT in group format. In S. C. Hayes & K. D. Strosahl (eds). *A Practical Guide to Acceptance & Commitment Therapy*. New York: Springer.

Wilson, K. G., Sandoz, E. K., Kitchens, J. & Roberts, M. E. (2010). The valued living questionnaire: Defining and measuring valued action within a behavioural framework. *The Psychological Record*, 60(2), 249–272.

Wykes, T., Steel, C., Everitt, B. & Tarrier, N. (2008). Cognitive behavior therapy for schizophrenia: effect sizes, clinical models, and methodological rigor. *Schizophrenia Bulletin*, 34(3), 523–537.

Yalom, I. (1995). *The Theory and Practice of Group Psychotherapy* (4th edn). New York: Basic Books.

16

Group Person-based Cognitive Therapy for Distressing Psychosis

Clara Strauss and Mark Hayward

16.1 Introduction

Person-based cognitive therapy (PBCT) (Chadwick, 2006) integrates traditional cognitive therapy with a mindfulness- and acceptance-based approach. This chapter will first summarise the PBCT model (for a full description, see Chapter 10), before advocating the potential benefits of a group approach. The 12-session group PBCT programme will then be outlined. The chapter will end with an overview of the state of the evidence base for group PBCT for psychosis.

16.2 Person-based Cognitive Therapy

Figure 16.1 illustrates the four domains of the PBCT model. On the left-hand side, the two domains that are derived from traditional cognitive therapy for psychosis can be seen: 'symptomatic meaning' (where beliefs about psychotic and other experiences are identified and evaluated) and 'schema' (where positive self-schema are recognised and strengthened). The right-hand side shows the two mindfulness- and acceptance-based domains: 'relationship with internal experience' (where mindfulness practice and principles help to develop a different way of relating to psychotic and other experiences) and 'symbolic self' (where the emphasis in on conceptualising the self as complex, contradictory and changing).

Acceptance and Commitment Therapy and Mindfulness for Psychosis, First Edition.
Edited by Eric M. J. Morris, Louise C. Johns and Joseph E. Oliver.
© 2013 John Wiley & Sons, Ltd. Published 2013 by John Wiley & Sons, Ltd.

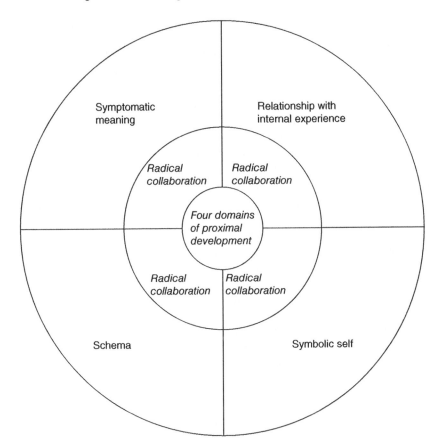

Figure 16.1 Four domains of proximal development (Chadwick, 2006, p. 10)

Chadwick draws on Vygotsky's (1978) concept of the zone of proximal development (ZoPD) to describe the importance of the therapeutic relationship in PBCT. Vygotsky was interested in the finding that a child could learn more with the guidance of an adult than when on their own. Applying this to therapy, Chadwick views the therapeutic relationship as the vehicle through which greater learning can occur compared to working on one's own.

Finally, Chadwick emphasises the importance of 'radical collaboration', particularly when working with people who are experiencing distressing psychosis. Although a collaborative working relationship is at the heart of cognitive therapy, Chadwick argues that when working with people distressed by, for example, hearing voices or paranoid ideas, we need to be aware of our own potential therapy-interfering beliefs and assumptions (e.g. 'I'm a bad therapist if my client doesn't change') and we can learn to bring acceptance to what we encounter during the course of therapy. Socratic dialogue and guided discovery facilitate the development of a radically collaborative therapeutic relationship.

Table 16.1   Yalom's (1995) eight therapeutic factors, and examples from group PBCT

Therapeutic factor	*Example from group PBCT*
1. Altruism	Group members supporting each other when someone is feeling distressed
2. Catharsis	Group members being supported to talk about distressing feelings resulting from psychosis in a safe environment, perhaps for the first time
3. Guidance	Someone in the group giving advice or suggestions to another group member
4. Group cohesion	A sense of being and working together
5. Instillation of hope	Increasing hope for the future by seeing other group members who are further along their journey of recovery
6. Interpersonal learning	Having experience of positive social interactions in the group, which help to challenge core beliefs about others (e.g. 'No one can be trusted')
7. Self-understanding	Through a schema focus, developing a greater awareness of how the self has been constructed and moving towards a sense of the symbolic self
8. Universality	Group members realising that other people have psychotic experiences, and experiencing a sense of belonging and being accepted by others

16.2.1   Group PBCT

In his seminal 2006 chapter on group PBCT, Chadwick focuses on the group process in PBCT and the considerations that can be taken into account when setting up and running groups in different contexts. In order to complement this, the current chapter will focus more on the content of group PBCT, by outlining the session-by-session protocol.

In Chapter 10, Lyn Ellett describes PBCT as it is applied in individual therapy. However, the notions of the ZoPD and radical collaboration lend themselves well to group therapy. In a group context, the ZoPD does not just exist between the group facilitators and group members, but also between members of the group, allowing greater learning and change to occur when participants work together within one of the PBCT domains.

16.3   The Importance of the Group Process in PBCT

Chadwick draws on the work of Yalom (1995) to consider the therapeutic factors that can facilitate learning and change in group PBCT (see Table 16.1). While some of these factors may be present in individual therapy, many are either dependent on a group approach or are enhanced by group therapy.

Universality is a theme that frequently emerges in group therapy in general and in group therapies for psychosis in particular (e.g. Goodliffe *et al.*, 2010). It is not uncommon for people who are, for instance, hearing voices to believe that they are alone in their experience. Attending a group and meeting other people who are hearing voices can be an important opportunity to challenge this belief and to realise that hearing voices is not an uncommon experience.

People experiencing psychosis often hold suspicious or mistrustful core beliefs about others. Being in a group where members listen to each other with respect and without judgement can provide evidence to challenge the accuracy of these beliefs and help to develop alternative beliefs that other people can be trusted. While these beliefs may be challenged to some extent through the experience of a respectful individual therapeutic relationship, it is likely that the effect is more powerful when someone experiences multiple, positive interpersonal relationships in a group setting with their peers.

16.4   Facilitating a PBCT Group

16.4.1   Inclusion Criteria

In our research team, headed by Paul Chadwick, we have been running groups specifically for people distressed by hearing voices for the past few years. Diagnosis is not an inclusion criterion; rather, the primary criterion for inclusion is that the person has been hearing voices for at least a year and reports that they find this experience distressing. Our experience has been of running these groups with adults (18 years or older), and we do not have experience with younger participants. The primary exclusion criterion is being unwilling to participate in or being unsuitable for a group-therapy approach. Being 'psychologically minded' is not an inclusion criterion, and we have plenty of anecdotal examples of people who have benefitted from the universality and group-cohesion aspects while perhaps struggling to engage fully with the conceptual ideas.

16.4.2   The 12-week Programme

Group PBCT is a 12-week programme, with one session per week of 90 minutes each, including a 10-minute break halfway through. The groups are run with up to 12 participants and with two group facilitators, at least one of whom is a cognitive therapist or an applied psychologist with a cognitive therapy background and has experience of teaching mindfulness practice.

Yalom (1995) recommends against unstructured groups for people experiencing psychosis. He suggests that having a consistent and predictable structure to each group session can ameliorate feelings of anxiety and apprehension and thus enable participants to engage more fully in the therapeutic process. Because of this, each of the 12 sessions of group PBCT has the same broad structure, and participants are introduced to this consistent structure in Session 1:

- Welcome and introduction to session: 5 minutes.
- Mindfulness practice:[1] 10 minutes.
- Socratic discussion about mindfulness practice: 20 minutes.
- Break: 10 minutes.
- Exploring beliefs about voices and/or self:[2] 30 minutes.
- Socratic discussion about the session (learning about voices and self): 10 minutes.

A brief synopsis of the protocol is given in Table 16.2.

16.4.3   Mindfulness Practice in PBCT

Mindfulness practice in PBCT is distinct from mindfulness practice in other forms of mindfulness-based therapy, such as mindfulness-based cognitive therapy (MBCT) (Segal *et al.*, 2002). Practices are never longer than 10 minutes, as mindfulness practice can sometimes heighten feelings of distress. There is verbal guidance throughout the practice and silences are kept to a minimum, so that participants are able to keep returning to the verbal guidance. The practice itself involves initially bringing awareness to the body and then to the breath. As is usual in mindfulness practice, participants are encouraged to use the breath as an anchor to the present moment. When the mind wanders (which it will) to thoughts, feelings and voices, participants are encouraged to notice where it has wandered to and to gently bring their awareness back to the breath. The practice ends with a brief period of choice-less awareness (where awareness is brought to whatever happens to arise in the moment), before awareness is brought back to the body and the room.

Importantly, the same practice is used through the 12 sessions. Just as predictability and consistency are important in terms of session structure, so we have found that having the same mindfulness practice throughout adds to the predictability of the session. An audio recording is provided for each participant with 5- and 10-minute versions of the practice, and they are encouraged to practise daily throughout the 12 weeks. At the end of each session, this encouragement is reinforced.

The instruction to notice when the mind wanders to voices is threaded throughout the middle and end of the practice, and participants are guided to notice voice comments and then gently but surely bring attention back to the

Table 16.2   Group PBCT for distressing voices: session-by-session protocol summary

1	1.	10-minute mindfulness practice
	2.	Socratic discussion about mindfulness practice
	3.	Hopes and concerns
	4.	Shared group rules
	5.	Socratic discussion about what has been learnt about voices and self
	6.	Home task (listen to mindfulness practice CD daily)
2	1.	10-minute mindfulness practice
	2.	Socratic discussion about mindfulness practice
	3.	Sharing of voice-hearing experiences
	4.	Socratic drawing out of ABC model of distress at hearing voices
	5.	Socratic discussion about what has been learnt about voices and self
	6.	Home task (mindfulness practice CD)
3	1.	10-minute mindfulness practice
	2.	Socratic discussion about mindfulness practice, linking to beliefs about voices
	3.	Revisiting of ABC model
	4.	Identification and rating of beliefs about voices using the ABC model (especially power and control beliefs)
	5.	Socratic discussion about what has been learnt about voices and self
	6.	Home task (mindfulness practice CD)
4	1.	10-minute mindfulness practice
	2.	Socratic discussion about mindfulness practice, linking to beliefs about voices
	3.	Revisiting of ABC formulation from Session 3
	4.	Gathering of evidence that supports and does not support unhelpful beliefs about voice
	5.	Socratic discussion about what has been learnt about voices and self
	6.	Home tasks (mindfulness practice CD and noticing of evidence not supporting beliefs about voices)
5	1.	10-minute mindfulness practice
	2.	Socratic discussion about mindfulness practice, linking to beliefs about voices and self
	3.	Reframing of beliefs about voices as positively framed beliefs about self in relation to voices
	4.	Gathering of evidence that supports beliefs about self in relation to voices
	5.	Socratic discussion about what has been learnt about voices and self
	6.	Home tasks (mindfulness practice CD and data log to gather evidence)
6	1.	10-minute mindfulness practice
	2.	Socratic discussion about mindfulness practice, linking to beliefs about voices and self
	3.	Revisiting of beliefs about self in relation to voices
	4.	Gathering of further evidence in support of beliefs about self in relation to voices
	5.	Socratic discussion about what has been learnt about voices and self
	6.	Home tasks (mindfulness practice CD and continuing to use data log to gather evidence)

(continued)

Table 16.2   (*continued*)

7	1.	10-minute mindfulness practice
	2.	Socratic discussion about mindfulness practice, linking to beliefs about voices and self
	3.	Drawing out of the global, stable experience of negative self-schema
	4.	Identification of weakly held positive self-schema
	5.	Socratic discussion about what has been learnt about voices and self
	6.	Home tasks (mindfulness practice CD and data log about self in relation to voices)
8	1.	10-minute mindfulness practice
	2.	Socratic discussion about mindfulness practice, linking to beliefs about voices and self
	3.	Noting of evidence in support of beliefs about self in relation to voices
	4.	Gathering and writing down of evidence in support of positive self-schema
	5.	Socratic discussion about what has been learnt about voices and self
	6.	Home tasks (mindfulness practice CD, data logs and acting 'as if' beliefs are true)
9	1.	10-minute mindfulness practice
	2.	Socratic discussion about mindfulness practice, linking to beliefs about voices and self
	3.	Noting of new evidence in support of beliefs about self in relation to voices
	4.	Continued gathering of evidence in support of positive self-schema
	5.	Socratic discussion about what has been learnt about voices and self
	6.	Home tasks (mindfulness practice CD, data logs and acting 'as if' beliefs are true)
10	1.	10-minute mindfulness practice
	2.	Socratic discussion about mindfulness practice, linking to beliefs about voices and self
	3.	Noting of evidence in support of beliefs about self and voices
	4.	Socratic drawing out of the notion of a symbolic self
	5.	Socratic discussion about what has been learnt about voices and self
	6.	Home tasks (mindfulness practice CD, data logs and acting 'as if' beliefs are true)
11	1.	10-minute mindfulness practice
	2.	Socratic discussion about mindfulness practice, linking to beliefs about voices and self
	3.	Noting of evidence in support of beliefs about self and voices and rating of conviction
	4.	Identification of individual key learning points from Sessions 1–10
	5.	Socratic discussion about what has been learnt about voices and self
	6.	Home tasks (mindfulness practice CDs, data logs and acting 'as if' beliefs are true)
12	1.	10-minute mindfulness practice
	2.	Socratic discussion about mindfulness practice, linking to beliefs about voices and self
	3.	Noting of new evidence in support of beliefs about self and voices
	4.	Identification of 6-month goals, drawing on individual key learning points from Session 11
	5.	Socratic discussion about what has been learnt about voices and self
	6.	Home tasks (identification of ongoing home tasks for progress towards 6-month goals)

ABC = A (antecedent event: voice comments), B (beliefs and thoughts about A, especially beliefs about voices power and control), C (emotional and behavioural consequences of A + B). See Section 16.4.4.2.

sensations of breathing. Therefore, voices are explicitly brought into the practice and are treated just as any other experience is treated in mindfulness practice.

For participants, this guidance to sit with and observe voice experiences can be unsettling at first. They are usually well practised in a range of distraction techniques, often recommended by other mental-health professionals, and these usually work to a greater or lesser extent to reduce distress at hearing voices (as outlined in Chapter 2). Thus the belief that the only way to manage distress at hearing voices is to distract oneself can be strongly held. The first few attempts at sitting mindfully with voices can result in increased distress for some people, which we can anticipate and normalise. However, in our experience, after half a dozen or so practices, most participants have a 'lightbulb' moment, where they notice an unpleasant voice comment during the practice and are able to bring awareness back to the breath without getting lost in thinking about it. These experiences can be drawn out during Socratic discussion following each mindfulness practice, which can facilitate evaluation of beliefs about voices and self and the development of metacognitive insight. For instance, experiences such as this can add to the evidence (see later) that voices do not always have control.

16.4.4   Cognitive Therapy in PBCT

The latter half of each session (apart from Session 1) is devoted to a cognitive therapy for psychosis approach. Sessions 2–6 focus on identifying and evaluating beliefs about voices (the top left-hand corner of the PBCT model), Sessions 7–10 focus on identifying and strengthening positive self-schema and exploring the notion of symbolic self (the bottom left-hand corner of the model, moving into the bottom right-hand corner) and Sessions 11 and 12 focus on consolidation across all four domains. A brief summary of the cognitive therapy aspects of each session follows, starting at Session 2.

16.4.4.1   *Session 2*
Participants are given the opportunity to talk about their voice-hearing experiences in pairs, both currently and looking back to when voices first started. They are invited to say as much or as little about these experiences as they wish and are advised to consider what they will choose to disclose and not to disclose. In the wider group, participants are invited to share these experiences, with facilitators beginning to verbally draw out As, Bs and Cs Socratically (see Session 3). This session is important in establishing group cohesion and a sense of universality (Yalom, 1995) and in beginning to draw out the importance of beliefs about voice power and control in determining distress.

16.4.4.2   *Session 3*
The ABC model is introduced: A (antecedent event: voice comments), B (beliefs and thoughts about A, especially beliefs about voices power and control), C (emotional and behavioural consequences of A + B). This is done Socratically (i.e. it is not

Table 16.3 ABC table

A (Antecedent event)	B (Beliefs and thoughts about A)	C (Consequences of A + B)
Voice comments	Especially beliefs about voice power and control	Feelings Behaviour

presented in a psychoeducation fashion). Participants are invited through Socratic questioning to share their experiences of voices, and these experiences are drawn out by the therapists, using a written ABC table (see Table 16.3).

In Socratic discussion about a specific voice-hearing experience (A), participants are first invited to talk about the emotional and behaviour consequences of the experience (C) through asking questions such as, 'How did you feel when the voices told you not to go out?', 'What did you notice in your body?' and 'What did you do?' It can be helpful to draw out consequences before beliefs, as emotional and behavioural consequences are often more readily accessible than beliefs and thoughts about voices.

Once the consequences of the experience have been identified and written down, participants are asked about their beliefs and thoughts through questions related to the consequences, such as 'When you were feeling anxious, what went through your mind?' Finally, participants are asked what sense they make of the ABC formulation and what they see as the association between the Bs and Cs. Completing two or three ABC formulations for different group members can facilitate participants to discover that beliefs and thoughts about voices shape their consequences, rather than the voices themselves.

This session ends with unhelpful beliefs about voices being explicitly named, especially beliefs about voice power and control. For instance, the belief that 'voices have control over me' might be highlighted as a shared belief amongst group members. Participants are invited to individually rate their conviction in these beliefs using a percentage scale. To facilitate hope, participants are informed that the accuracy of these beliefs will be explored in the following sessions.

16.4.4.3 Session 4

Using standard cognitive therapy techniques, each of the beliefs identified in Session 3 is brought to Session 4 in order to gather and evaluate evidence. For each belief, evidence in its support is gathered and written down (first in pairs and then as a whole group), followed by evidence that does not support it. This is where the power of the group comes to the fore, as a number of group members come forward to suggest supporting and challenging evidence. When no more evidence emerges, group members are invited to consider all the evidence gathered and come to a conclusion. As a home task, participants are invited to notice evidence that does not support these beliefs and to write this down using a data log (Table 16.4)

Table 16.4 Example evidence-gathering chart

Belief about voices: *Voices have control over me*	
Evidence supporting belief	*Evidence not supporting belief*
Voices told me not to go out on Tuesday and I didn't go out even though I needed to get shopping in	Voices told me to cut myself and I didn't do it
Voices told me on Thursday afternoon to stop doing the crossword because I was too stupid to get it right, and I stopped	On Friday I started doing a crossword again and I carried on even when voices told me to stop because I was too stupid

Conclusion from evaluating the evidence: *Voices do not have total control over me* I currently believe this is true with 20% certainty

16.4.4.4   *Session 5*

Evidence is added to the data logs from Session 4, first discussing this in pairs and then as a whole group. However, whereas the conclusion from evaluating the gathered evidence in Session 4 was framed in terms of voices (e.g. 'Voices have control over me'), participants are invited to reframe this conclusion in terms of self (e.g. 'I have some control, even when voices are active'), in order to pave the way for a schema focus. It can be seen how although these two statements are largely synonymous, the second statement emphasises the self as having some control (rather than voices having less control). Conviction in these newly framed beliefs can be rated using a percentage scale, which can be returned to in subsequent sessions. Participants are given a data log in which to write down evidence in support of these newly framed beliefs as a home task in the coming week, and they are invited to bring particular attention to any experiences that support these new beliefs about self in relation to voices.

16.4.4.5   *Session 6*

The aim of Session 6 is to consolidate new learning about self in relation to voices, and participants are invited to identify evidence in support of their new beliefs about themselves in relation to voices (e.g. 'I have some control, even when voices are around'). Although no longer the main focus of Sessions 7–10, participants are encouraged to continue adding evidence to the data log as a home task. To support this, 5 minutes can be spent in reviewing the data log in each of the coming sessions.

16.4.4.6   *Session 7*

This is the first session in which self-schema becomes the main focus. In line with Chadwick (2006), the emphasis is not on identifying and challenging negative self-schema, but rather on identifying and strengthening weakly held positive self-schema. The rationale for this is that strongly held, fact-like, negative core beliefs about the self can be difficult to shift, particularly in a group setting with relatively few sessions.

The cognitive therapy section of the session begins with a drawing out of the global and stable experience of negative self-schema. Their origin in early childhood or as a result of later trauma is noted, and their tendency to become reinforced through processes such as the confirmatory bias is explored. It is acknowledged that negative self-schema often go hand in hand with distressing voices, but participants are not invited to identify their own negative self-schema. Instead, they are invited to identify an existing but weakly held positive belief about themselves, working in pairs or small groups. This is done by first inviting them to bring to mind a recent (or as recent as possible) event in which they felt okay or good about themselves as a person – ideally in a social situation. This might be a recent outing with a friend or family member, for example. Participants are then encouraged to recollect the event as well as possible by bringing to mind their thoughts, feelings and bodily sensations at the time (with eyes closed if this helps and feels okay). The primary question is how participants saw themselves as a person in that moment. What we are looking for here is a positive core-belief statement about the self, such as 'I am okay as I am', 'I am likeable' or 'I am capable'.

Once again, this can be an exercise that is facilitated by working in a group. Some group members will struggle to identify a relevant situation and it is not unusual for someone to bring to mind a positive social experience of being in the group itself – a sense of being accepted and liked by the other group members. In terms of what Yalom calls 'guidance', group members can help each other put words to a positive experience of the self. However, this work might initially be conducted most helpfully within pairs or small groups, given its deeply personal nature and the feelings of discomfort or shame that might emerge when sharing self-schematic statements with the group as a whole.

For this session, the home task is to continue adding evidence to the data log in support of new beliefs about the self in relation to voices. Participants are invited to notice evidence supporting positive self-schema.

16.4.4.7 Session 8

A new data log is introduced, in which participants are invited to gather and write down evidence in support of their identified positive self-schema. Again, working in pairs or small groups, participants are encouraged to recall evidence or experiences suggesting their positive self-schematic beliefs are accurate. This might be recent or from the more distant past, into childhood. A sheet recording weekly ratings of conviction in the positive core belief (on a percentage scale) can be helpful in enabling participants to chart how the strength of their chosen belief or beliefs changes over time.

The home task is to add evidence to the data logs. In addition, participants are invited to identify one activity they are not currently doing which they would be doing if they believed their positive core belief with more conviction. Once such an activity is identified, participants are invited to engage in it (or take a small step towards it) during the week. This acting 'as if' the positive core belief were true can in itself generate evidence to support its accuracy.

16.4.4.8   Session 9
The focus is to review the previous week, including the home tasks, with a view to adding more evidence to the positive self-schema data logs and to re-rating conviction in the positive self-schema. Some participants may choose to add one or two additional positive self-schema beliefs and to repeat exercises from the previous couple of sessions. As a home task, participants are again invited to act as if their positive self-schematic belief were true, and to continue adding evidence to the data logs.

16.4.4.9   Session 10
The bottom right-hand corner of the PBCT model shown in Figure 16.1 refers to the 'symbolic self'. This is where participants move from a fixed, narrow and unchanging concept of self, defined entirely in terms of negative self-schema ('I am bad', 'I am worthless') to a view of self which acknowledges that experiences of the self change over time, from situation to situation, and are contradictory (negative self-schema and positive self-schema can co-occur and contradict each other). This new learning is greatly facilitated by the previous 10 weeks of mindfulness practice, as participants come to notice that their experience of self is not fixed, but changing, and can include contradictory views of self. Participants may begin to realise that although negative self-schematic experiences feel true when they are strongly present, this does not mean that they are accurate. The experience, drawing on mindfulness practice, of thoughts and feelings of self seeming true in one moment but then fading and passing to different ones, can facilitate participants' learning and enable them to notice experiences of self in the moment, without becoming overly attached to them.

In this session, participants are invited to bring their newly strengthened positive self-schema to mind, as well as (with some care) a contradictory negative belief about themselves that can sometimes seem true. Socratic questioning can enable participants to wonder about the meaning of holding two opposing views of self at different times – to wonder what implications this has for their view of themselves. This can be a conceptually challenging step for anyone, and many participants struggle at this stage. However, some participants are able to come to a sense of self that is more fluid than it was previously, and to begin to let go of their previously held negative, fixed and narrow concept of self.

16.4.4.10   Session 11
The final two sessions involve consolidating learning across the first 10, and no new conceptual material is introduced. In this session, participants are invited to work in pairs or small groups to look back at the previous 10 sessions and what they have

learned. It is acknowledged that the key learning points will be different for different members of the group – there are no right or wrong answers. Using a worksheet, participants are asked to discuss and consider three or more key learning
points in terms of (1) what they have learned about voices, (2) what they have
learned about themselves and (3) what they have learned about other people.

16.4.4.11   Session 12

Drawing on the worksheet from Session 11 and staying in the same pairs or small
groups, participants are now asked to look forward over the next 6 months. The
tasks are (1) to describe what – if things go as well as possible – they will be doing,
in concrete and specific behavioural terms, in 6 months' time, (2) to look back at
their worksheet from Session 11 and identify which aspects of what they have
learned during the group might enable them to make progress towards their
6-month goals and (3) to write down at least three specific and concrete tasks or
activities that will help them to continue on their journey of recovery ('To continue
adding evidence to my positive data log').

16.5   PBCT: An Integrated Model

Although group PBCT sessions are divided into a focus on mindfulness practice
and discussion and a focus on beliefs about voices and self, it is important to
emphasise the conceptual links between the two. Rather than being conceptually
distinct, a core aspect of group PBCT is continually making links between what is
learned through mindfulness practice and what is learned through evaluating
beliefs about voices and self.

   During mindfulness practice, participants will often notice that voices come and
go, and naturally fade and pass. They will find that they are sometimes able to
notice unpleasant voice comments and then bring awareness back to the breath.
Socratic questioning about these experiences can facilitate the development of
metacognitive insight. Thus, through mindfulness practice, participants often have
the direct, in-the-moment experience that they have some control even when
voices are active. Indeed, this evidence, when noticed, can be added to data logs to
support beliefs about personal control in the face of voices.

   Just as mindfulness practice and discussion can facilitate the evaluation of beliefs
about voices and self, so can the process of evaluating beliefs about voices and self
facilitate mindfulness practice. As participants notice experiences in their daily
lives that support beliefs about personal control and positive self-schema, they are
more able to sit in mindfulness practice with unpleasant voice comments and
negative self-schematic experiences. Through developing and strengthening
alternative beliefs about voices and self, participants are better able to adopt a
decentred position during mindfulness practice and to observe voice comments

and negative self-schematic experiences without attaching to these experiences. In PBCT, therefore, although the sessions may be divided between mindfulness practice and cognitive therapy, it can be seen that these two aspects serve reciprocal functions in facilitating change, and that in combination the sum is greater than the parts.

16.6 Group PBCT: The Evidence

The evidence for the effectiveness of group PBCT is still in its infancy. Starting with efficacy studies of group cognitive behaviour therapy for psychosis (CBTp) (i.e. without mindfulness practice), Wykes *et al.* (2008) found that in seven trials there was a modest effect size in comparison to treatment as usual. However, the effect size of the most well controlled and well designed trials of group CBTp was negligible in terms of psychotic symptom reduction and small in terms of improvements in psychological well-being.

The evidence for the effectiveness of purely mindfulness-based groups for psychosis is limited. In their 2005 pre–post designed study, Chadwick and colleagues reported significant improvement on a measure of psychological well-being (CORE; Evans *et al.*, 2000) over time for 10 participants. This was followed by a pilot randomised controlled trial (RCT) in 2009, in which Chadwick and colleagues again found significant improvement over time on the CORE. The between-group effect size was in the medium range but failed to reach significance. Thus, while there is emerging evidence for the effectiveness of mindfulness-based groups for psychosis, the existing studies are small in size and limited in design and so firm conclusions about effectiveness are not yet warranted.

When it comes to group PBCT, an RCT for chronic depression found significant improvements in depression and mindfulness for PBCT participants in comparison to the control group (Strauss *et al.*, 2012). There is one published quantitative study of PBCT groups for distressing voices (Dannahy *et al.*, 2011). This was a pre–post design, with a stable baseline established for a subset of the 62 participants. Significant improvements over time were found on the CORE, as well as on a measure of voice-related distress and beliefs about voice control. Moreover, these improvements were maintained at 1-month follow-up. A thematic analysis of participant experiences of group PBCT for distressing voices supported the importance of all four PBCT domains in facilitating change (May *et al.*, 2012). While these are encouraging and promising findings, the Dannahy *et al.* (2011) study employed a relatively weak design, limiting its conclusions about effectiveness. In response to this, our research team is currently conducting an RCT of group PBCT for distressing voices and we will submit our findings for publication in 2013. Findings from our qualitative studies of PBCT groups are discussed in Chapter 12.

16.7 Conclusion

Group PBCT for distressing psychosis integrates cognitive therapy for psychosis with a mindfulness- and acceptance-based approach, giving equal weight to each. Progress is made within a radically collaborative therapeutic relationship and within a therapeutic ZoPD (Vygotsky, 1978), whereby participants make more progress in collaboration than they could make on their own. Each group session is clearly and consistently structured in order to provide a predictable and anxiety-lessening environment that can facilitate learning.

Although this therapy may be intuitively appealing, evidence for its effectiveness is still limited. The evidence for the effectiveness of purely CBTp-based groups for psychosis suggests that this approach on its own may be of limited benefit to participants. Studies evaluating the effectiveness of purely mindfulness-based groups for psychosis are limited in number and in their design, and although initial studies suggest the groups are effective, it is really too soon to advocate their widespread rollout. Further research is needed. Group PBCT, which combines these two approaches, has one pre–post study to support its effectiveness, and an RCT is currently underway to test this therapy using a more robust design. Until findings from this RCT are available, we suggest caution in running these groups clinically (as we do not yet know if they are effective), but we would welcome further research into this form of therapy, in terms of both evaluating outcomes and exploring potential mechanisms of change.

Notes

1   This is specially adapted for working with people who are experiencing psychosis (see Chadwick, 2006 for details).
2   In Session 1, this is replaced by an exploration of therapeutic hopes, concerns and goals and collaborative setting of group rules.

References

Chadwick, P. (2006). *Person-based Cognitive Therapy for Distressing Psychosis*. Chichester: John Wiley & Sons.
Chadwick, P., Newman-Taylor, K. & Abba, N. (2005). Mindfulness groups with psychosis. *Behavioural and Cognitive Psychotherapy, 33*, 351–359.
Chadwick, P., Hughes, S, Russell, D, Russell, I. & Dagnan, D. (2009). Mindfulness groups for distressing voices and paranoia: a replication and feasibility trial. *Behavioural & Cognitive Psychotherapy, 37*, 403–412.

Dannahy, L., Hayward, M., Strauss, C., Turton, W., Harding, E. & Chadwick, P. (2011). Group person-based cognitive therapy for distressing voices: pilot data from nine groups. *Journal of Behavior Therapy and Experimental Psychiatry*, 42, 111–116.

Evans, C., Mellor-Clark, J., Margison, F., Barkham, M., Audin, K., Connell, J. *et al.* (2000). CORE: clinical outcomes in routine evaluation. *Journal of Mental Health*, 9, 247–255.

Goodliffe, L., Hayward, M., Brown, D., Turton, W. & Dannahy, L. (2010). Group person-based cognitive therapy for distressing voices: views from the hearers. *Psychotherapy Research*, 20, 447–461.

May, K., Strauss, C., Coyle, A. & Hayward, M. (in press). Person-based cognitive therapy groups for distressing voices: A thematic analysis of participant experiences of the therapy. *Psychosis*, doi: 10.1080/17522439.2012.708775.

Segal, Z., Teasdale, J. & Williams, M. (2002). *Mindfulness-based Cognitive Therapy for Depression*. New York: Guilford Press.

Strauss, C. Hayward, M. & Chadwick, P. (2012). Group person-based cognitive therapy for chronic depression: a pilot randomized controlled trial. *British Journal of Clinical Psychology*, doi: 10.1111/j.2044-8260.2012.02036.x.

Vygotsky, L. S. (1978). Mind in society: the development of higher psychological processes. Boston: Harvard University Press.

Wykes, T., Steel, C., Everitt, B. & Tarrier, N. (2008). Cognitive behavior therapy for schizophrenia: effect sizes, clinical models, and methodological rigor. *Schizophrenia Bulletin*, 34, 523–537.

Yalom, I. D. (1995). *The Theory and Practice of Group Psychotherapy* (4th edn). New York: Basic Books.

Appendix A

Chessboard Metaphor

Hayes, S. C., Strosahl, K. & Wilson, K. G. (1999)
Acceptance and Commitment Therapy: An Experiential Approach to Behavior Change.
New York: Guilford Press, pp. 190–191

Imagine a chessboard that goes out infinitely in all directions. It's covered in black pieces and white pieces. They work together in teams, as in chess – the white pieces fight against the black pieces. You can think of your thoughts and feelings and beliefs as these pieces; they sort of hang out together in teams too. For example, 'bad' feelings (like anxiety, depression, resentment) hang out with 'bad' thoughts and 'bad' memories. Same thing with the 'good' ones. So it seems that the way the game is played is that we select the side that we want to win. We put the 'good' pieces (like thoughts that are self-confident, feelings of being in control etc.) on one side, and the 'bad' pieces on the other. Then we get up on the back of the black horse and ride to battle, fighting to win the war against anxiety, depression, thoughts about using drugs, whatever. It's a war game. But there's a logical problem here, and that is that from this posture huge portions of yourself are your own enemy. In other words, if you need to be in this war, there is something wrong with you. And because it appears that you're on the same level as these pieces, they can be as big or even bigger than you are – even though these pieces are in you. So somehow, even though it is not logical, the more you fight the bigger they get. If it is true that 'if you are not willing to have it, you've got it,' then as you fight these pieces they become more central to your life, more habitual, more dominating, and more linked to every area of living. The logical idea is that you knock enough of them off the board that you eventually dominate them – except that your experience tells you that the exact opposite happens. Apparently, the white pieces can't be deliberately knocked off the board. So the battle goes on. You feel hopeless, you have a sense that you can't win, and yet you can't stop fighting. If you're on the back of that black horse, fighting is the only choice you have, because the white pieces seem life threatening. Yet living in a war zone is no way to live.'

Appendix B

Leaves-on-the-Stream Metaphor

Adapted from Luoma, J. B., Hayes, S. C. &
Walser, R. D. (2007)

Learning ACT: An Acceptance and Commitment Therapy Skills-training Manual for Therapists.
Oakland: Context Press

(1) Find a comfortable position and either close your eyes or fix them on a spot, whichever you prefer. Get in touch with the experience of sitting on the chair, with your feet in contact with the floor.

(2) Now I'd like to invite you to imagine that you are standing by the bank of a gently flowing stream, watching the water flow past. Imagine feeling the ground beneath your feet, the sounds of water flowing past, the way that the stream looks as you watch it (pause briefly).

(3) Imagine that there are leaves from trees, all different shapes and sizes and colours, floating past on the stream. And you are just watching these float on the stream, this is all you need to do for the next few minutes (pause).

(4) Now, I'd like you to notice each sensation, feeling and thought that you become aware of, and imagine placing it on a leaf, and letting it float on by. Do this regardless of whether the thoughts and feelings are positive or negative, pleasurable or painful. Even if they are the most wonderful thoughts, place them on the leaf and let them float by (pause).

(5) If your thoughts stop, just watch the stream. Sooner or later your thoughts will start up again (pause).

(6) Allow the stream to flow at its own rate. Notice any urges to speed up or slow down the stream... and let these be on leaves as well. Let the stream flow how it will.

(7) If you have thoughts or feelings about doing this exercise, place these on leaves as well (pause).

Acceptance and Commitment Therapy and Mindfulness for Psychosis, First Edition.
Edited by Eric M. J. Morris, Louise C. Johns and Joseph E. Oliver.
© 2013 John Wiley & Sons, Ltd. Published 2013 by John Wiley & Sons, Ltd.

(8) If a leaf gets stuck or won't go away, let it hang around. For a little while, all you are doing is observing this experience – there is no need to force the leaf down the stream (pause).

(9) If you find yourself getting caught up with a thought or feeling, and the stream disappears, just notice what you got caught up with, and gently turn this into a leaf and let it float on the stream. You are just observing each experience as a leaf on the stream. It is normal and natural to lose track of this exercise, and it will keep happening. When you notice it does, just bring yourself back to watching the leaves on the stream.

(10) Gently let the image of the stream and leaves dissolve and bring your awareness back to sitting in the chair, in the room.

Appendix C

Passengers-on-the-Bus Metaphor

Hayes, S. C., Strosahl, K. & Wilson, K. G. (1999)

Acceptance and Commitment Therapy: An Experiential Approach to Behavior Change.
New York: Guilford Press, pp. 157–158

Suppose there is a bus and you're the driver. On this bus we've got a bunch of passengers. The passengers are thoughts, feelings, bodily states, memories, and other aspects of experience. Some of them are scary. What happens is that you're driving along and the passengers start threatening you, telling you what you have to do, where you have to go. 'You've got to turn left,' 'You've got to go right,' and so on. The threat they have over you is that if you don't do what they say, they're going to come up front from the back of the bus.

It's as if you've made deals with these passengers, and the deal is, 'You sit in the back of the bus and scrunch down so that I can't see you very often, and I'll do what you say pretty much.' Now, what if one day you get tired of that and say, 'I don't like this! I'm going to throw those people off the bus!' You stop the bus, and you go back to deal with the mean-looking passengers. But you notice that the very first thing you had to do was stop. Notice now, you're not driving anywhere, you're just dealing with these passengers. And they're very strong. They don't intend to leave, and you wrestle with them, but it just doesn't turn out very successfully.

Eventually, you go back to trying to calm the passengers down, trying to get them to sit way in the back again where you can't see them. The problem with this deal is that you do what they ask in exchange for getting them out of your life. Pretty soon they don't even have to tell you, 'Turn left' – you know as soon as you get near a left turn that the passengers are going to crawl all over you. In time you may get good enough that you can almost pretend that they're not on the bus at all. You just tell yourself that left is the only direction you want to turn. However, when they eventually do show up, it's with the added power of the deals that you've made with them in the past.

Acceptance and Commitment Therapy and Mindfulness for Psychosis, First Edition.
Edited by Eric M. J. Morris, Louise C. Johns and Joseph E. Oliver.

Now the trick about the whole thing is that the power the passengers have over you is 100% based on this: 'If you don't do what we say, we're coming up and we're making you look at us.' That's it. It's true that when they come up front they look as if they could do a whole lot more. They do look pretty scary. The deal you make is to do what they say so they won't come up and stand next to you and make you look at them. But what if it was a little different to this? Imagine that the driver (you) has control of the bus, but you trade off the control in these secret deals with the passengers. What if, in other words, by trying to get control, you've actually given up control! What if it were the case that these passengers can't make you do something against your will.

Appendix D

Person-in-the-Hole Metaphor

Hayes, S. C., Strosahl, K. & Wilson, K. G. (1999)
Acceptance and Commitment Therapy: An Experiential Approach to Behavior Change.
New York: Guilford Press, pp. 101–102

The situation you are in seems a bit like this. Imagine that you're placed in a field, wearing a blindfold, and you're given a little tool bag to carry. You're told that your job is to run around this field, blindfolded. That is how you are supposed to live life. And so you do what you're told. Now, unbeknownst to you, in this field there are a number of widely spaced, fairly deep holes. You don't know that at first. So you start running about and sooner or later you fall into a large hole. You feel around and sure enough, you can't climb out and there are no escape routes you can find. Probably what you would do in such a predicament is take the tool bag you were given and see what is in there; maybe there is something you can use to get out of the hole. Now suppose the only tool in the bag is a shovel. So you dutifully start digging, but pretty soon you notice that you're not out of the hole. So you try digging faster and faster. But you're still in the hole. So you try big shovelfuls, or little ones, or throwing the dirt far away or not. But still you're in the hole. All this effort and all this work and oddly enough the hole has just gotten bigger and bigger and bigger. Isn't that your experience? So you come to me thinking, 'Maybe he has a really huge shovel – a gold plated steam shovel.' Well, I don't. And even if I did I wouldn't use it, because digging is not a way out of the hole – digging is what makes holes. So maybe the whole agenda here is hopeless – you can't dig your way out, that just digs you in.

Acceptance and Commitment Therapy and Mindfulness for Psychosis, First Edition.
Edited by Eric M. J. Morris, Louise C. Johns and Joseph E. Oliver.

Appendix E

Polygraph Metaphor

Hayes, S. C., Strosahl, K. & Wilson, K. G. (1999)
Acceptance and Commitment Therapy: An Experiential Approach to Behavior Change.
New York: Guilford Press, p. 123

Suppose I had you hooked up to the best polygraph machine that's ever been built. This is a perfect machine, the most sensitive ever made. When you are all wired up to it, there is no way you can be aroused or anxious without the machine's knowing it. So I tell you that you have a very simple task here: All you have to do is stay relaxed. If you get the least bit anxious, however, I will know it. I know that you want to try hard, but I want to give you an extra incentive, so I also have a .44 Magnum, which I will hold to your head. If you just stay relaxed, I won't blow your brains out, but if you get nervous (and I'll know it because you're wired up to this perfect machine), I'm going to have to kill you. So, just relax!... What do you think would happen?... Guess what you'd get?... The tiniest bit of anxiety would be terrifying. You'd naturally be saying, 'Oh, my gosh! I'm getting anxious! Here it comes!' BAMM! How could it work otherwise?

Acceptance and Commitment Therapy and Mindfulness for Psychosis, First Edition.
Edited by Eric M. J. Morris, Louise C. Johns and Joseph E. Oliver.
© 2013 John Wiley & Sons, Ltd. Published 2013 by John Wiley & Sons, Ltd.

Appendix F

See the Wood for the Trees
(And Other Helpful Advice
for Living Life)

Dr Ross White

Clinical Research Fellow, Mental Health and Well-being, University of Glasgow, UK,
Ross.White@glasgow.ac.uk

In developing an ACT protocol for distress following psychosis, the allegory featuring a character called 'Jeremy' was created to help produce some coherence between various metaphors that are used by practitioners of ACT. The protocol has been influenced by the Matrix approach pioneered by Kevin Polk, Mark Webster and colleagues. It is hoped that the use of an extended metaphor featuring Jeremy will help the patient retain a memory of the information discussed in the sessions and the various learning points. The allegory also serves as a story of hope, which the individual may be able to relate to when thinking about their own journey towards a meaningful life.

Chapter 1   The Difference between Sensory
Experience and Mental Experience

Jeremy has been travelling with a party of tourists through the rainforests of Brazil. The vehicle on which they have been travelling has broken down. Wandering into the forest to check out some of the exotic plant life, Jeremy slips off a ridge and tumbles down 100 feet into the dense jungle. He lies there unconscious for some time. Coming round, he calls out for other members of his party, but no one

Acceptance and Commitment Therapy and Mindfulness for Psychosis, First Edition.
Edited by Eric M. J. Morris, Louise C. Johns and Joseph E. Oliver.
© 2013 John Wiley & Sons, Ltd. Published 2013 by John Wiley & Sons, Ltd.

calls back. He is bruised and sore, lost and disorientated. He has only what he is carrying with him: his pen-knife with a built-in compass. For 2 days, Jeremy wanders around the jungle without water trying to find his friends. Although he is able to eat fruit from the jungle trees, he is absolutely parched. All he can do is think about water. In his head, he can imagine what running water sounds like; how it feels when you drink it down; and how it runs away from you when you try to hold it in your hands. But, unfortunately, no matter how much Jeremy runs these thoughts about water through his head, the water never reaches his throat. Desperately dehydrated, he suddenly stumbles on a stream. Dropping to his knees, he hurriedly drinks down the cold, pure water flowing in the stream. He sits back and thinks about how the experience of thinking about drinking water differs from actually drinking the water.

The purpose of this extract is to highlight the distinction that Kevin Polk and colleagues make when socialising people to the Matrix between internal mental experience (imagining, worrying, dreaming, thinking etc.) and five-sense experience (seeing, tasting, hearing, touching and smelling). Whereas we can get lost in internal mental experience (cognitive fusion), engaging with our five-sense experience can help connect us with the present moment. Kevin Polk introduces this notion by asking if the individual can distinguish between these two types of experience. Jeremy is able to clearly make this distinction between what it is like to imagine water and the actual experience of having water.

Chapter 2   The Drawbacks of Trying to Avoid the Things we Struggle With

Jeremy follows the stream that he had been drinking from. Now that he has found it, he wants to stay close to this source of drinking water. He makes slow progress, but he eventually comes to a point where the stream meets a mighty river. He remembers that the truck on which they were travelling had taken a small ferry across a big river. He knows that he should try to cross the river, but he fears that the river might be infested with crocodiles. He is also concerned that the river current might be unpredictable and dangerous. Rather than risk swimming across the river, he decides instead to journey along the river bank. The undergrowth is dense and the branches scrape at him as he tries to get through them.

This section of Jeremy's journey demonstrates how we can all get caught living our lives in the confines of fear. In discussions with patients, it is important to acknowledge that worrying – and the avoidant behaviours that stem from this – might keep us safe in the short-term, but you should also point out that these avoidant behaviours (e.g. isolating ourselves, taking drugs or alcohol) can cause problems of their own and only serve to keep us distant from our values.

Chapter 3 Moving towards Your Values and Carrying the Anxiety with You

Jeremy is sore from where the thick undergrowth has been scraping at his face, arms and legs. He knows that his best chance of getting back to civilisation lies with him heading east to the coast. He consults the compass on his Swiss army knife and sees that by following the river, he is actually heading north. He knows that, despite the dangers, he has to cross the river. Looking around, he finds an old hollowed-out tree trunk. He decides to try and use this to float across the river.

This extract illustrates the importance of taking stock of the direction in which our lives are moving. This can provide an opportunity to appreciate what it is that we consider important in life. We will all face anxiety, worry and discomfort at times (that is part of what it is to be human). Maybe this anxiety, worry and discomfort will be worth having if we are moving towards what it is we value in life. By committing to act in a way that is consistent with our values, we can lead a life that is vital.

Chapter 4 Getting Distance between You and the 'Story of your Life'

Jeremy kneels on the tree trunk and pushes himself out in the river. He uses a couple of branches as paddles and attempts to cross the river. As he crosses, all kinds of fearful thoughts enter his head: 'I'm a fool for getting myself into this situation', 'I'm going to fail', 'I don't know what's beneath me'. Jeremy notices that he is nervously saying these thoughts aloud. To help himself cope, he decides to sing these thoughts out loud, mixing the fearful words with a happy tune. He notices that this helps take some of the sting out of the thoughts. Changing the way you think about worrying thoughts can help change their impact.

As Jeremy floats across the river, a beautiful tropical bird flies low over the river's surface. As it passes right before Jeremy, it seems to tip its wing as if to say hello to him. For a split second, Jeremy forgets all his worries. The brilliant blue feathers of the Macaw and the gracefulness of its flight have taken his breath away. Jeremy reflects on how appreciating the beauty of this moment seems to leave no room in his mind for worry.

This section of the story provides an opportunity to demonstrate how patients might cope with acute experiences of anxiety and worry. This can be done by either defusing with the content of the anxious thoughts (through changing the context in which this content is experienced, for example by singing the thoughts to a happy tune) or connecting with the present moment through engaging with five-sense experience (e.g. getting out of your head by really noticing what it is that you are seeing).

Chapter 5   Control is the Problem, not the Solution

A little shaken, but still in one piece, Jeremy finally reaches the other side of the river. Clambering off the tree trunk on to the muddy river bank, Jeremy realises to his horror that he is sinking into the mud. He is in quicksand. Jeremy struggles against the rising quicksand and tries to step out of it. However, the instinctive response of struggling against the quicksand only increases the downward pressure and worsens the situation. A memory from a distant documentary on the Discovery Channel flashes into Jeremy's head. Jeremy recalls that the only way to get out of quicksand is to stop struggling against it. Relaxing, Jeremy stops resisting, and as he lies back into it, his legs gently start to rise. As if swimming across the top of the quicksand, he grabs at a branch of a tree and moves free to safety.

Jeremy's experiences in this section of the story are intended to illustrate to patients how struggling with their suffering can inadvertently drive them deeper into it. The counterintuitive approach of leaning into the suffering and exploring it can help free them to move on with their lives.

Chapter 6   Letting Go of Thoughts

Jeremy sits under a tree to rest. As he looks out over the river, he watches the leaves that have fallen from the trees floating on the water's surface. His eyes follow the leaves as they flow downstream. Jeremy notices that as quickly as these leaves disappear around the bend of the river, they are replaced by a seemingly never-ending stream of other leaves. Jeremy reflects on how the anxious thoughts that he was experiencing not so long have now floated out of sight, just like the leaves on the surface of the river. Other thoughts have flowed in to take the place of the anxiety. Jeremy concludes that he much prefers to watch the flow of the leaves down the river than to get caught up in the current and being carried away by it. Similarly, noticing your thoughts can be a better position to take than being swept away with them.

It is hoped that this passage of Jeremy's story, incorporating the 'leaves-on-the-stream' metaphor (Appendix B), will illustrate to patients that we are constantly experiencing a stream of consciousness and that at times we can all get caught up in this and swept up by our thoughts. Noticing the flow of our thoughts can free us from getting caught up in them. Mindfulness exercises are highlighted as a way of observing our thoughts without getting caught up in reacting to them.

Chapter 7   Seeing the Wood for the Trees

Lying back on the forest floor, Jeremy glances up to see a beautiful bird perched atop a very tall tree. If only Jeremy had wings, perhaps he could fly out of this place and get back to his own life... With a jolt, Jeremy sits up, a smile spreading across his face. He can't fly, but he can try to get a bird's eye view. Why hasn't he thought of this before? Jeremy grabs the trunk of the nearest tree and slowly but surely begins to climb. Nearing the top, he is able to see for miles over the surrounding area. Looking east, he can see the coastline in the distance. Running his eyes along the coast in a northerly direction, he sees a town. From this new way of looking at things, he is able to broaden his horizon and see how where he has been relates to where he wants to go. Jeremy now has a sense of being able to place himself within the wider scheme of things. At long last, Jeremy is able to see the wood despite the trees.

See the wood... not just the trees.

This extract of the story is intended to illustrate the 'observer self/self as context' perspective that patients are encouraged to develop over the course of acceptance and commitment therapy (ACT). Rather than becoming disorientated by the immediacy of the suffering that the person may be experiencing, this is about helping them to see how this suffering might relate to the larger picture of where they want to take their life.

Chapter 8   Coping with Worries

Jeremy is wandering in the forest and the wind has picked up. The trees sway and bend in the wind. He can hear the boughs creaking and he worries that a branch might break off and fall on his head. This brings back a memory from Jeremy's childhood. He was about 9 years old and he was out walking with his father. It was a wet and windy day, but they needed to take the family dog out for its evening walk. In an attempt to get some shelter from the wind and the rain, Jeremy's dad suggested to Jeremy that instead of walking along the main road they should take the slightly longer route of walking through the wood. A bit worried about this, Jeremy turned to his dad and protested: 'We shouldn't do that. The wind might blow a tree over and knock it on our heads.' Smiling down at his son, Jeremy's father replied, 'Yes, but it might not'. Thinking about this memory, Jeremy smiles to himself. There are so many things in the world that we could worry about, but worrying about them won't make them any less – or more – likely to happen.

This passage is intended to highlight how fruitless an endeavour worrying can be. For all the energy that patients invest in worrying, sometimes circumstances are outside their control, and this energy could instead be directed towards achieving goals consistent with their values.

Chapter 9   Review of the Importance of Values and Committed Action

To help stay on track, Jeremy climbs trees twice a day – once in the morning and once in the afternoon. Sometimes when he is up a tree, the wind blows and the tree sways. At these times, Jeremy finds it difficult to look out over the horizon, because he has to cling to the tree for safety. But when the wind settles, he is able to look out once again. Being able to get a broader perspective on things, rather than always staring at the trees straight in front of him, allows Jeremy to make good progress towards the sea. When Jeremy climbs a tree, he picks out certain features in the landscape that he can aim for. This helps to break his journey into manageable blocks and lets him know that he is still on course. For example, he might set himself the task of getting over a hill that lies between him and the ocean, or he might try to get to a particular clearing in the forest that he sees up ahead before nightfall. Sometimes he achieves these goals, other times he does not. The most important thing however is that he continues to let his journey be guided by a desire to get back to his friends and family.

This passage is intended to reiterate to the patient the importance of utilising the 'observer self' / 'self as context' perspective. It should be emphasised that this will be an ongoing process that the patient can engage in as they move forward with life. There will be difficulties and stress at times, but this is part of living a vital life and should not detract from the task at hand.

Chapter 10   Review of 'Noticing We Can Notice' Work

Reaching the sea shore, Jeremy has some troubling thoughts to contend with. All the difficulties that he has experienced over the last few days seem to run through his head. Jeremy wonders what his recent experiences say about him as a person. Is he someone who has managed to get themselves lost? Is he someone who struggles to overcome challenges put in front of him? Is he someone who makes bad decisions? As he ponders these thoughts, he looks up and sees a rainbow rising up from the sea. Seeing this rainbow helps Jeremy find an answer to these questions. Smiling to himself, he realises that just as a rainbow is a blend of different colours, he is a blend of many different qualities. Focusing on one particular colour doesn't capture the richness of the rainbow. Similarly, Jeremy's dwelling on things that he feels he hasn't coped with well doesn't do him justice as a person.

This extract is aimed at helping patients to see how a preoccupation with the labels that have been used by themselves and others to describe their lives can never do them justice. A narrow focus on particular aspects of our selves prevents us from appreciating the wonder of all the other aspects of our lives.

Chapter 11   Looking to the Future

Walking along the shore, Jeremy spots a collection of brightly coloured fishing boats pulled up on the beach. The palm trees that line the shore arc over the boats, protecting them from the hot sun. A sense of relief washes over Jeremy. He has managed to find his way out of the jungle and for the first time in a week he can see other people. Although his journey may not be quite finished yet, he knows that he is another step closer to where he wants to be. Jeremy is offered hospitality by the residents of the fishing village that he has stumbled across. Over the next few days he gets an opportunity to rest and recuperate. The inhabitants of the village use their radio to contact the coast guard, who send a boat down the coast to pick Jeremy up. Jeremy is looking forward to seeing his family and friends again. Reflecting back on the adventure he has been on, Jeremy wonders for a moment what other adventures might lie ahead. The future will always be uncertain, but after what Jeremy has been through, he is able to see that there is no clear path to leading a meaningful life – leading a meaningful life is the path!

Jeremy's progress in this passage is intended to highlight to patients that there will always be uncertainties in life. But rather than getting too preoccupied with this uncertainty, it's about appreciating that the uncertainty is part of leading a life that is meaningful.

The end (…of the beginning).

Appendix G

Skiing Metaphor

Hayes, S. C., Strosahl, K. & Wilson, K. G. (1999)
Acceptance and Commitment Therapy: An Experiential Approach to Behavior Change.
New York: Guilford Press, p. 220

Suppose you go skiing. You take a lift to the top of a hill, and you are just about to ski down the hill when a man comes along and asks where you are going. 'I'm going to the lodge at the bottom,' you reply. He says, 'I can help you with that,' and promptly grabs you, throws you into a helicopter, flies you to the lodge, and disappears. So you look around kind of dazed, take a lift to the top of the hill, and you are just about to ski down it when that same man grabs you, throws you into the helicopter, and flies you to the lodge. You'd be upset, no? Skiing is not just the goal of getting to the lodge, because any number of activities can accomplish that for us. Skiing is how we are going to get there. You notice that getting to the lodge is important because it allows us to do the process of skiing in a direction. If I tried to ski uphill instead of down, it wouldn't work. Valuing down over up is necessary in downhill skiing. There is a way to say this: outcome is the process through which process can become the outcome. We need goals, but we need to hold them lightly so that the real point of living and having goals can emerge.

Acceptance and Commitment Therapy and Mindfulness for Psychosis, First Edition.
Edited by Eric M. J. Morris, Louise C. Johns and Joseph E. Oliver.

Appendix H

Tug-of-War-with-the-Monster Metaphor

Hayes, S. C., Strosahl, K. & Wilson, K. G. (1999)
Acceptance and Commitment Therapy: An Experiential Approach to Behavior Change.
New York: Guilford Press, p. 109

The situation you are in is like being in a tug-of-war with a monster. It is big, ugly, and very strong. In between you and the monster is a pit, and as far as you can tell it is bottomless. If you lose this tug-of-war, you will fall into the pit and be destroyed. So you pull and pull, but the harder you pull, the harder the monster pulls, and you edge closer and closer to the pit. The hardest thing to see is that our job here is not to win the tug-of-war … Our job is to drop the rope.

Acceptance and Commitment Therapy and Mindfulness for Psychosis, First Edition.
Edited by Eric M. J. Morris, Louise C. Johns and Joseph E. Oliver.
© 2013 John Wiley & Sons, Ltd. Published 2013 by John Wiley & Sons, Ltd.

Index

Printed and bound by CPI Group (UK) Ltd, Croydon, CR0 4YY

16/04/2025

14658466-0004